PERINATAL NURSING

PERINATAL NURSING

Care of Newborns and Their Families

Florence Bright Roberts, R.N., M.N.
Doctoral Student
University of Tennessee, Knoxville
Formerly, Assistant Professor
Nursing of Children
University of Tennessee College of Nursing, Memphis

With Clinical Consultation and Editorial Assistance from
Judy Cox Chapman, R.N., M.N.
Associate Professor
Maternal and Child Nursing
Vanderbilt University School of Nursing, Nashville

McGraw-Hill Book Company
A Blakiston Publication
New York St. Louis San Francisco Auckland Bogotá
Düsseldorf Johannesburg London Madrid Mexico Montreal
New Delhi Panama Paris São Paulo Singapore
Sydney Tokyo Toronto

NOTICE

Medicine is an ever-changing science. As new research and clinical experience broaden our knowledge, changes in treatment and drug therapy are required. The editors and the publisher of this work have made every effort to ensure that the drug dosage schedules herein are accurate and in accord with the standards accepted at the time of publication. Readers are advised, however, to check the product information sheet included in the package of each drug they plan to administer to be certain that changes have not been made in the recommended dose or in the contraindications for administration. This recommendation is of particular importance in regard to new or infrequently used drugs.

PERINATAL NURSING

1234567890DODO7832109876

This book was set in Times Roman by National ShareGraphics, Inc.
The editors were Sally J. Barhydt and Michael LaBarbera;
the cover was designed by Joseph Gillians;
the production supervisor was Dennis J. Conroy.
The drawings were done by J & R Services, Inc.
R. R. Donnelley & Sons Company was printer and binder.

Library of Congress Cataloging in Publication Data

Roberts, Florence Bright, date
Perinatal nursing.

"A Blakiston publication."
Includes index.
1. Infants (Newborn)—Care and hygiene. 2. Pediatric nursing. I. Title. [DNLM: 1. Infant, Newborn—Nursing texts. 2. Pediatric nursing. WY159 R644p]
RJ253.R76 610.73'62 76–13570
ISBN 0–07–053125–0

To Kathleen and Nancy,
Who taught me how to love newborns

And to Paul,
Who shares that love with me
Who not only encouraged this work but also
shared child care and household responsibilities
to make it possible.

Contents

Foreword

The increased emphasis on health and wellness, as well as the continuing adequate attention to illness care, provide great opportunity for professional nurses to play more significant roles in health care delivery.

Preparation for these roles includes among other things a broad knowledge of (1) normal physiology, (2) deviations from normal, and (3) social influences on wellness and illness. This publication is directed toward providing information which can contribute to this broad knowledge for the improvement of patient care. Also, the material can be useful to individuals who are beginning students in nursing and to those who are engaged in the practice of nursing.

The students of Florence Roberts have long known that she respects the role of students in the learning process and that this process is an individual matter. They are also aware that she strives to spark the imagination and interest of learners, and utilizes creative approaches for doing this, and reflects the joy of learning by her actions. This publication carries these messages which have already been received by many students.

Ruth Neil Murry, R.N.
Dean, College of Nursing
University of Tennessee, Memphis

Preface

The writing of a textbook requires initial decisions about emphasis and style. In keeping with our philosophy that only with a thorough knowledge of the normal can one hope to understand the abnormal, special emphasis in this book is on the normal infant. This emphasis should enable one to acquire the foundation needed for the development of nursing care competencies. We feel that to provide even minimally adequate care, the nurse must view the neonate (as well as other patients) within the context of the family; a second emphasis, then, is on the family. Several aspects of the family are discussed in detail in the text and the student is provided with a list of suggested readings which consider special family constellations and problems to be used as needed for specific clinical situations.

Throughout this text, theory from both the biological and social sciences has been presented to provide a basis for planning nursing care. By applying the theory in the problem-solving process, the nurse can tailor care to individual newborns and their families. For the most part, this book does not attempt to provide the "how to" approach to the care of the newborn but instead focuses upon the basic theories which the nurse will continue to use as settings and resources, i.e., equipment and support systems, change. Clinical skills are discussed, but it is felt that textbook presentation of such skills serves at best as a guide for learning them through clinical practice under the supervision of expert practitioners.

The approach used in presenting much of the information in this book differs from that in many nursing texts. Particularly in the early chapters where the emphasis is on normal physiology, research data are presented along with a range of opinion, especially where controversy exists. The nursing implications of these data are frequently but not always specified. This approach was chosen to encourage the student to use the material creatively and imaginatively. Though the inclusion of controversies may be somewhat disconcerting to some students, it is felt that practitioners today and in the future must be able to handle ambiguities and uncertainties. It is hoped that the student will be stimulated to identify areas for future investigation in which nurses may make a significant contribution. In this way, nursing knowledge and theory may be expanded, and patient welfare improved.

A developmental and nursing care frame of reference is used for the organization of the content. This leads to a more scattered presentation of disease content than would be found in a systems or pathology orientation, but the index should facilitate retrieval of specific content when it is needed. The student is encouraged to read the chapters in sequence, as the later ones build upon the first several. The content is structured carefully so that beginning students can use it without prior knowledge of either pediatrics or obstetrics. A special section on the nursery care of the full-term infant describes in detail techniques used in the care of newborns. These are designed for use by students who have had no experience with infants, and they are in direct response to our observations of problems encountered by students as they approach newborns for the first time.

Every attempt has been made to ensure accuracy, relevancy, and currency of clinical data. To supplement the author's personal experiences and study of the current literature in neonatology, special clinical consultation was sought from Mrs. Judy Cox Chapman, associate professor of maternal and child nursing at Vanderbilt University School of Nursing. Mrs. Chapman has not only taken her consultation role seriously, but has gone far beyond the call of duty, poring over textbooks to validate and document her suggestions and consulting clinical personnel whenever a question was not resolved to her satisfaction. More than this, she has become a personal friend as she has reviewed, page by page, the entire manuscript and offered suggestions and encouragement throughout.

Special thanks also go to Mrs. Susan DeVane, senior student at Vanderbilt University School of Nursing, and to Mrs. Carol Dalglish, clinical specialist in maternity nursing and assistant professor of maternal and child nursing at Vanderbilt University Hospital, who reviewed parts of the manuscript as critical readers.

Because no one book can adequately serve the needs of all students today, we urge the use of suggested references to complement and supplement this volume. Our hope is that nursing students will recognize and accept the challenge of caring for newborns and their families and that both the students and the childbearing families will benefit from the availability of this book.

Florence Bright Roberts
Judy Cox Chapman

PERINATAL NURSING

Chapter 1

Fetal Development

In the Western world, age is counted from the moment of birth. In China, on the other hand, the infant is considered to be 1 year old at birth. Where *does* life begin? This question has been argued through the ages. In one sense it can never be answered; for, even if one could decide when life begins for an individual, that individual springs not from inanimate substance but from *life* itself.

This study of the newborn, then, will begin with a brief review of gametogenesis, the production of the reproductive cells each containing half the genetic material which the new individual will inherit.

GAMETOGENESIS

Meiosis, the process through which the gametes are produced, requires *two* separate cell divisions. In the formation of spermatozoa, these two divisions result in four fully functional spermatozoa of approximately equal size, each containing 23 chromosomes. In the production of ova, however, the cellular material becomes concentrated in one large cell containing 23 chromosomes. The first cell division results in one large cell and one very small nonfunctional polar body which is cast off. In the second division a second polar body is produced and discarded.

The remaining single functional ovum is much larger than a spermatozoon, as it contains supplies to nourish the new individual until external nutritional sources can be established.

Anatomy of Spermatozoa

After the second meiotic division, the sperm cells, which look like other body cells at first, undergo a striking change in shape (see Figure 1-1). Extraneous cytoplasm disappears, and the chromosomes of the cell form a very compact unit called the *head.* A cap, or *acrosome,* covers the anterior part of the head, and a thin flagellar structure called the *tail* is attached posteriorly. The acrosome is thought to contain an enzyme which helps dissolve the outer covering of the ovum, making penetration possible. The tail provides the propulsion necessary for movement of the spermatozoon in the female reproductive tract. Between the head and the tail is a very small section called the *neck* which contains a centriole, a subcellular unit essential to cell division.

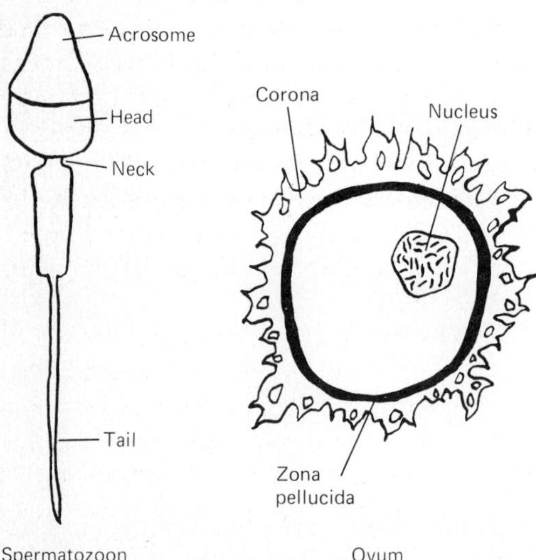

Figure 1-1 The spermatozoon and ovum (not drawn to scale). *(Spermatozoan adapted from B. M. Patten, Human Embryology, McGraw-Hill, New York, 1968, p. 15, by permission. Ovum redrawn and adapted from G. Scipien et al., Comprehensive Pediatric Nursing, McGraw-Hill, New York, 1975, p. 88, by permission.)*

Anatomy of Ova

During its development, the ovum is housed in a special site on the ovary called a follicle. Each ovum has its own follicle, and a study of an adult ovary will show many follicles in different stages of maturity. Within the follicle the ovum grows in size until it is much larger than the cells around it. Inside the ovum, its cytoplasm develops granules of food substance called yolk, which in the human ovum is dispersed throughout the cell. The cell is surrounded by a clear noncellular layer called the *zona pellucida,* whose function is not known, though it may be related to the exchange of materials between the developing ovum and the tissues around it.[1] Beyond the zona pellucida is the *corona radiata,* a ring of elongated cells which radiate from the ovum like the corona around the sun caused by gases erupting from its surface. Before the ovum is discharged from the follicle, it undergoes a first meiotic division and the second one is begun but stops before completion. When the ovum is released, there is a sudden rupture of the follicle and the ovum bursts forth, carrying with it some of the cells of the corona radiata, which it keeps around it until after penetration by a spermatozoon (see Figure 1-1).

FERTILIZATION

Union of the spermatozoon and ovum occurs in the upper end of the *oviduct* (also called the uterine tube or fallopian tube), where the ovum becomes surrounded by spermatozoa. The cells of the corona radiata are held together by a substance called *hyaluronidic acid.* In order for a sperm to reach the ovum, this acid must be dissolved. Each spermatozoon is thought to carry in its acrosome a minute amount of *hyaluronidase,* an enzyme that breaks down the hyaluronidic acid. It is only after many spermatozoa have released the enzyme that enough of the acid is dissolved for one spermatozoon to work its way through the corona to reach the ovum. At the moment of penetration of the ovum, changes in the outer membrane of the ovum occur which prohibit multiple penetrations.

Only the head and neck of the spermatozoon penetrate the ovum, carrying with them the concentrated chromosomes and the centriole. The tail is discarded at the time of entry. Soon after entry, the head of the sperm begins to form distinct chromosomes and the centriole begins the formation of a spindle apparatus in preparation for the first *mitotic* division of the fertilized ovum, or *zygote.* In the meantime, the second *meiotic* division has been completed in the nucleus of the ovum, and the second polar body is extruded from the ovum. At this stage the chromosomes from the male and the female gametes are called the male and female *pronuclei.* The two pronuclei migrate toward each other, and the chromosomes arrange themselves in the equatorial zone of the newly formed spindle apparatus. Fertilization is complete with the mingling of the chromosomes from both parents.

DEVELOPMENT OF THE NEW INDIVIDUAL

The study of the development of the new individual is, in itself, a very complex and difficult subject. For our purposes, a discussion of basic concepts and a summary of major events and important landmarks of development will suffice. The processes of implantation and placentation will be discussed separately.

Basic Concepts

Phylogenic Recapitulation A striking phenomenon which becomes evident as one studies embryology is the *phylogenic recapitulation* which the embryo demonstrates. Essentially, this is the human embryo's progression through stages in development shared by other creatures. Certain stages in human embryonic development, for instance, are identical to some stages in the chick, the frog, and the pig. It is fortunate for the embryologist that this is true because only an occasional human embryo becomes available for study. As these human embryos have become available, however, they have substantiated findings from research on lower forms of life.

Cell Differentiation During the first few hours after fertilization, the zygote divides rapidly to form new cells, all of which seem to be exactly alike. Then, mysteriously, the cells begin to differentiate. First, there are two distinctly different kinds of cells, and then three, and then more. Nobody knows exactly how the cells "know" when and how to become different, but it happens. In studying lower forms of life, notably the frog, it has been found that during very early differentiation, a nucleus taken from a differentiated cell and injected into an ovum whose nucleus has been removed can stimulate normal development from the beginning stages.[2] In a sense, the nucleus "starts over." However, nuclei taken from cells in later stages of differentiation have lost the ability to "start over." Just why one nucleus can stimulate complete development and another cannot is not at all clear. Some embryologists think that the mechanism which allows such differentiation of tissues and reversals of this ability is carried in the regulator and structural genes.[3] Structural genes carry genetic information for the formation of proteins. Regulator genes somehow determine when particular structural genes will be functional. (See Chapter 7, Genes; Chromosomes.)

Tissue Differentiation *Induction,* a process through which cells in one part of an embryo influence the cells around them to develop in a specific way, is very important in tissue differentiation. It is thought that this process is controlled by chemical substances, probably rather simple in nature. The cells that cause the reaction of the surrounding cells are called *inductors,* the substances that are produced are called *evocators,* and the reacting cells' capacity to respond is called their *competence.* The effect of the inductors is not limited to the area in which they are normally found. If, for instance, an optic cup, which normally forms the rear wall of the eye, is removed from the cephalic end of the embryo and implanted in the caudal end at a certain time in its development, the cup will induce the formation of a lens from the tissues of the caudal end of the embryo.[4] A little later in its development, if the optic cup is removed and transplanted, a lens will form both at the original site and at the site of transplantation. Later still, if the optic cup is transplanted, a lens will form in the original site but not in the transplanted site. It is not known whether the inductor loses its potency or whether for some reason the recipient cells lose their competence. One important fact is known, however: *Correct timing is absolutely essential.* If something interferes at the normal time for induction, there is no way for the embryo to "do it later." This fact becomes very important when considering the origins of some congenital defects. Induction occurs very early in embryonic life. All the organs of the body have begun development by the time the embryo is 10 weeks old.

Cell Migration Another peculiar thing that happens in the early development of the embryo is that some of the cells move around. They actually migrate from one site to another in a fashion similar to the movement of an amoeba. These special cells, called *mesenchymal cells,* first appear just after the embryo has become a two-layered organism. The two layers, the *ectoderm* and the *entoderm,* separate, and a new layer, the *mesoderm,* forms. It is the cells of the mesoderm which move. One investigator studying these cells removed some and put them into a fluid culture medium.[5] The cells rolled up into balls and sank to the bottom of the culture medium as though "sulking." When he put a cobweb into the medium, the cells began crawling along its fibers! Descendents of these cells, the fibroblasts, react similarly in later life when they crawl along fibrin mesh to aid in the formation of blood clots. Patten believes strongly that there is a collagen mesh network similar to fibrin in the space between the ectoderm and entoderm in the embryo upon which the mesenchymal cells migrate.[6] Such a network has been found in the chamber where the heart forms.

Shaping the Embryonic "Body" In considering the interaction of groups of cells within the embryo, it is necessary to understand that different groups of cells are growing at different rates. This fact makes possible the phenomenon of *invagination.* In this process, cells which are growing more slowly than those around them appear, over a period of time, to be sinking into the tissues. Actually, the cells around them are overtaking them in growth and building up tissue around them. The oral cavity is formed in this way, as are the nostrils, for example.

Besides the uneven growth rate, it is important to note that the embryo is growing in a confined space. This causes the curving of the embryonic body and accounts for another very important process, *folding*. The embryo begins life as a straight line of cells. As new cells are formed, they are forced to conform to the sphere in which the embryo is growing. As the sides of the "body" grow, they are folded downward until they meet on the ventral side and fuse at the midline. As structures within the body grow, they undergo folding as they conform to the space available to them. Thus, both the heart and the intestinal tract begin formation as straight tubes, later folding to fit into the spaces available to them.

Cephalocaudal Maturation Most students of growth and development are aware of the concept of *cephalocaudal maturation* in an infant's development after birth. The infant learns to control the head before the hands, and the hands before the feet. This "direction" of maturation is apparent during embryonic development as well. In the very early stages of cell differentiation, when the mesoderm first forms, the newly formed mesodermal cells migrate to one end of the embryo, where they begin forming what will be the head. As new cells are formed, they more or less line up behind these first cells down the length of the "body." Thus, the cells that eventually form the head are "older" than the ones forming the tail.

Differential Maturity One last concept is that the various tissues and groups of tissues are at different stages of maturity throughout their development. Thus, the infant's long bones do not reach maturity for several years, but the bladder is essentially structurally complete at birth.

Early Embryonic Development

Immediately after fertilization, the fertilized egg, now called the zygote, begins rapid cell division, a process called *cleavage.* During this period, the number of cells increases so rapidly that there is no growth period between cell divisions. Consequently, individual cells in each succeeding generation are smaller than those in the last, and the total volume of protoplasm remains approximately the same as was contained in the fertilized egg. All these cells, called *blastomeres,* appear to be alike. Since they are dividing within the confines of the zona pellucida, which is a sphere, the mass of cells is spherical. The resulting ball of cells is called the *morula* because of its resemblance to a mulberry, genus *Morus.* About 3 to 4 days after fertilization, the morula enters the uterus from the uterine tubes where fertilization took place. In the next 2 to 3 days, the internal cells of the morula gradually become rearranged to form a hollow ball called a *blastula.* The cells by this time have begun to show differentiation, and an increase in their total volume is occurring as the zona pellucida disintegrates. There are three distinct parts to the blastula (see Figure 1-2). The *inner cell mass* is an

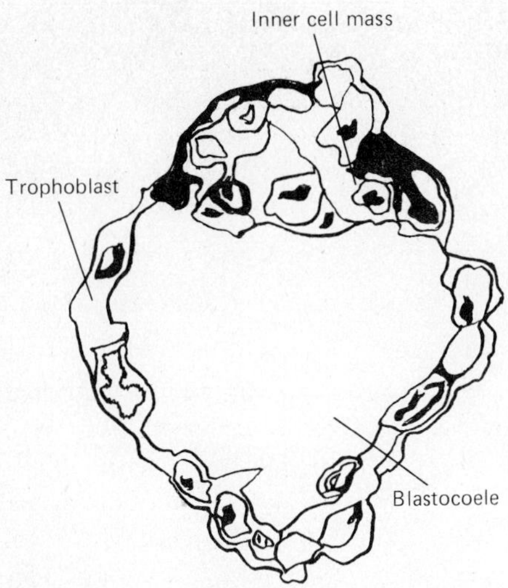

Figure 1-2 The blastula. *(After Carnegie Collection photograph no. 8663 ×600 as shown in B. M. Patten, Human Embryology, McGraw-Hill, New York, 1968, p. 50, by permission.)*

aggregation of cells at one side of the blastula; the *trophoblasts* (trophectoderm) are the cells which form the outer wall of the sphere; and the *blastocoele* is the cavity in the interior of the sphere. The inner cell mass will eventually become the embryo and its protective membranes. The trophoblasts will invade the uterine mucosa to provide the early embryo with nourishment until the placenta can be established (*tropho-* is a prefix meaning nutrition). The blastocoele is the space into which the embryo will grow (*coele-* is a suffix meaning cavity).

About 1 week after fertilization, the inner cell mass has differentiated into an *embryonic disk* of two layers, the ectoderm and entoderm, from which the embryo itself will develop. In addition, there is a small cavity above that disk, the *amnionic cavity.* The blastula is now partially buried (implanted) in the uterine mucosa (see Figure 1-3).

By 10 days after fertilization, the amnionic cavity has developed a layer of cells around it called the *amnion* (see Figure 1-4). These cells represent the origins of the amnionic membrane which surrounds the fetus during its development. The embryonic disk still appears to be two-layered, but projecting from the disk is the beginning of a circle of entodermal cells which will enclose the *yolk sac* or *primitive gut.* The trophoblasts have differentiated into two types of cells. An interior cellular layer that forms the definitive wall of the blastula is now called the *cyto*trophoblast (*cyto-* is a prefix meaning cell). Exterior to this is a nebulous mass called the *syn*trophoblast, which derives its name from the characteristic obliteration of distinctive cell boundaries (*syn-* is a prefix meaning together). These two types

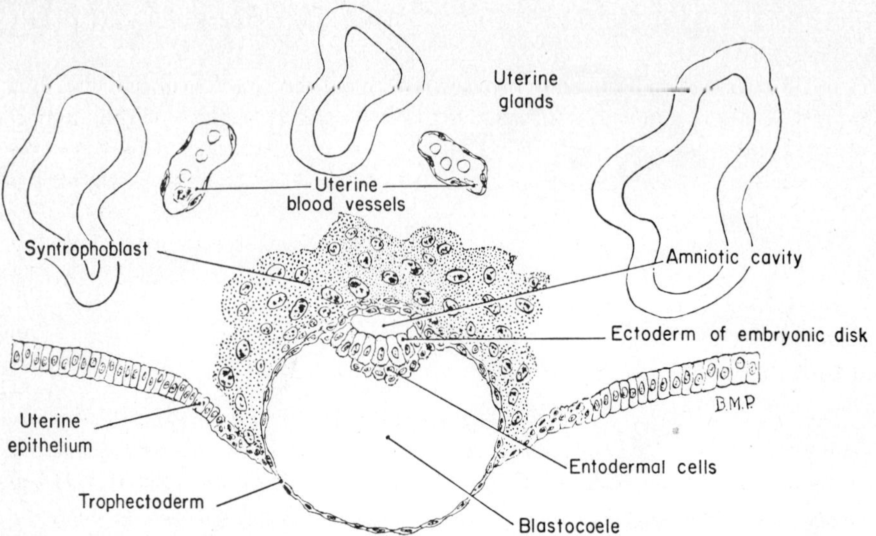

Figure 1-3 The blastula partially implanted in the uterine mucosa. *(From B. M. Patten, Human Embryology, McGraw-Hill, New York, 1968, p. 52, by permission.)*

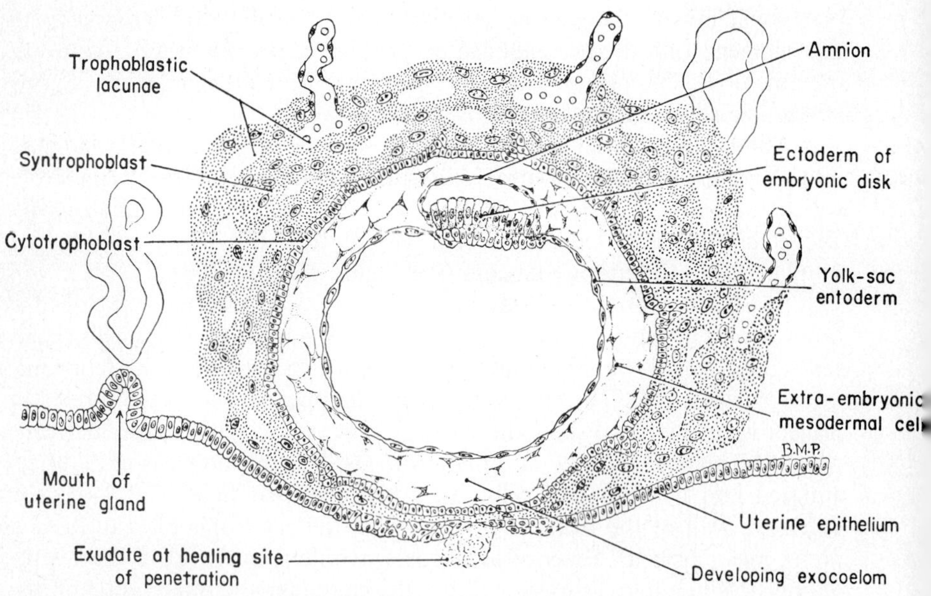

Figure 1-4 The blastula fully implanted, showing especially the development of the amnionic membrane and the yolk sac. *(From B. M. Patten, Human Embryology, McGraw-Hill, New York, 1968, p. 53, by permission.)*

of cells serve particular functions in the process of implantation that will be discussed later.

By 13 days a *mesodermal* layer has appeared in the embryonic disk (between the ectoderm and entoderm). The exterior surface of the amnion is also lined with mesodermal cells, and some mesodermal cells have collected at the caudal end of the embryonic disk, where they are beginning to form the *body stalk,* later to become the umbilical cord. The cytotrophoblast is forming projections into the syntrophoblast. These projections are the forerunners of the *chorionic villi,* which will provide the early embryo with nutrition from the lining of the uterus.

Early Embryonic Landmarks

The first distinctive landmark appearing on the embryonic disk is a line of cells which will form the longitudinal axis of the body. This line of cells, approximately half the length of the embryonic disk, has been named the *primitive streak.* It is an area of very rapid growth from which the embryonic mesodermal (mesenchymal) cells arise. At one end of the primitive streak, near the middle of the embryonic disk, is a thickened projection called *Hensen's node,* around which mesodermal cells migrate on their journey from the primitive streak to the cephalic end of the embryo (see Figure 1-5). There is a vacant space between the entoderm and ectoderm anterior to Hensen's node where a third early landmark, the *notochord,* will form. The notochord is a cylindrical group of cells which marks the location of the vertebral column. The embryo at this stage has been implanted for about 1 week, and the walls of the blastula have expanded considerably, giving the embryo more room to develop.

Soon after the notochord is formed, it causes (by induction) the ectoderm above it to become thickened to form the *neural plate,* which folds

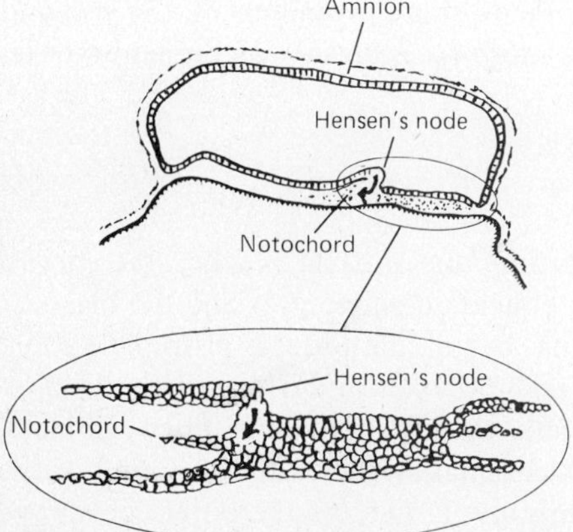

Figure 1-5 Cell migration from the primitive streak. *(Redrawn from B. M. Patten, Human Embryology, McGraw-Hill, New York, 1968, pp. 56–57, by permission.)*

inward to form the *neural groove.* The anterior part of the neural plate will thicken and increase in size to form the brain, while the posterior portion will become the spinal cord.

By the end of 3 weeks of development, the cephalic end of the embryo is readily identifiable. On the lateral surfaces of the head, thickened areas of epithelial tissues called *placodes* form, marking early development of the inner ears. These placodes sink into the tissues by invagination and form the auditory vesicle (blister), which is less conspicuous. Later the outer ear will form close to the site of the original auditory placodes. About the same time, anterior and ventral to the auditory placodes, another pair of vesicles appear, the *optic vesicles,* which are the forerunners of the eyes. Ventral and caudal to the eyes, the other facial features begin to form. Most prominent of the landmarks are the paired *maxillary processes,* which will form the upper jaw, the *mandibular arch,* which will form the lower jaw, and the *stomodaeal depression* between these two, which will become the mouth. Above the maxillary processes two small depressions form. These are the *nasal pits,* which mark the location of the nose. By 6 weeks a primitive face is identifiable (see Figure 1-6).

Meanwhile, in the middle of the embryonic body, the *body cavity,* which will become the thoracic and abdominal cavities, is forming. The early embryo seen from the outside shows a prominence just under the mandibular arch. This bulging, the *cardiac prominence,* marks the cavity in which the early heart is developing. Caudal to the cardiac prominence is the *hepatic prominence,* in which the liver is developing. At about the fourth week after fertilization, there appears a slight groove between the cardiac and hepatic prominences. This groove indicates where the diaphragm will develop and thus indicates the boundary between the thoracic and abdominal cavities. The *mesonephric prominence,* beside the "backbone" of the embryo, indicates the formation of a primitive kidney.

During the fifth week of development, small prominences, the arm and leg buds, appear. These will become more recognizable as the embryo develops.

IMPLANTATION

Approximately 3 days after fertilization, the morula reaches the uterus. After another 3 to 4 days, the zona pellucida disintegrates and the blastula, which has developed from the morula, begins the process of implantation. When the zona pellucida disintegrates, the exterior surface of the trophoblastic cells is sticky to touch, especially directly above the inner cell mass. Usually the surface above the inner cell mass adheres to the lining of the uterus, and the trophoblasts begin to grow larger. As the outer cells grow, they lose their distinctive cell boundaries, thus differentiating into the syn-

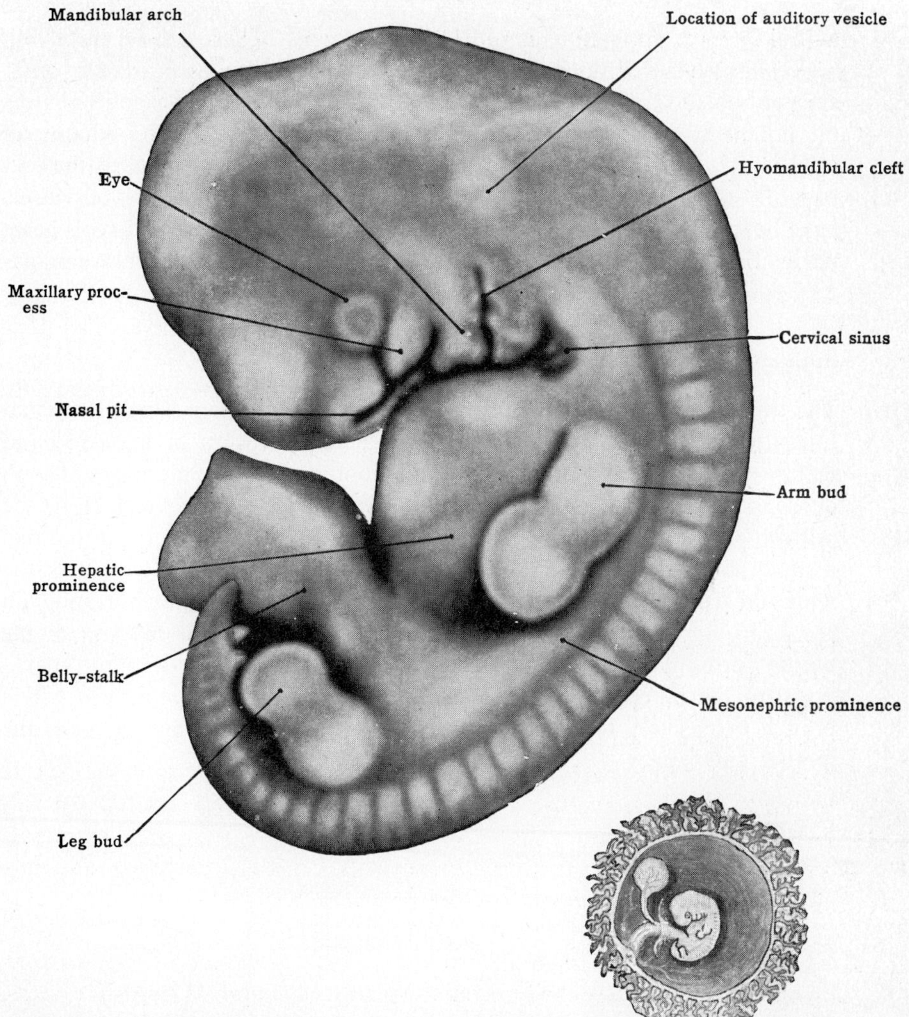

Figure 1-6 By the middle of the sixth week of development, the face is identifiable and arm and legs buds are apparent. *(From B. M. Patten, Human Embryology, McGraw-Hill, New York, 1968, p. 73, by permission.)*

trophoblast mentioned earlier. As the syntrophoblast expands, it erodes maternal tissues, probably by means of enzymes produced by the cells. The resulting liquid material is thought to be used as a nutrient for the growing blastula until a more sophisticated feeding system can be established. A substance is also thought to be produced which prevents blood clotting; thus, as the syntrophoblast erodes through small blood vessels, blood pools form around the blastula as a ready food supply.[7] The cytotrophoblasts gradually form projections into the syntrophoblast. These are the early villi, which have two cell layers: an inner cytotrophoblastic layer and the outer syntrophoblast. At about the beginning of the third week, mesoderm enters the hollow space of the villi to form a connective tissue core, which will eventually contain the blood vessels needed to carry nutrients to the embryo. By the end of the third or early in the fourth week, the blood vessels have been established in the villi. About this same time, the embryo's heart begins functioning and blood cells begin moving through the early circulatory paths.

PLACENTATION

The third week of development also marks the beginning of true placental formation. The placenta is an organ formed by fusion of maternal and embryonic tissues. The tips of the developing villi become covered with dense masses of cytotrophoblasts called *cell columns* (see Figure 1-7). As the syntrophoblast erodes the maternal tissue, the cell columns come into direct contact with maternal tissue. The cytotrophoblasts spread out to cover the maternal tissues, and the inner connective mesoderm of the chorionic villi grow through the cell columns to become fused with the mucosa of the uterus, forming *anchoring villi,* which will eventually form the septa (partitions) of the placenta. Between the anchoring villi are *floating villi* which branch extensively to form the functional units of exchange between the mother and fetus.

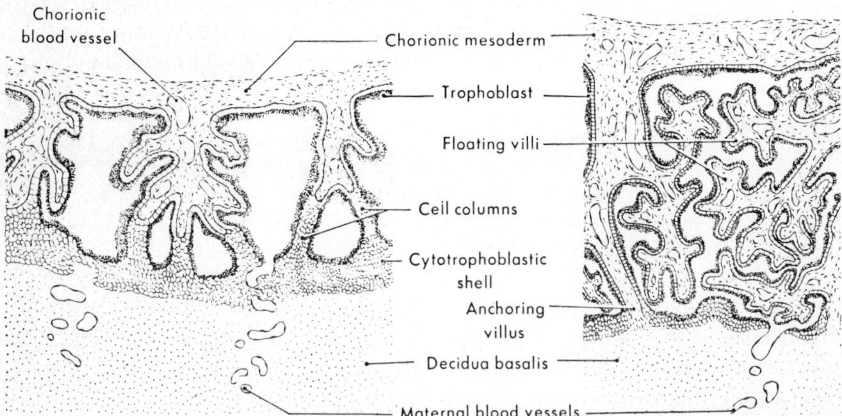

Figure 1-7 The formation of anchoring and floating villi in early placental development. *(From B. M. Patten, Human Embryology, McGraw-Hill, New York, 1968, p. 122, by permission.)*

Placental Partitions

As the placenta becomes established, the anchoring villi enlarge to form recognizable partitions dividing the placenta into 15 or 16 segments called *cotyledons.* In each segment, the branching villi form highly complex, branched vascular systems through which the actual exchange of gases and nutrients between mother and infant takes place (see Figure 1-8). Around the villi in these cotyledons are microscopic spaces through which maternal blood flows. The two circulatory systems are separated by the so-called *placental barrier,* which is simply the cell layers through which the molecules must pass on their way to and from maternal and embryonic circulatory systems.

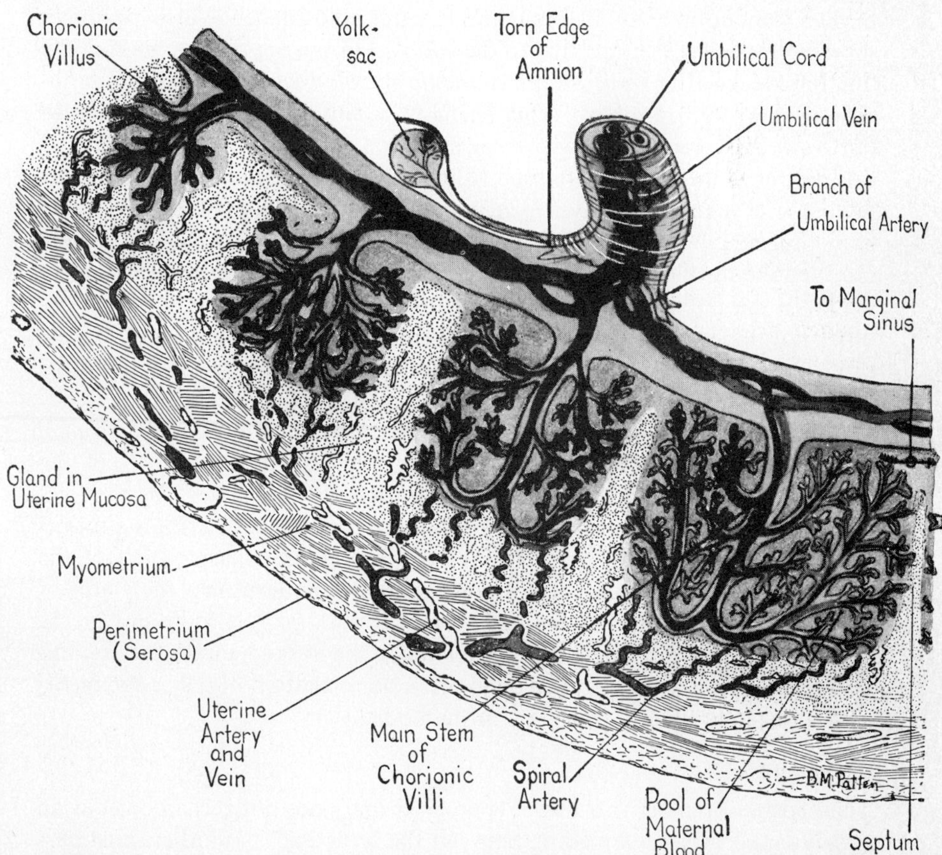

Figure 1-8 The developing placenta. Fetal villi are illustrated in progressively greater development (branching) from left to right in the drawing. *(From B. M. Patten, Human Embryology, McGraw-Hill, New York, 1968, p. 123, by permission.)*

The Placenta As an Organ of Transfer

The placenta is a highly complex organ which functions as a means for transporting nutrient substances from the mother to the fetus and for eliminating waste products from the fetus into the maternal cardiovascular system. Depending on their nature, substances pass through the placenta by *simple diffusion,* by *facilitated transport* (faster movement than simple diffusion), by *active transport* (movement across the placenta against electrochemical gradients), or by *pinocytosis* (materials are engulfed by amoebalike cells). Materials may cross in either direction, from mother to fetus or from fetus to mother, by these means.

Placental Hormones

Besides functioning as an organ of transfer, the placenta also produces some hormones which are vital to the survival of the pregnancy. During the first few weeks after fertilization, *chorionic gonadotrophin* is produced, probably by the syntrophoblast. This hormone maintains the *corpus luteum* in the ovary and stimulates *progesterone* secretion there until the placenta itself can produce enough progesterone to maintain the pregnancy. (The corpus luteum is a yellowish body which functions as an endocrine gland during early pregnancy. It develops from the follicular cells that formerly provided food for the developing ovum before ovulation.) Progesterone functions to maintain the lining of the uterus and to decrease uterine excitability. Another hormone, *placental lactogen,* is also thought to be produced by the syntrophoblast. This hormone stimulates key maternal metabolic adjustments to make more protein and glucose available for the fetus.

Estrogens also are produced by the placenta. Two estrogens, *estradiol* and *estrone,* seem to be produced by the placenta independently of the fetus. However, a third, *estriol,* must have precursors produced by the fetal adrenal glands. It has been suggested that the synthesis of estriol is a means of metabolizing fetal adrenal hormones.[8] Therefore, measurement of the presence of this estrogen provides one means of determining the status of the fetus before delivery. A final hormone, *relaxin,* is also found in the blood of pregnant women. The placenta is the suspected source for this hormone. Its function seems to be to promote relaxation of pelvic ligaments and connective tissues elsewhere in the body.

Placental Barrier

The placental barrier is a useful concept if one does not rely upon it as an absolute. All materials passing between the fetus and its mother must pass through several layers of cells and noncellular materials as they traverse the space between the maternal bloodstream and that of the fetus. Many substances are thus prevented from passing from one system to the other, notably the blood cells themselves. However, the barrier is not totally exclusive, and an occasional blood cell crosses from one circulatory system to the other.[9] (The importance of this phenomenon is discussed in Chapter 9, Hemolytic Disease of the Newborn.) Drugs are known to cross the placenta freely, as are viruses and at least one spirochete, *Treponema pallidum,* the causative organism in syphilis. As the pregnancy progresses, some of the cells between the maternal and fetal blood pools disappear and others decrease in number so that the "placental barrier" actually decreases in thickness and its permeability increases accordingly. Never, however, is there wholesale mixing of maternal and fetal blood.

Regression of Chorionic Villi

At first, the chorionic villi are distributed equally around the blastula. The only villi to remain by the end of the fourth month, however, are those contained within the placenta. To trace the regression of the remaining villi, some areas inside the uterus must be delineated. The lining of the pregnant uterus is called the *decidua.* The decidua directly adjacent to the inner cell mass is the *decidua basalis;* the decidua covering the rest of the (implanted) blastula is the *decidua capsularis;* the remainder of the decidua is the *decidua parietalis* (see Figure 1-9). After the blastula is completely implanted, it grows within the decidua, pushing the decidua capsularis farther and farther away from its maternal blood supply. The villi in that region stop growing from lack of nutrition. With further growth of the embryo, the decidua capsularis is compressed against the decidua parietalis, and the nonfunctional villi disappear because of the pressure. The area of the cho-

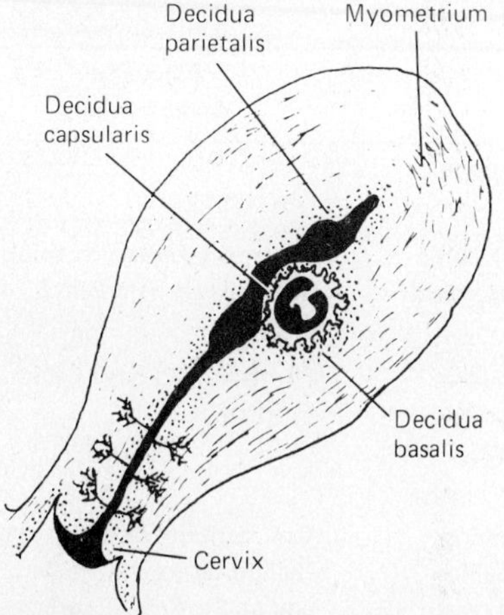

Figure 1-9 The uterus in early pregnancy, showing the different areas of the decidua. *(Adapted from B. M. Patten, Human Embryology, McGraw-Hill, New York, 1968, p. 115, by permission.)*

rion which has highly developed villi is called the *chorion frondosum.* The smooth chorion that has lost its villi is called the *chorion laeve.*

THE UMBILICAL CORD

While the placenta is being established, the umbilical cord is also being formed. The portion of the yolk sac which connects it to the embryo is called the *yolk stalk.* This yolk stalk fuses with a highly vascularized diverticulum of the caudal end of the gut to form the belly stalk. This in turn eventually fuses with the embryonic portion of the developing placenta to provide circulatory pathways connecting the chorionic villi and the embryo. As the body stalk elongates, it becomes known as the *umbilical cord.*

OVERVIEW OF EMBRYONIC AND PLACENTAL DEVELOPMENT

Table 1-1 provides an overview of anatomical development during embryonic and fetal periods. This table should not be considered an exact timetable of development, but rather an aid for grasping relative sequential development of the various systems of the body and of the placenta before birth.

Table 1-1 Gestational Development

Fertilization age	Significant embryonic/ fetal development	Placental development
3–4 days	Fertilized ovum, having undergone cleavage, enters the uterus.	
1 week	Implantation has begun. Embryonic disk has differentiated into ectoderm and entoderm.	Syntrophoblastic invasion of maternal tissues has begun.
2 weeks	Embryonic "body" is 1.5 mm long. Three germ layers have been established. The primitive streak and notochord are present.	Primitive villi have begun to form.
3 weeks	Tubular heart has begun twitching. Primitive red blood cells are being formed. Pronephritic tubules have appeared. Primordia of ear and eye are present.	Villi contain vascular core. Cell columns are present, and anchoring villi are being formed. Placenta covers about one-fifteenth of the internal surface of the uterus.

Table 1-1 Gestational Development (Cont.)

Fertilization age	Significant embryonic/ fetal development	Placental development
4 weeks	Crown-rump measurement of body is now 3.6 mm. Blood is being propelled through the circulatory system. Brain has differentiated into forebrain, midbrain, and hindbrain. Mesonephros (functional primitive kidney) has begun forming. Stomodaeal plate (membrane) has ruptured to make the oral cavity continuous with the foregut. Elongation of the tube which will become the intestines is just beginning.	Placenta has begun functioning as a means of metabolic exchange between mother and baby. Floating villi continue to develop and branch.
5 weeks	Appendage buds are present. Brain has differentiated into five regions. Ten pairs of cranial nerves are recognizable. Mesonephros is functional. Metanephric ducts (final kidney) begin forming.	
6 weeks	Nasal pits appear on the "face." Red blood cells begin to be adult form. Trachea has been formed, and its caudal end is bifurcated (beginning of lung formation). Optic vessicle has invaginated to form optic cup. Local dilation indicates location of stomach. Intestines have become looped. Proctodaeum (membrane between hindgut and anal region) has ruptured so that hindgut is continuous with anal region.	
7 weeks	Eyelids begin to form.	
8 weeks	Fetus is now 1 inch long. Heart chambers have been established. External genitalia are now recognizable as male or female.	Placenta covers one-third of internal surface of uterus.
12 weeks	Fetus now weighs 1 oz.	
16 weeks	Fetus is 6½ inches long and weighs 4 oz. Bladder takes adult form.	
20 weeks	Fetus is 10 inches long and weighs ½ lb. Small amount of "woolly" hair on head.	Placenta covers one-half of internal surface of uterus.
24 weeks	Fetus is 12 inches long and weighs 1½ lb. Eyebrows and lashes are forming.	Placental growth now occurs in thickness rather than width.

Table 1-1 Gestational Development (Cont.)

Fertilization age	Significant embryonic/ fetal development	Placental development
28 weeks	Fetus is 15 inches long and weighs 2½ lb. Lungs are functional. Lanugo is present. Survival rate is less than 50% if delivered now.	
32 weeks	Fetus 16 inches long and weighs 6 lb. Fingernails and toenails are at the ends of the digits. Lanugo is being shed.	
40 weeks	Fetus is 20 inches long and weighs 7–7½ lb. Lanugo is mostly shed. Fetus is now full term.	Placenta is 3 to 4 times as thick as it was at 20 weeks.

Compiled from several sources.

REFERENCES

1 Bradley M. Patten, *Human Embryology,* McGraw-Hill, New York, 1968, p. 20.
2 Elizabeth D. Hay, "Embryonic Origin of Tissues," in Roy O. Greep (ed.), *Histology,* McGraw-Hill, New York, 1966, p. 67.
3 Ibid., p. 71.
4 Patten, op. cit., p. 181.
5 Ibid., p. 69.
6 Ibid., p. 68.
7 Ibid., p. 114.
8 Allan B. Weingold, "The Fetus and Fetal Environment," in Edward Wasserman and Lawrence B. Slobody (eds.), *Survey of Clinical Pediatrics,* McGraw-Hill, New York, 1974, p. 190.
9 Ibid., p. 188.

BIBLIOGRAPHY

DeCoursey, Russell Myles: *The Human Organism,* McGraw-Hill, New York, 1968.

Hay, Elizabeth D.: "Embryonic Origin of Tissues," in Roy O. Greep (ed.), *Histology,* McGraw-Hill, New York, 1966.

Langley, L. L., Ira R. Telford, and John B. Christensen: *Dynamic Anatomy and Physiology,* McGraw-Hill, New York, 1969.

Patten, Bradley M.: *Human Embryology,* McGraw-Hill, New York, 1968.

Weingold, Allan B.: "The Fetus and Fetal Environment," in Edward Wasserman and Lawrence B. Slobody (eds.), *Survey of Clinical Pediatrics,* McGraw-Hill, New York, 1974.

Chapter 2

The Term Infant at Birth

THE ONSET OF LABOR

The exact mechanisms that initiate labor are not known, although several factors which seem to play a part have been identified. Langley et al. suggest that the stretching of the uterus as the fetus grows causes reflex uterine contractions throughout pregnancy which increase in strength as term approaches.[1] They also suggest that the stretching of the uterus early in labor as the fetus moves down into the birth canal sends nerve impulses to the posterior pituitary gland, causing the release of *oxytocin,* a hormone known to strengthen uterine contractions.[2]

Hellman agrees that stretching of the uterus may contribute to the onset of labor, especially when more than one fetus is present.[3] He also states that a sudden decrease in uterine size, as occurs when the amnionic membrane ruptures and fluid rushes out, may precipitate labor. He seems, however, to place more emphasis on the effects of hormonal relationships. He suggest that the muscle of the uterus (*myometrium*) demonstrates increasing sensitivity and reactivity to oxytocin during pregnancy due to increasing levels of estrogen (a uterine-stimulating hormone). The stimulating effects of the estrogen and oxytocin are blocked, however, until late pregnancy by the presence of *progesterone* in the myometrium. Progesterone is a hormone produced by the placenta and deposited in the myometrium adjacent to it throughout pregnancy. It has been demonstrated that the part of the uterus adjacent to the placenta is less responsive to stretch stimuli and less active electrically than the remainder of the organ. Just before term, the production of progesterone decreases. At this time, the muscle again becomes responsive to oxytocin and labor begins, according to this theory. Hellman also states that psychic factors seem to be important in some cases, citing profound grief and psychic shock from an automobile accident as examples.

On the other hand, Dawes, an English physiologist, feels that his work with animals rules out stretching of the uterus as a major factor in the initiation of labor.[4] He has found that there is a pattern of increasing uterine activity throughout pregnancy and that this pattern remains constant even in those rare situations in which the fetus is developing outside the uterus (as in the fallopian tube). He has demonstrated in animals that if the fetus is removed during gestation but the placenta left intact in utero, the placenta is delivered at the time the fetus would normally be expected to be born. In addition, he has found that although oxytocin facilitates labor, labor can progress without it. Finally, he states that the presence of an observer in the room with laboring animals delays delivery. (This should not be confused with the helping presence of another person when a woman is in labor.)

Thus, there are theories, arguments, and evidence leading to no definite conclusions about the initiation of labor. The cause is probably a combination of factors and indeed may, in the end, be a somewhat individualized phenomenon, as are so many human responses.

THE EVENTS OF LABOR AND DELIVERY

Whatever the cause, the events of labor and delivery have been clearly described. It is certain that uterine contractions do occur throughout pregnancy. These may become rather strong and at times rhythmic toward term before the onset of labor. True labor, however, is identified not by the presence of contractions, but by progressive changes produced in the cervix by these contractions. The *cervix* is the narrow neck of the uterus opening into the vagina. During pregnancy, it is about 5 cm (2 inches) long and its tiny opening is occluded by a mucus plug. During labor, the cervix is stretched laterally until it forms an opening about 10 cm (4 inches) in diameter. As it is stretched, its length gradually decreases until it becomes only a thin rim. Although the two events are interrelated, two separate criteria are used in evaluating the progress of labor. *Dilation* (dilatation) is the gradual *increase* in the *width* of the cervical opening; *effacement* is the progressive *decrease* in *length* of the cervix. See Figure 2-1 for a diagrammatic representation of these changes. The cervix is said to be completely dilated when its opening is 10 cm in diameter. Effacement is complete when only a paper-thin rim of the cervix can be felt by an examiner.

The Stages of Labor

Traditionally, labor is described in three stages. *Stage one* lasts from the beginning of true labor contractions (those which produce cervical changes) until complete dilation and effacement of the cervix has been reached. For most women having their first babies (*primigravida*) the first stage of labor lasts from 12 to 14 hours. In *multigravida* (women who have already had two or more babies) the first stage of labor varies considerably, but it is generally shorter than that of the primigravida. (The exception to this rule

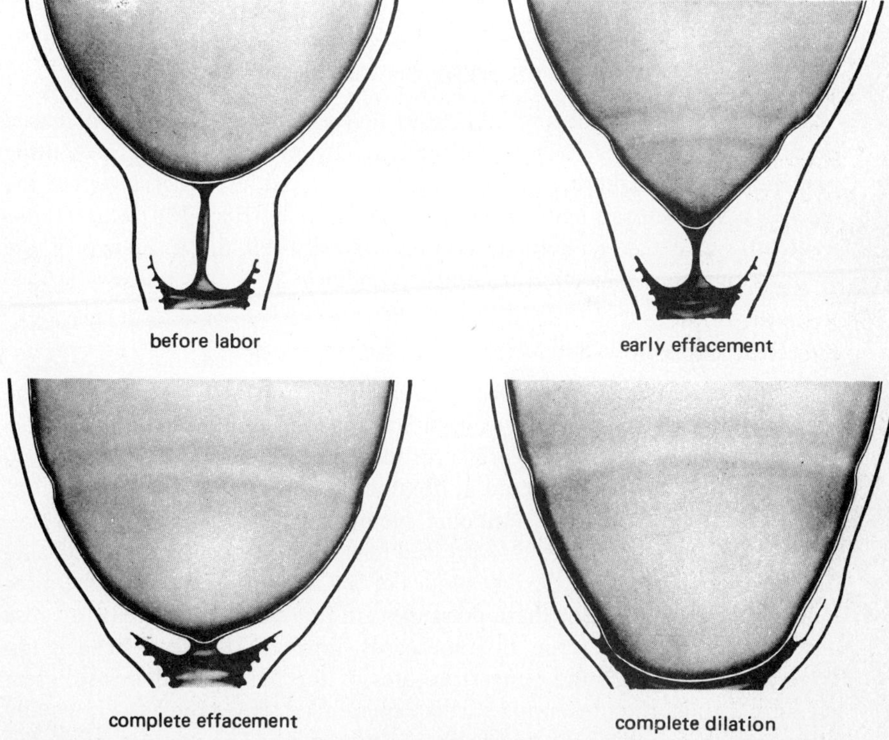

Figure 2-1 During labor the cervix shortens (effacement) and its opening becomes wider (dilation or dilatation). (*From Mechanisms of Normal Labor, Ross Clinical Education Aid # 13, Ross Laboratories, Columbus, Ohio, by permission.)*

is the woman who has had many babies and for whom labor may be prolonged because of an "overused" uterine muscle which can no longer contract effectively.)

The *second stage of labor* is defined as that period of time from complete dilation and effacement of the cervix to the actual delivery of the infant. During this time the fetus must move down through the birth canal and pass through the vaginal orifice. This process usually lasts for a few minutes in the multigravida and up to 2 hours in normal labor for the primigravida.

The *third stage of labor* is that time from the birth of the baby to the delivery of the placenta. This event usually takes place in the first half hour after delivery of the baby, very often within 5 or 10 minutes of the baby's delivery.

It is becoming more common to consider a *fourth stage*: the first hour after delivery of the placenta. This time is critical both because it is the time when the mother is most likely to hemorrhage after childbirth and because it is an important time for the early establishment of the family unit.

EFFECTS OF LABOR AND DELIVERY ON THE FETUS

The fetus is affected during labor and delivery directly by the increased intrauterine pressures during contractions, by pressure of the presenting part against the structures of the birth canal, and by drugs given to the mother which subsequently cross the placental barrier. The fetus is also frequently affected, sometimes very profoundly, by the influence of the contractions upon placental respiratory function.

Effects of Pressure

The fetus experiences two types of pressure during labor. First, when the uterus contracts, pressure is exerted internally as the size of the uterus decreases. These contraction pressures may reach levels as high as 50 to 60 mmHg in normal labor without abdominal pushing.

In addition, after the amnionic membranes have ruptured, the presenting part, usually the head, is pressed first against the cervix as it is being dilated and later against the soft tissues of the perineum to stretch them for delivery. In normal labor these pressures are not sufficiently great to cause any problems for the fetus. In some cases, however, the fetal head is too large to pass through the bony structures of the pelvis. In this case, great pressure against the presenting part is experienced. Since the head is usually the presenting part, severe brain damage can result. The episiotomy (surgical incision of the perineum to widen its aperture) and/or the use of low forceps for the actual delivery eliminates most of the pressure which would result from stretching the perineum.

The fetus does respond to pressure physiologically, even when only normal pressure is experienced. The fetal heart rate may decrease in response to contractions during labor. This response, called *early deceleration,* is thought to be due to pressure on the head which affects vagal nerve stimulation of the heart.[5] The slowing of the heart begins during the very early phases of the contraction and lasts usually less than 30 seconds, never more than 90 seconds. It returns to the baseline rate by the end of the contraction. Placental gas exchange during this period is enhanced by the pooling of blood in the intervillous spaces, so that there is no accompanying hypoxia nor hypercapnia.

Passage through the Pelvis

In considering the total effects of pressure upon the fetus, it is necessary to describe, briefly, the passage of the fetus through the pelvis. For convenience, the passage of the presenting part through the pelvis is expressed in terms of its *station.* The station of the presenting part is considered to be 0 when it is even with the ischial spines. The distance of the presenting parts from the ischial spines is measured in centimeters and expressed as negative numbers (−1, −2, etc.) if the part is above the level of the ischial spines and as a positive number (+1, +2, etc.) when it is below the ischial spines (see Figure 2-2). The head enters the pelvis through the pelvic inlet, which is usually about 10 cm (4 inches) in diameter. The head must then pass between the ischial spines, which represent the narrowest plane of the pel-

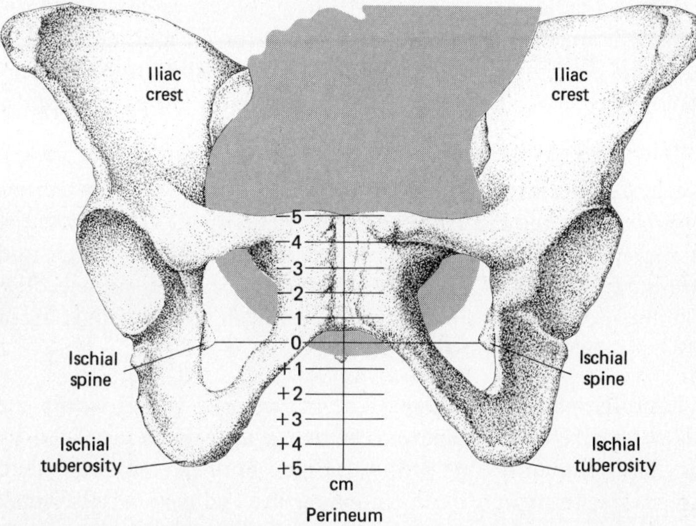

Figure 2-2 Station marks the infant's progress through the pelvis. (*From Mechanisms of Normal Labor, Ross Clinical Education Aid # 13, Ross Laboratories, Columbus, Ohio, by permission.*)

vis, normally 9.5 to 10 cm.[6]

To facilitate passage of the fetus through the pelvis, the fetus usually assumes a head-down (vertex) position with the chin flexed upon the chest. This position allows the smallest possible diameter of the fetal head (suboccipitobregmatic diameter) to pass through the pelvis, thus decreasing the risk of undue pressure on the head. Any deviation from the normal flexed fetal position increases the diameter of the head which must pass through the pelvis and thus increases the risk of injury of the baby.

Molding A mechanism which is protective for the fetus is the process of molding the fetal head to fit the shape of the pelvis. This is a process through which the fetal head may be somewhat elongated and narrowed. The cranial bones are pushed closer together, and the edges may even overlap at the suture lines (see Figure 4-3). This process decreases the diameter of the fetal head without damaging the brain tissue because it occurs slowly over a period of hours. Babies whose heads are molded at birth are usually products of relatively long labors. The heads resume their normal shapes in the first few days following delivery. Rapid deliveries which do not allow for molding may cause brain damage by exerting too much pressure on the head.

Analgesia and Anesthesia during Labor and Delivery

The common types of obstetric analgesia and anesthesia used are systemic, conduction, and psychoprophylactic. The judicious employment of psychoprophylactic techniques, whether used exclusively or in conjunction with pharmacological agents, decreases the need for drugs during labor and delivery. Since there is no drug which is totally safe for all mothers and infants, the use of the psychoprophylactic methods is certainly to be encouraged. Let us consider now, however, fetal reactions to drugs commonly given.

Transplacental Transmission of Drugs It is thought that most drugs cross the placenta by simple diffusion and that virtually all drugs cross the placenta to some extent.[7] Some drugs pass the placental barrier faster and with more ease than do others. Of particular importance, here, are narcotics and their antagonists, ultrashort barbiturates, and inhalation drugs, all of which cross the placenta very readily.

General Fetal Responses to Drugs The life of drug action within the body depends primarily upon the rate at which a drug is metabolized by liver enzymes and excreted by the kidneys. Since both liver function and renal function in the fetus and young neonate are reduced, drugs which enter fetal circulation may remain active longer and at higher doses than would ordinarily be expected from studies on adult patients. This is particularly important when considering drug-related depression in the newborn. Moore notes that depressed neonates may have a depressed sucking effort for up to 4 days after delivery, accompanied by a decrease in both visual attentiveness and overall activity.[8]

Another phenomenon which is of interest in considering depressed infants is that the fetal brain receives a greater percentage of cardiac output than the brain of the newborn infant does.[9] During intrauterine stress which causes hypoxia and hypercapnia, the *percentage* of blood volume flowing to the brain increases still further because the blood is shunted past some of the less vital organs. The dosage of drugs carried to the brain of an hypoxic fetus is thus increased, compounding an already bad situation, since drug depression in the infant is directly related to the concentration of drug in the central nervous system. In addition, the blood-brain barrier is more permeable in the young neonate than it will be later in life, further increasing the dosage of medication carried to the central nervous system.[10]

Some drugs can be helpful to the fetus by stimulating enzyme systems to greater efficiency. The noted example is phenobarbital, which stimulates the enzyme system involved in the metabolism of bilirubin. Phenobarbital has been given to mothers late in pregnancy in limited trials to decrease bilirubin levels in their infants after birth.[11] Such use of drugs is advised only with caution, however, because the total action of the drugs is not known, and it is feared that some unwanted side effects may accompany the desired ones.

Systemic Drugs Used in Labor As will be noted later, nearly all drugs, even those used for local anesthetic blocks, do indeed have systemic effects; however, here we shall focus on those systemic drugs ordinarily used to provide pain relief or to decrease anxiety in the early stages of labor. It should be emphasized, again, that good nursing care and use of psychoprophylactic techniques will reduce the dosage of drugs needed.

One drug commonly given in labor is meperidine hydrochloride (Demerol), often combined with hydroxyzine pamoate (Vistaril) to potentiate its effects. These drugs do cross the placenta readily and appear to sedate the infant, decreasing respiratory efforts at delivery. There is disagreement about the safe time to administer such drugs to the laboring woman. Hellman cites an interval of at least 4 hours between the last dose of the medication and delivery of the infant as the minimum safe interval,[12] but he also states that firm evidence to support this hypothesis is lacking. Shnider and Moya, on the other hand, report that depression of study infants was not found to be significantly different from that of control groups when meperidine was given to the mother less than 1 hour or more than 3 hours before delivery time.[13] Peak depression occurred when the baby was born during the second and third hours after administration of the drug. The size of the dose given to the mother, its route of administration, and its combination with other drugs did influence its effect on the infant.

The narcotized infant is likely to be suffering from hypoxia, hypercapnia with its accompanying acidosis, and a decrease or even abolition of the reflexes which normally prevent aspiration of amnionic fluid or mucus. Hellman cites secondary apnea (the baby gasps once or twice and then ceases respiratory activity) as a probable result of narcotic depression.[14]

The two narcotic antagonists currently in use, nalorine (Nalline) and levallorphan (Lorfan), are commonly given either to the laboring woman close to delivery time or to the infant immediately after birth. This practice is not without controversy, however. Bauer states that these drugs have analgesic effects of their own and that their use compounds the drug problems the infant is already experiencing.[15] He feels, contrary to popular belief and current practice, that the dosage of narcotics given to laboring mothers is not likely to be the cause of respiratory depression in infants and that depressed infants are better treated with assisted ventilation and oxygen administration than with narcotic antagonists.

Barbiturates and tranquilizers are sometimes given to laboring mothers to allay anxiety. Moore feels that this is an unwise practice because both of these drugs can depress the infant, and if drug depression occurs, there are no drug antagonists to counteract it.[16] Bauer stresses the importance of avoiding the administration of *any* mixtures of drugs because of the unknown effects of drug interaction.[17] He especially cautions against the use of diazepam (Valium) and barbiturates together, citing long-term untoward effects (12 to 36 hours), such as abnormal reflexes, hypertension or hypotension, and inappropriate responses, as sequelae of this particular combination.

Regional Anesthetics Regional anesthetics are drugs injected with the intention of anesthetizing only a portion of the body. Regional anesthetics are basically of two types: (1) local anesthetics injected directly into the tissues to deaden them and (2) spinal anesthetics, injected into the spinal canal to deaden nerve pathways (see Figure 2-3).

Local anesthetics, although generally safer than systemic drugs, are not without hazard for the fetus. Bauer states that so long as anesthetics are used in doses which result in analgesia, they are safe for both mother and child; however, he implies that they are frequently used in larger, anesthetic doses.[18] These, he contends, are not so safe as once thought. No matter how they are administered, paracervically, peridurally (as in caudal anesthesia), or intramuscularly, maternal blood levels reach significant levels. The drugs, of course, can then cross the placenta to the baby. He feels that there is a special hazard when aromatic amino local anesthetics (lidocaine, Mepivacaine) are used, presumably because they are absorbed by the blood-

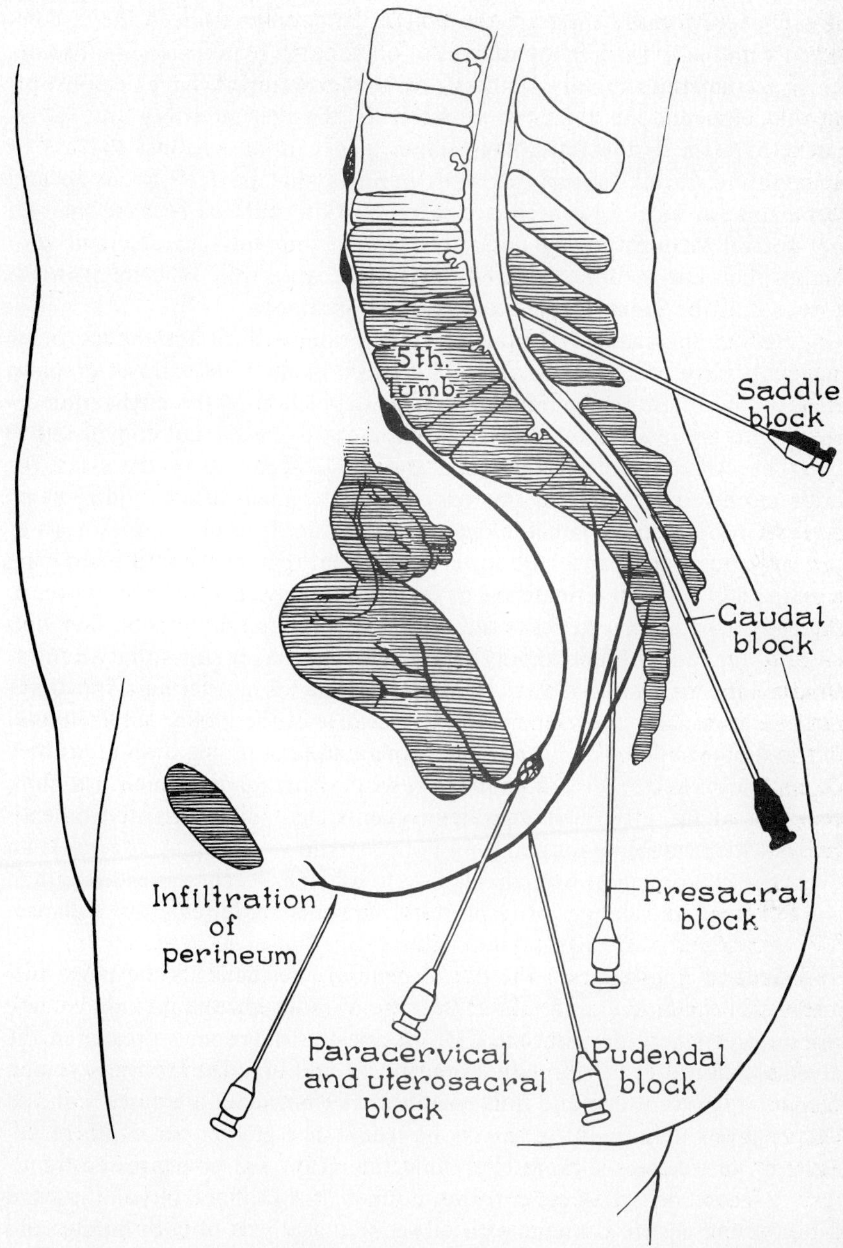

Figure 2-3 Several methods may be used for regional anesthesia during labor. (*From L. M. Hellman and Jack A. Pritchard, Williams Obstetrics, 14th ed., Prentice-Hall, Englewood Cliffs, 1971, by permission.*)

stream more rapidly than are the others. Sometimes epinephrine is combined with these drugs in an attempt to prevent the hypotension that sometimes accompanies spinal anesthesia. Animal experiments have demonstrated that epinepherine causes constriction of the uterine artery and subsequent hypoxia in the fetus, thus Bauer also cautions against the use of epinephrine during labor.[19] He does indicate that he feels procaine and tetracaine for local anesthesia are safer than other drugs because they do not spread throughout the tissues so rapidly, but this characteristic also makes their use technically more difficult because their placement in the tissues must be exact if pain relief is to be obtained.

Besides the hazards of systemic absorption of local anesthetics, other accidents have occurred, notably penetration of the fetal scalp or cranium with the injection needle and subsequent deposition of the medication directly into the fetal circulation, resulting in bradycardia and convulsions.[20]

The classic saddle block spinal anesthesia seems to be the safest for both mother and child. In this procedure, the medication is introduced directly into the spinal canal in the lumbar region. It results in anesthesia of the legs and of the pelvic and lower abdominal regions without interfering significantly with either maternal or fetal physiology. The greatest danger in the use of spinal anesthetics is the possibility of maternal hypotension with its resulting loss of blood supply to the placenta. Bauer states that an intravenous infusion should always be started before administering a spinal anesthetic, especially in pregnant women because of the additional likelihood of the supine hypotension syndrome (explained later in this chapter) as they lie on their backs.[21] Greiss cautions also that pregnant women are more sensitive to the effects of anesthetic agents than nonpregnant women.[22] Doses which would be normal for a nonpregnant woman may constitute an overdose in a pregnant woman, leading to a higher level of anesthesia than was intended and danger of respiratory paralysis and circulatory collapse.

General Anesthetics The use of general anesthetics is the most hazardous for the mother and infant. Because of reduced residual lung volume in late pregnancy, the concentration of anesthesia becomes greater in the alveoli than would be normally expected. In addition, the laboring woman tends to hyperventilate and thus becomes anesthetized more quickly and to deeper levels than might otherwise be true.[23] The greater her depth of anesthesia, of course, the more likely that the infant will be depressed by it.

A second hazard of general anesthesia is the likelihood of vomiting and aspiration of gastric contents with subsequent asphyxia of both mother and infant. Gastric emptying time is increased during pregnancy, and gastric emptying almost ceases during labor. Therefore, if the laboring woman has had anything to eat even several hours before delivery, the use of a general anesthetic is risky. The American College of Obstetricians and Gynecologists' Committee on Obstetrical Anesthesia and Analgesia recommends that a woman should have been NPO (i.e., nothing taken orally) at least 6 hours before a general anesthetic can be administered.[24] However, Greiss states that food may stay in the stomach for 24 to 48 hours after labor has begun and that no pregnant woman should be considered free from the hazard of vomiting and aspiration.[25]

Effects of Labor on Placental Respiratory Function

For the fetus, the organ of respiration is the placenta rather than the lungs. However, the principles of gas exchange are essentially the same as in the lungs after birth. The primary difference is that the oxygen comes to the fetus not directly from air but from maternal blood as it flows through the intervillous spaces of the placenta.

Partial Pressure In discussing respiratory function, the concentrations of oxygen and carbon dioxide in the lungs or in the blood are expressed in terms of their *partial pressures.* Gases exert pressure in all directions. At sea level, atmospheric gases exert a total pressure of 760 mmHg. Partial pressure is that part of the total pressure exerted by a single gas in a mixture; thus, if the percentage of oxygen present in a given sample of gas at sea level is 20.94 percent, then its partial pressure at sea level is 760 mmHg multiplied by 20.94 percent, or 159.1 mmHg. Partial pressure of a gas is usually written as *P* followed by the chemical symbols for the gas; thus, the partial pressure of oxygen just calculated would be written: $P\text{o}_2$ 159.1. In physiology, partial pressures become important because they determine the direction of exchange of gases from one tissue to another. Gases, like other substances, move from an area of higher concentration to an area of lower concentration.

Several factors affect the rate of exchange. For instance, if the blood, which transports gases, is moving very slowly through the tissues, it is exposed to the differences in pressure for a longer time, and the pressures can more nearly equalize. If it becomes stagnant, however, exchange ceases after equalization has been reached. If the blood is moving too fast, the pressures may not have time to completely equalize; thus, incomplete exchange occurs.

In addition, each gas has a *diffusion coefficient,* which is essentially the *rate* at which it moves across tissue barriers (capillary walls, interstitial fluid, and the like). Oxygen has a much lower diffusion coefficient than does carbon dioxide; hence it crosses tissue barriers more slowly than does carbon dioxide in similar circumstances.

Maternal blood in the intervillous spaces carries a $P\text{o}_2$ of 40 mmHg and a $P\text{co}_2$ of 38 mmHg. The blood entering the villi from the fetus has a $P\text{o}_2$ of approximately 16 mmHg and a $P\text{co}_2$ of approximately 46 mmHg. Hence, oxygen moves from the mother's bloodstream into the fetal blood, and CO_2

moves from fetal blood into maternal blood. Because of its low diffusion coefficient, oxygen reaches only partial pressure of approximately 29 mmHg in the umbilical vein, a level much lower than is normally obtained in extrauterine existence. (Po_2 reaches approximately 100 mmHg in the blood as it leaves the lungs postnatally.) This low Po_2 in the intrauterine environment has been likened to the atmosphere on the top of Mount Everest.[26] However, this condition is normal for intrauterine existence and poses no threat to the fetus. The fetal partial pressure of carbon dioxide more nearly approximates extrauterine conditions, reaching 42 mmHg in the umbilical vein. (Pco_2 levels in blood leaving the lungs postnatally are usually about 40 mmHg.)

Factors Affecting Placental Gas Exchange

Of primary importance in determining gas exchange in the placenta are the rate of maternal blood flow through the placenta and the level of maternal blood pressure. During a uterine contraction, the maternal veins and arteries supplying the placenta are squeezed shut and blood is thought to pool in the intervillous spaces.[27] It is thought that a relatively larger volume of blood is trapped in these spaces during a contraction than is present at any other time, because the thinner-walled veins are shut before the arteries are occluded. The exchange of gases is thus enhanced by this phenomenon, and normal labor poses no threat to the fetus. However, prolonged contractions (longer than 90 seconds) or a series of contractions with insufficient relaxation of the uterus between them to allow for circulation of maternal blood to resume can become life-threatening. Fetal hypoxia and acidosis are common sequelae of these occurrences because the stagnant maternal blood is soon depleted of its oxygen stores, and it becomes saturated with carbon dioxide and unable to remove any more from fetal circulation.

A drop in maternal blood pressure also presents a potential threat to the fetus. Systemic hypotension causes a decrease in the volume of blood available for placental circulation; hence, it decreases proportionately the supply of oxygen available to the fetus and the means for removing fetal carbon dioxide. During labor, maternal hypotension is most likely to occur as a result of anesthesia, from maternal hemorrhage due to premature separation of the placenta, or from *supine hypotension syndrome.* In supine hypotension syndrome, a sudden drop in maternal blood pressure may occur when a pregnant woman lies on her back. The blood return to the heart is decreased by the weight of the uterus on the inferior vena cava, and the decreased circulating blood volume results in a lowering of the blood pressure. Usually, turning the mother to one side will relieve the pressure and rapidly restore normal blood pressure. If the maternal hypotension is severe or prolonged, however, the baby may experience hypoxia and acidosis.

ADAPTATION TO EXTRAUTERINE LIFE

Normal newborns exhibit generalized reactions to delivery. They are at first very wide-awake, alert, and active as they react to the stresses of labor and the sudden change in environment. This period of wakefulness is called the *first period of reactivity.* It usually lasts from 10 to 60 minutes after birth. Irregularity and increased activity are characteristic of both motor and smooth-muscle responses. Respiratory movements are rapid and irregular, and the heart rate increases to an average peak of 180 beats/minute at 3 minutes after birth. Bowel sounds become audible and oral mucus may be produced. The infant exhibits exploratory behavior such as flaring of the nares or sniffing in the absence of respiratory distress, movements of the head and limbs, sucking, chewing, pursing of the lips, blinking of the eyes, and periods of crying interspersed with sudden periods of quiet.[28]

Following this period of activity, the infant quiets down and goes to sleep. During this time, the respiratory and heart rates slow down and become more regular and the infant's color should show adequate oxygenation of tissues. The infant usually sleeps from 2 to 6 hours, depending upon many factors which have not yet been identified.

A *second period of reactivity* follows the period of sleep. During this period, as in the first, the infant's heart and respiratory rates increase and become unstable. Bowel activity increases and meconium is usually expelled. Oral mucus often becomes a problem, and the infant may gag or vomit because of it. Rudolph likens this period to the recovery period following anesthesia, and he stresses that close observation and knowledgeable care during this time are vitally important.[29] The second period of reactivity may last a few minutes or several hours. Following this, the infant again becomes quiet, but may not go back to sleep. The infant may then be ready for the first feeding.

Establishing Respiratory Function

The first and most dramatic physiologic adaptation which must occur after birth is the establishment of respiratory function. To understand this phenomenon better, let us review briefly fetal lung development.

Fetal Lung Development The fetal lung first appears as an invagination of the foregut which develops into a glandlike organ with many internal branches to its structure. Beginning at about the fifth month of fetal life, this tissue receives an increasingly complex vascular network which comes to lie directly beside the terminal ends of the branches. By a gradual growth of the terminal "air spaces" of the branches accompanied by closer and closer apposition of the capillaries, the familiar alveolar structures of postnatal life are formed. The fetal lungs at birth are filled with fluid. It was thought at one time that this was amnionic fluid inhaled in utero. Although there seem to be respiratory movements before birth, available evidence now denies any tidal movement of amnionic fluid in and out of the lungs. Instead, the fluid in the lungs seems to have its origin in the vascular system.[30]

The First Breath As delivery occurs in the usual vertex position, the upper airway, having been delivered first, has a lower pressure than the thorax, still in the birth canal. This condition aids in the escape of some of the fluid from the lungs. Then, as the thorax is delivered, there is an automatic elastic recoil of the lungs which expands them somewhat and draws air into them. The diaphragm also begins to function, performing its main duty of decreasing the intrathoracic pressure by enlarging the thoracic cavity and thus providing for the inspiratory phase of the respiratory cycle. According to Karlberg, it is the action of the diaphragm which is primarily responsible for establishing respiration of the newborn.[31] Animal studies indicate the following factors as possible initiators of the first diaphragmatic contractions: a decrease in body temperature, the tying of the umbilical cord, a combination of low $P\text{o}_2$ and increased $P\text{co}_2$, and tactile stimulation.[32] Korones feels that the biochemical changes and the decrease in temperature are of major importance, although he stresses that extreme cooling of the infant contributes detrimentally to overall functioning.[33]

Establishment of Residual Air Volume Normally, the exhalation which follows the first breath does not remove all the inhaled air from the lungs, thus beginning the establishment of a residual air volume. According to Dawes, neonatal residual air reaches near-adult proportions within 15 minutes after birth.[34] Karlberg, on the other hand, states that this "adult" level of function is not reached until the infant is several days old.[35] The important point here, however, is that residual air volume is established from the first breath.

The Work of Respiration Because contraction of the diaphram is involved in the initiation and continuation of respiration, a certain amount of energy is expended. It is important, especially for later consideration, to realize how much effort is needed to expand the lungs of the newborn infant. It has been shown with lambs that at term the pressure required to expand the lungs for the first breath may be as much as 30 mmHg higher than that needed for subsequent breaths.[36] The reasons for this difference are rather complex, but they can be illustrated with a balloon. The air pressure needed to begin inflating a balloon is much greater than that needed to continue expanding it once it contains a little air. In a sphere, the molecules of the walls of the sphere have an attraction for each other and hence toward the center of the sphere. This attraction, *surface tension,* is a force which is inversely proportional to the radius of the sphere; thus, the smaller the radius, the greater the attraction of the molecules for each other, and vice versa. Therefore, when the walls of the balloon are close to each other, the initial inflation of the balloon requires a greater force than will be required to enlarge it once expansion has begun. Similarly, the first breath requires a greater force than later breaths when a residual volume of air is being established in the alveoli. As might be reasoned, anything which increases surface tension increases the force required for expansion of a sphere, and likewise, anything that decreases surface tension decreases the force required for expansion.

Surfactant A material of protein and lipid content that lowers the surface tension in the alveoli is produced in the fetal lungs from about the twenty-third week of gestation. This substance, *surfactant,* is probably produced by cells that line the alveoli. It is usually present in sufficient quantities to facilitate normal respiration by the thirtieth week of gestation in most infants, and earlier for some.[37] When surfactant is absent from the lungs or in insufficient quantities, the surface tension of the alveoli may be so great that the lungs collapse almost totally after each breath, preventing the accumulation of residual air. This in turn requires the infant to expend as much energy for every breath as is required normally only for the initial inflation. Atelectasis is also a common finding in surfactant-poor lungs.

Removal of Lung Fluid The infant's lungs must be cleared of the fluid before adequate air exchange can occur. Some of this fluid is evacuated during the birth process. The remainder is thought to be removed via the lymphatics.[38] Besides interfering with aeration, the lung fluid also increases the work of respiration by increasing the resistance to air flow into the lungs.

Maintenance of Respiratory Function The newborn infant tends to gasp once or twice and then gradually to assume a rhythmic respiratory pattern, although the rate and depth of respirations may be quite variable for several days. Characteristically, the abdomen rises and falls at the same time as the chest during inhalation and exhalation. All newborns are nose breathers. They are unable to breathe through their mouths, and any interference in the passage of air through the nostrils can threaten the airway.

The Fetal Erythrocyte In considering the total respiratory function, the erythrocyte, which carries the oxygen, merits some attention. The erythrocyte of the newborn is somewhat different from that of the adult. It has a higher metabolic rate and contains different proportions of enzymes than are found in the adult. These differences make the red blood cells of the infant under 3 months of age susceptible to damage by substances (benzocaine for instance) which are not harmful to older children or adults.[39] Even contact with substances on diapers may be sufficient to cause alteration in red blood cell function.[40]

The hemoglobin carried by the newborn's erythrocyte is also different. It is fetal hemoglobin, which has a greater affinity for oxygen and which oxidizes faster than does adult hemoglobin. This characteristic was of importance in fetal life, where the oxygen resources were lower than those in inhaled air (recall the "Mount Everest environment" of the uterus). In postnatal life, fetal hemoglobin does not seem to be needed, and it is gradually replaced by adult hemoglobin.

The concentration of hemoglobin and its change in the first 3 months of life represent an interesting phenomenon. At birth the concentration of hemoglobin is, on the average, 17 g/100 ml of blood. By 3 months this concentration has dropped for most infants to approximately 12.5 g/100 ml of blood. One explanation for this drop is that when the infant is born, the oxygen saturation is only about 65 percent, so that while the concentration of hemoglobin is 17 g/100 ml, the concentration of *oxyhemoglobin* is only about 11 to 12 g/100 ml. At birth or soon after, the oxygen saturation of the blood reaches about 95 percent, raising the concentration of oxyhemoglobin to something over 16 g/100 ml. (From this time on, the concentration of hemoglobin and oxyhemoglobin are essentially equal.) It is thought that this is such a high level of oxyhemoglobin that the production of new red blood cells ceases until the level of oxyhemoglobin again drops to the 11 to 12 g/100 ml range at 3 months.[41]

Postnatal Circulatory Changes

Of equal importance to the establishment of respiratory effort and the oxygenation of hemoglobin is the transport of oxygen to the tissues. Let us now consider the circulatory system and the changes that occur in it at birth, beginning with an overview of fetal circulation.

Fetal Circulation The umbilical arteries arise at the caudal end of the aorta. As the caudal portion of the embryo grows, the umbilical arteries are carried caudally away from the aorta, but they retain their paired condition; thus, there are *two umbilical arteries* in the umbilical cord.

The umbilical veins also arise as paired structures, but during early embryonic development they fuse in the belly stalk to form a single channel, thus the resulting *single umbilical vein* in the umbilical cord. Internally, the left umbilical vein enlarges and the right one atrophies and becomes nonfunctional.

As the single umbilical vein enters the fetus from the umbilical cord, it goes to the liver, where a portion of the blood enters hepatic circulation. The remainder of the blood is carried through a "bypass" vessel, the *ductus venosus,* past the liver and directly into the inferior vena cava. The blood that enters hepatic circulation is carried eventually to the inferior vena cava by way of the hepatic vein. In the inferior vena cava, the blood from the umbilical vein is mixed with blood from the lower part of the systemic circulation.

Blood Flow Schematically, fetal blood enters the right atrium from the inferior vena cava and flows from there through an opening in the septum, the *foramen ovale,* into the left atrium (see Figure 2-4). Actually, the anatomical relationship of the inferior vena cava to the foramen ovale is not completely clear and has been the subject of debate for some time.[42] For our purposes, however, the usual schematic representation will suffice.

As a result of relative pressures and anatomic relationships, most of the blood from the inferior vena cava enters the left atrium, with only a little remaining in the right atrium. In contrast, *all* the blood entering the heart from the superior vena cava is collected by the right atrium.

From the left atrium, blood enters the left ventricle and then the ascending aorta in the usual adult pattern, as it leaves the heart. It flows through systemic circulation and into the umbilical arteries to be returned to the placenta.

Blood entering the right atrium from the superior vena cava mixes with a small amount of blood entering the right atrium from the inferior vena cava and flows into the right ventricle. From there it flows into the pulmonary arteries. Because of the high vascular resistance of the pulmonary circulation during fetal life, however, most of this blood bypasses the smaller vessels of the pulmonary circulation and enters a short, wide vessel, the *ductus arteriosus,* which connects the pulmonary artery directly with the descending portion of the aortic arch.

Oxygen Saturation It is important to note that the oxygen saturation of the blood varies from one part of fetal circulation to another. The highest oxygen saturation occurs in the umbilical vein, with the next greatest in the upper inferior vena cava as blood coming directly from the placenta mixes with blood from the lower systemic circulation. This blood flows to the left side of the heart and into the ascending aortic arch, from which blood is supplied to the head and upper body. In this way, vital brain tissues receive the blood with the highest possible levels of oxygen saturation, a protective mechanism. The blood coming from the superior vena cava, having lost much of its oxygen to the tissues, is mixed with a smaller amount of blood from the inferior vena cava, raising its oxygen saturation somewhat but not so high as that of blood which flows into the left atrium. This less oxygenated blood eventually joins the blood from the left atrium at the descending aortic arch, from which it flows to the tissues of the lower body.

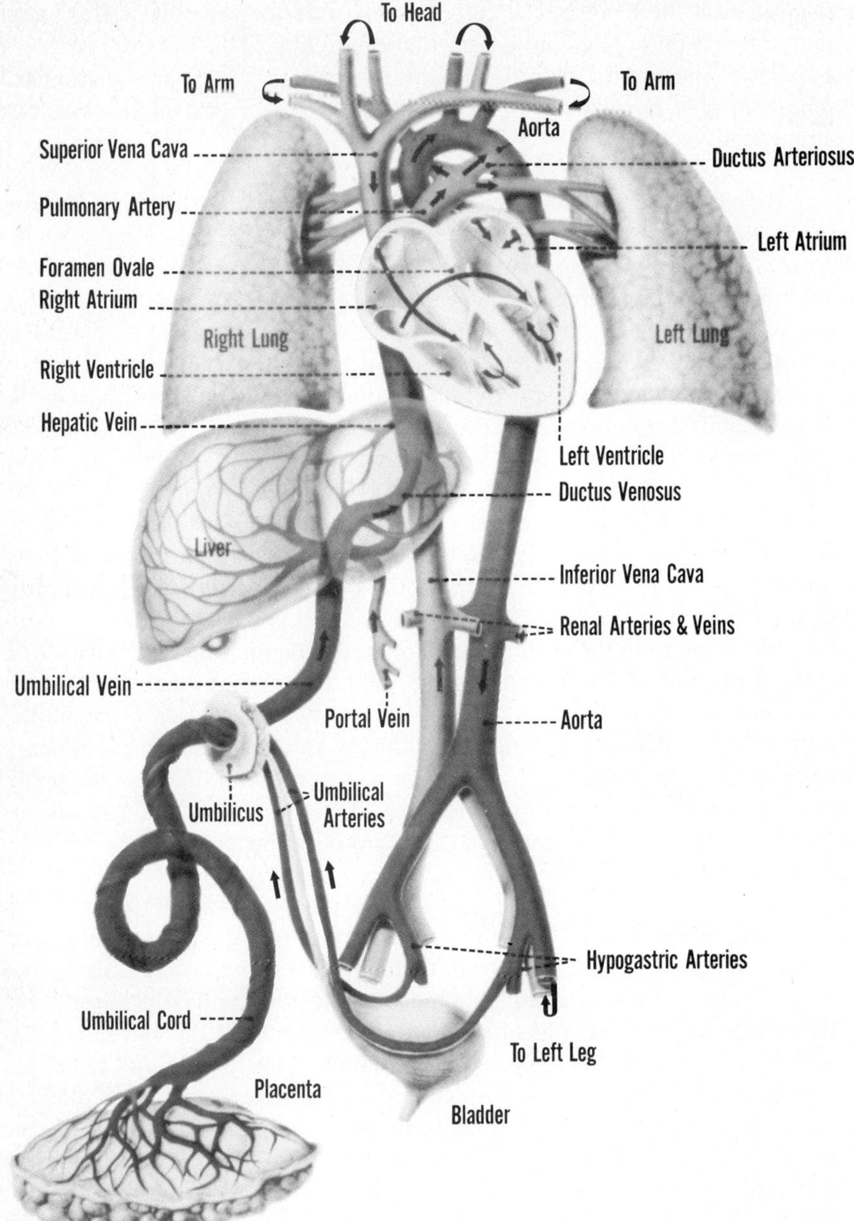

Figure 2-4 Fetal circulation. (*From Fetal Circulation, Ross Clinical Education Aid #1, Ross Laboratories, Columbus, Ohio, by permission.*)

Circulatory Changes after Birth After birth, the foramen ovale, the ductus arteriosus, and the ductus venosus must be closed. The entrance of air into the lungs lowers the resistance of the pulmonary vessels to blood flow through them. As a result of this lowered resistance, some of the blood that was flowing through the ductus arteriosus is channeled through the lungs. This, then, increases the blood return to the left atrium. As the blood pressure in the left atrium increases above that in the right atrium, the flap which lies on the left side of the foramen ovale closes, and the blood from the inferior vena cava takes the path of least resistance, entering the right atrium and being routed to the right ventricle and on to the lungs.

The ductus arteriosus closes in two stages. The first is a constriction of the vessel, thought to occur in the first hour after birth. The factors that cause this constriction are not definitely known, but Dawes seems to feel that constriction of the ductus is a peculiar response of that vessel to oxygen and that the increased oxygen tension in the blood after birth is one important factor in its closure.[43] Constriction occurs during a period of a few hours, followed by anatomical closure (due to fibrosis) in 1 to 8 days. There is evidence that hypoxia in the first few hours after birth may cause the ductus to redilate, after which its sensitivity to oxygen decreases, and thus it may not again constrict as it should.[44]

It is not known exactly what causes the ductus venosus to close after birth, but it is thought to be functionally closed within 1 to 3 hours after delivery.[45] The umbilical vein and arteries cease to function after the cord is clamped, and they eventually become obliterated to form ligaments.

Acquisition and Utilization of Energy

Maintenance of body temperature and glucose metabolism are two additional adaptations the infant must make after birth. They are both a part of a larger concept: the acquisition and utilization of energy. Let us turn our attention first to some basic physiological concepts.

Energy Sources Energy in all its forms comes ultimately from the sun. It is transformed from radiant energy to chemical energy by plants in the process of photosynthesis. From plants, it is passed on to animals and human beings in this form, chemical energy, which can be released by the process of metabolism. Basically, the energy is stored in the form of chemical bonds, that force required to keep atoms of a molecule attached to each other. Some bonds are called *low-energy bonds.* They require relatively little force to keep them in place. When they are broken, relatively little energy is released. Hydrogen bonds are examples of low-energy bonds. Hydrogen ions can change the shapes of molecules (such as large proteins), but they are split off relatively easily to be shifted from one molecule to another. Others are called *high-energy bonds.* Phosphate radicals (PO_4) require much energy to keep them attached to their molecules. An example of a high-energy compound is *adenosine triphosphate* (ATP), which could be considered to be the storage battery for cellular energy. When it is broken down, much energy is released. Energy is used as chemical energy (for the formation of new compounds), as mechanical energy (for muscle movement), as electrical energy (for nerve conduction), as electrochemical energy (for active transport of materials across membranes), and as thermal energy (for the maintenance of body temperature).

Glucose Metabolism The cell obtains its energy basically from the breakdown of glucose. Glucose is supplied to the body primarily from carbohydrates, but it can also be obtained from the glycerol component of fats and from some amino acids. In addition, fatty acids (which do not contain glucose) can be metabolized to provide energy.

In the cell, the mitochondria are the particles that contain the enzymes necessary for metabolism. As glucose is metabolized through the Krebs cycle, energy is released. About 60 percent of it is given off as heat, and the remainder is captured by the cell in the form of high-energy bonds in ATP. Substances other than glucose can enter the Krebs cycle (to be metabolized by the same process) if they can be converted into one of the substances metabolized by Krebs cycle enzymes. Fatty acids, for instance, enter the Krebs cycle after they have been split from the larger fat molecule and converted into a simpler substance. It is important to note that very large quantities of oxygen are used in the completion of the Krebs cycle.

When an excess of glucose is available to the body, some of it is stored in the cardiac muscle and in the liver in the form of glycogen, which can be readily converted back to glucose. The glycogen in the cardiac muscle is utilized for contractile energy. That stored in the liver is available for general body use when glucose in the blood is consumed. There is no glycogen stored in the brain, which has a very high glucose utilization rate; therefore, the glycogen stored in the liver is vital to maintaining normal neurological function by maintaining a constant blood glucose level. Normally, in the adult only enough glycogen is stored in the liver to supply the body's energy needs for 12 to 48 hours of total fasting.[46] The amount available to a newborn infant may vary depending upon the state of nutrition in utero and how much intrauterine stress the infant has experienced, but it is generally less than is found in the adult.

Fat Metabolism After the body's supply of glycogen is spent, or nearly so, the body begins to metabolize fats in order to supply needed glucose. Fats are composed of glycerol and fatty acids. Glycerol is converted into glycogen in the liver, and from there it is converted into glucose. The fatty acids called *free fatty acids* can be metabolized directly by the cells. In their metabolism, they are converted to a substance that can enter the Krebs cycle to be metabolized, but this can occur *only* if there is a sufficient quantity of a special carbohydrate (oxaloacetic acid) produced by glucose metabolism to supply energy for completion of the Krebs cycle. When insufficient amounts of this special carbohydrate are present, fatty acid metabolism is diverted to the formation of ketone bodies. This diversion of the metabolic process can lead to the development of ketosis, or diabetic acidosis, which is a very serious clinical condition.

Several factors may stimulate fat metabolism. These include the influence of hormones (growth hormone and ACTH, for instance), diabetes, starvation, and exposure to cold. Of these, *exposure to cold,* is particularly important to the neonate, and it will be discussed later in this chapter.

Fetal Metabolism Shortly before and Immediately after Birth In utero, the fetus receives a continuous supply of glucose from its mother, transplacentally, unless the mother is hypoglycemic, in which case the fetus can utilize its own body resources for the needed supply of energy. Near term, umbilical vein levels of glucose are about 70 to 90 mg/100 ml.[47] About 2 hours after birth, the infant's blood glucose level has fallen to about 50 mg/100 ml, and then it gradually rises to about 70 mg/100 ml by the third or fourth day, where it stabilizes.[48] The brain is probably adapted to relatively low levels of blood glucose during fetal development, so that there is a rather wide margin for safety after birth. Blood glucose concentrations have been studied in infants in varying circumstances. It has been found in one study that shortly after birth, infants who have been kept warm have a glucose level of about 60 mg/100 ml; those who have been allowed to cool have levels averaging about 45 mg/100 ml; and preterm infants may have levels as low as 30 mg/100 ml or less.[49] (More detail about hypoglycemia will follow in Chapters 8 and 9.)

Cold Stress and Metabolic Processes Reference has been made to the effects of cooling of infants upon blood glucose levels and fat metabolism. Let us now consider the problem of exposure to cold.

Human infants are *homeotherms*; that is, to survive infants must maintain their body temperatures at a constant level in spite of environmental changes. It is as though there were an internal thermostat. There is, in fact, a physiological concept called *set point,* which is just that. There seems to be a regulatory center that governs the level of the "normal" body temperature for an individual. Interestingly, preterm infants, who are greatly handicapped in maintaining their body temperatures, seem to have a lower set point than do full-term babies.[50]

Heat Production In utero, the temperature of the fetus is approximately 0.5°C (0.9°F) higher than that of its mother. Upon delivery, the infant is thrust into an environment which drains much of this body warmth away. To survive, the infant must produce enough heat to replace what is lost to the environment. In adults, shivering contributes greatly to heat production. In the newborn infant, however, heat production comes essentially from a release of chemical bonds during metabolism (*nonshivering thermogenesis*). Approximately 60 percent of the energy released by metabolic activity is cast off in the form of heat. Basal metabolism, however, does not produce enough heat to compensate for heavy losses in the unprotected environment. Compensation requires great increases in metabolic activity, which in turn utilize large quantities of energy (glucose) and oxygen.

Metabolic rate changes can be measured by the rate of oxygen consumption. The higher the metabolic rate, the more oxygen required by the baby. For instance, a decrease in body temperature of 3.5°C (6.3°F) has been found to require a 100 percent increase in oxygen consumption for more than 1½ hours just to replace the heat lost during the temperature drop.[51] It becomes obvious that subjecting a baby to cold stress is detrimental. It can be fatal for infants who have difficulty maintaining high metabolic rates either because of low energy stores or because of difficulty in obtaining or transporting oxygen.

Brown Fat and Heat Production In the adult body, the adipose tissue is primarily white fat, that is, cells containing a single large vacuole for the storage of fat and a thin rim of cytoplasm at the edge of the cell. In newborn infants, as in many animals, there is also a substance called *brown fat.*

In the infant, deposits of brown fat, constituting 2 to 6 percent of the total body weight, are located along the back between the scapulae, around the kidneys and adrenals, in the mediastinum, and at the nape of the neck, where during cold stress the skin may feel warmer to touch than elsewhere. In a well-nourished state, the brown fat is yellowish in color and contains many small fat vacuoles and a rich nerve and blood supply. When the fat becomes depleted, the tissue appears to become yellowish brown and then reddish brown. The color is due primarily to its rich blood supply.[52] Large quantities of mitochondria are also present in the cells, reflecting the higher metabolic rate which occurs there.

It has been hypothesized that the white fat is mobilized in times of starvation and that the brown fat is reserved and utilized for the production of heat during cold stress.[53] It is thought that the fat molecules stored in the fat vacuoles are the fuel used by the brown fat to produce heat.

Oxygen Consumption and Heat Production The relationship of oxygen to heat production has been clearly demonstrated by animal studies.[54] For instance, in rabbits, three thermometers were implanted, one in subcutaneous tissue over a deposit of brown fat, one subcutaneously over a lumbar muscle, and one into the colon. When the rabbit was maintained at a constant temperature of 35°C (95°F), all three thermometers registered equal readings. When the temperature was dropped to 25°C (77°F), all the thermometers registered a decrease in temperature, beginning with the one closest to the surface of the animal. After 30 minutes, however, the temperature of the thermometer over the brown fat began to rise, and it remained 1 degree higher than the colonic thermometer and 2 degrees higher than the thermometer in the lumbar region, thus demonstrating that heat is produced in the brown fat. Later, the inhaled oxygen given to the rabbit was drastically decreased, and when this happened, all three thermometers again registered a fall in temperature. When the inhaled oxygen was restored to normal, the temperature over the brown fat rose to its previous heights, thus demonstrating the need for oxygen in maintaining body temperature. In other studies by the same investigator, it has been shown that during cold stress the blood volume circulating through the brown fat more than triples, thus leading to the assumption that the blood is heated by metabolic activity and carries this heat to the rest of the body as it is circulated.

Brown fat hypertrophies for a few weeks after birth, and then it gradually disappears. Brown fat stores have been found to be totally depleted of fat stores within 36 to 48 hours of birth, however, in babies who have been cared for in environments which are too cold.[55] Recent findings indicate that once the fat stores in the brown fat have been depleted, the mitochondria there utilize glycerol and free fatty acids obtained from the circulation to continue their work of producing heat.[56] Again, the oxygen requirements of this process must be stressed. Healthy full-term babies cared for in an environment of 32 to 34°C (89.6 to 93.2°F) utilized oxygen at the rate of 5.4 ml/kg/minute. After exposure to environmental temperatures of 25 to 26°C (77 to 77.8°F), their oxygen consumption rose to 9.3 ml/kg/minute.[57]

It should be noted that when oxygen levels are inadequate to maintain normal glucose metabolism, anaeroblic metabolism of glycogen occurs. One of the consequences of this anaerobic process is an increase in lactic acid production, which can lead to the development of clinical acidosis.

Blood Glucose Levels and Heat Production The relationship between heat production and blood glucose levels is not so clear as that between oxygen consumption and heat production. It has been noted by many authors that blood glucose levels in infants subjected to cold stress tend to be lower than those of infants kept warm. The implication is that heat production utilizes the body's stores of glucose, thus causing hypoglycemia. Experimental evidence, however, contradicts this simple cause-and-effect relationship. It has been demonstrated in preterm babies who were unable to maintain body temperature, for instance, that infusions with glucose did not alter their body temperatures although their blood glucose levels did rise appreciably.[58] In contrast, other babies who were hypoglycemic did maintain their body temperatures satisfactorily in spite of very low blood glucose levels (below 20 mg/100 ml). It would seem, then, that the blood glucose level does not directly affect the baby's ability to maintain body temperature, although its importance in maintaining neurologic and general body function and in preventing acidosis during fat metabolism cannot be overstressed.

Conservation of Body Heat

Besides producing heat, the baby must conserve heat in order to maintain body temperature. In making this adaptation to extrauterine life, the infant must combat losses of heat to the environment.

Heat Transfer Heat is a fluid commodity, constantly in motion as it is transferred from areas of greater concentration to areas of lesser concentration, just as ions move from a solution of higher concentration to one with a lower concentration. Temperature is not constant throughout the body. It is higher at the body core where metabolic activity is occurring, and it gradually decreases toward the surface of the body; thus, rectal temperature is normally higher than axillary temperature. (The difference in readings from the two sites may be less marked for the newborn than for adults or older children, due probably to immaturity of the heat regulating system.) Similarly heat moves from one object to another, moving from a warm object to a cooler one; thus, objects in a room and its furniture and walls absorb heat from a warm body. Similarly, cool air surrounding a baby absorbs heat from the infant.

Modes of Heat Loss Heat is lost from the body primarily by four modes: *conduction, convection, radiation,* and *evaporation. Conduction* is the loss of heat through direct contact with cooler substances. Materials transfer heat by conduction at different rates. Metals are much better conductors of heat than are nonmetals; air is a less effective conductor of heat than are solid materials or water. Materials which are poor conductors of heat are called *insulators.* In the clinical area, heat can be lost if the infant is placed on a cold surface, especially a metal or plastic surface, as opposed to a surface covered by a sheet or blanket.

Convection is the transfer of heat through currents in moving bodies of liquids and gases. The quantity of heat lost depends upon the rate of motion and the relative differences in temperature between the object and the fluid in motion. In the clinical area, drafts, especially drafts of very cold air, can cause great heat losses.

Radiation is the transfer of energy which becomes heat when absorbed by a body. Radiant energy is transmitted without regard to air temperature and in fact can be transmitted in a vacuum. The main source of radiant energy is the sun, which of course transmits its energy through the vacuum of space. The energy moves from a warm body to a cooler one in proportion to the relative differences in temperature of the two bodies.

In considering radiant energy losses from the infant, it is important to note that the radiant energy from the sun is in the form of relatively short wavelengths which can pass through some solid objects, notably glass and plastic. Radiant energy which leaves an infant, on the other hand, is in the form of relatively long wavelengths which are absorbed by plastic but do not pass through it. An infant in an incubator, then, radiates heat to the walls of the incubator, which are always cooler than the infant's body temperature. The walls of the incubator in turn radiate heat to surrounding objects, such as the walls of the room and furniture in the room. Since the loss of heat due to radiation is not related to air temperature, it can be seen that maintaining the air temperature inside the incubator at a particular level will not decrease the loss of energy from the infant due to radiation. Placing an incubator next to a noninsulated outer window or a wall cooled by an air-conditioning vent can result in tremendous heat losses from the baby even though the air temperature inside the incubator is maintained at a recommended level. Sometimes a small plastic box, with openings for air circulation, is placed over an infant inside the incubator to decrease radiant heat losses.[59] The air around the heat shield warms the plastic to near the baby's temperature so that little heat is lost to the shield. Since the longer wavelengths of radiant energy do not pass through the shield, no heat is lost to the outer environment.

The infant may be warmed by radiant heat from the sun if placed in the sunlight, even though in an incubator. This phenomenon, called the "greenhouse effect," is due to the passage of the relatively short wavelengths of solar radiation through the window and the walls of the incubator. Such an infant may experience a febrile episode and be treated erroneously for an infection if the cause of the temperature increase is not correctly identified.

Evaporation is the process by which liquids are changed to gases by absorbing heat from surroundings. Evaporation can be a particularly important form of heat loss immediately after birth, since the infant is wet at birth.

Heat is also lost from the body by the loss of warmed body fluids or solids (urine or feces), and by the necessity of warming and adding water vapor to inhaled air.

Natural Means of Heat Conservation Anything which decreases the loss of heat decreases the amount of heat production needed to maintain body temperature. Among the natural mechanisms for conserving heat is a layer of fat under the skin. Fat is a relatively poor conductor of heat and thus decreases losses from the body core. Another natural means of heat conservation is constriction of the surface blood vessels. This may explain partially the typical cyanosis of the newborn's hands and feet. A third natural means for conserving heat is the term infant's tendency to assume the fetal position with arms and legs flexed on the body, thus decreasing the surface area for loss of heat.

Environmental Means for Conserving Heat The environment can be manipulated to minimize heat losses. This is a complex task, however, and one which will be discussed in detail in the next chapter when nursing care of the neonate will be considered. In the meantime, let us turn our attention to the final aspect of extrauterine adaptation, maintaining the internal environment.

Elimination of Waste Products and Toxins

In utero, the fetus depends almost entirely upon the mother to eliminate waste products and toxins and for protection against trauma and hostile organisms. After birth, however, newborns must eliminate their own waste products, metabolize toxins, establish hemostasis, and defend against invading organisms. Let us consider first the elimination of wastes.

Renal Function The embryonic kidney develops in three distinct stages. First a primitive *pronephros* is formed. A series of pronephric tubules develops beginning about the end of the third week of life. These tubules develop in a caudal direction, with the first ones formed beginning to degenerate before the last ones have become fully developed late in the fourth week. The pronephros never becomes functional in the mammal. Midway in the fourth week a new structure, the *mesonephros,* begins to form caudal to the pronephros. Its tubules attain a higher degree of development and do become functional in eliminating nitrogenous wastes. As in the pronephros, the tubules most cephalic in position begin to regress as new tubules are formed caudally, so that the mesonephros appears to migrate caudally. These tubules form a characteristic Bowman's capsule and glomerulus so familiar in mature kidneys. Finally, the *metanephros* or permanent kidney develops. By the thirty-fifth week of gestation, the formation of the metanephros is complete. It continues to grow in size by cellular hypertrophy, however, until the individual is about 20 years old.

Functionally, the kidney reaches adult levels of efficiency about the time the child is 2 years old. Until that time, there are several functional differences. In utero, the kidney begins to excrete very dilute urine at about 3 months. Even at birth, the infant's ability to concentrate urine is much less than that of the adult. This is especially important when the infant is dehydrated, since fluid continues to be lost through the kidneys out of proportion to that lost by an adult in the same circumstances.

The kidneys also have difficulty excreting acids. This characteristic is thought to be a contributing factor to the preterm infant's tendency to develop metabolic acidosis.[60]

Diet is of importance in considering kidney function. Cow's milk has a higher phosphorous content than breast milk. This causes greater acidity and thus a greater work load for the kidneys as they maintain the pH of body fluids. Babies who receive primarily cow's milk are slower to develop the ability to concentrate their urine than breast-fed babies.[61] This greater acid load is thought to be a contributing factor. However, these same babies seem to have a more efficient response in times of metabolic acidosis, perhaps because of an adaptation of general renal function.[62] Another problem associated with high phosphate content of cow's milk, however, is the development of hyperphosphatemia. This condition may result in tetany, since calcium levels fall when hyperphosphatemia is present. The development of hyperphosphatemia is thought to be due to a combination of immature renal function (a poor ability to excrete phosphorous) and a functional hypoparathyroidism.[63]

Intestinal Function The intestinal tract seems to function well from the beginning. Food is absorbed as needed, and wastes are eliminated readily. The first stools are composed of meconium, which is a sticky greenish-black substance composed of digested amnionic fluid, secretions from the intestinal tract and gall bladder, and epithelial cells from the inner walls of the intestine. After the infant begins to ingest milk, the stools become more yellowish-green (transitional stool), and finally they become pale yellow. The consistency of the stools will vary depending upon the composition of the infant's diet. These will be discussed more fully in Chapter 3.

Detoxification of Drugs Note should be made of the infant's difficulty in detoxifying drugs. Renal immaturity and a deficiency of liver enzymes contribute to this difficulty. Notably deficient in the first weeks of life is *glucuronyl transferase,* a liver enzyme central to the detoxification of bilirubin and many drugs, for example, chloramphenicol, thyroxine, and morphine. Many deaths occurred from the use of chloramphenicol before it was discovered that newborns could not metabolize it properly.

Other peculiarities also render the newborn especially susceptible to drug reactions. Some drugs which can be given with assurance to older children and adults may be fatal to the newborn. Sulfisoxazole is an example. It competes with bilirubin for attachment to albumin in the serum, forcing the bilirubin into the tissues where damage is done. (See Chapter 9, The Infant with Hyperbilirubinemia.)

Another factor to consider is that the blood-brain barrier is much more permeable in the newborn than in the older child, making the entire nervous system more susceptible to damage from toxins and drugs. It cannot be emphasized too strongly that the neonate is highly susceptible to toxic reactions to drugs, especially during the first month of life. No drug should automatically be considered safe for newborns just because it is safe for older children and adults. Some specifically neonatal reactions do not become apparent until drugs are tested either with newborn animals or in carefully controlled clinical trials with newborn infants.

Development of Hemostasis

The development of hemostasis is of relative unimportance in utero, where the infant is protected from trauma. After birth, however, it assumes great importance.

In the clotting process, thromboplastin is released from platelets and other injured cells. This substance is combined with prothrombin, which then unites with soluble fibrinogen to form insoluble fibrin. Fibrin forms the network upon which the clot is built. Vitamin K is necessary for the synthesis of prothrombin in the liver. In the adult, vitamin K is obtained from food and is synthesized by bacteria in the intestinal tract. Since the intestinal tract is sterile at birth and the newborn does not ingest foods containing vitamin K, prothrombin cannot be manufactured. For this reason, vitamin K is given by injection soon after birth. It should be noted, however, that large doses of water-soluble vitamin K have been found to cause hemolysis of the red blood cells.[64] This is true whether the doses are given directly to the infant or to the mother during labor, as was the practice at one time. Currently the use of a nonsoluble form, vitamin K_1, is recommended by the American Academy of Pediatrics (AAP).[65] Even with this therapy, however, the newborn's ability to coagulate blood may be significantly deficient for the first 24 hours of life.[66]

Defenses against Hostile Organisms

There are basically three types of responses to hostile organisms: (1) inflammation and phagocytosis, (2) a generalized physiological response, and (3) specific immological responses.

Inflammation and Phagocytosis In the adult, when organisms penetrate the natural barriers such as the skin, an immediate inflammatory response occurs. White cells rush to the scene, the local capillaries dilate, allowing protein-rich fluid to enter the area, and fibrin barries are established to localize the infection. In infants, a less dramatic reaction occurs. Leukocytes are reduced both in number and in efficiency, and fibrin barriers are less completely formed, resulting in a tendency to generalized rather than localized infections.

Phagocytosis, the second part of this response, also seems to be less well developed in the infant than in the adult. The presence of certain substances (opsonins) which increase the ability of the cells to phagocytize foreign matter seems to be necessary for efficient operation of this defense. Opsonins are transferred to the infant from the mother late in the pregnancy; thus preterm infants may be especially handicapped in this regard.

Generalized Physiologic Response A generalized response also occurs whenever an invasion of organisms occurs. In adults, a characteristic response to bacterial invasion, for instance, is fever. This response is absent in newborns. They may have severe infections without any fever at all. Other characteristic responses, such as stiff neck in meningitis, may also be absent, making the recognition of illness especially difficult.

Specific Immune Responses Antibodies which circulate in the blood are called *immunoglobulins.* There are three major ones: gamma-G (also designated immunoglobulin-G, or IgG), gamma-M (IgM), and gamma-A (IgA). Of these, gamma-G constitutes 90 percent of adult gamma globulin. It is the only one transferred transplacentally to the fetus, thus conferring upon the fetus temporary passive immunity to most of the organisms to which the mother is immune. It is important to note, however, that the infant will be susceptible to diseases against which the mother has no immunity. As with many other substances, the fetus receives most of its gamma-G globulins near term. This particular globulin has a half-life of 20 to 30 days; that is, one-half of it disappears in 20 to 30 days. Very little is produced in the infant until about the third or fourth month of extrauterine life.

Gamma-M, on the other hand, a much larger molecule, is produced by the infant from birth upon exposure to the environment. Production may begin in utero if an intrauterine infection has occurred, however, making the presence of significant levels at birth (cord levels more than 20 mg/100 ml) diagnostic of intrauterine infection.[67] Gamma-M has a high rate of synthesis but a short half-life (1.7 to 3 days). It is especially effective against bacterial infections and thus may have special importance in the first weeks.

Gamma-A is the only form of gamma globulin that is secreted in body fluids. It is found in colostrum (the substance produced by the breast prior to milk production), saliva, tears, and respiratory secretions. The infant who is breast-fed receives it from the mother, and infants can also produce it themselves.

The infant's immunity system has been compared to a library with empty shelves.[68] The potential is there, but specific responses do not occur until specific foreign proteins are contacted. Interaction of the infant with the total environment stimulates the ability to produce antibodies. It should be noted, however, that in animals, continuous use of antibiotics delays the

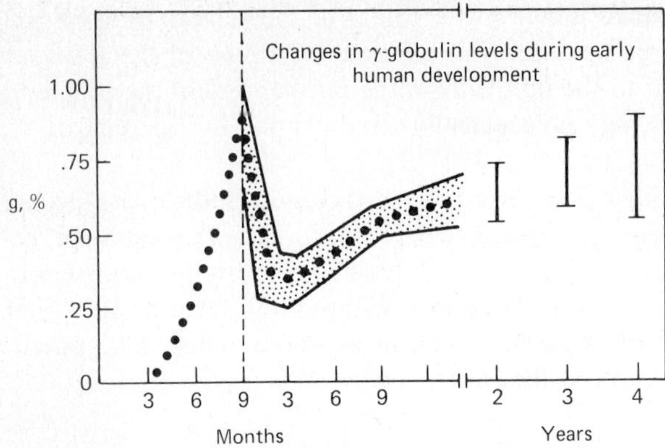

Figure 2-5 Total fetal gamma globulin levels before and after birth. Note the gradual rise in the level during the last months of pregnancy and the precipitous drop after birth. *(From Robert E. Cooke (ed.), The Biologic Basis of Pediatric Practice, McGraw-Hill, New York, 1968, p. 524, by permission.)*

development of this ability.[69] The infant's total level of all gamma globulins is significantly lower than that of the adult for 3 to 4 months after birth in spite of production of gamma-M and gamma-A types, because of failure to produce the gamma-G antibodies until about the third month. (See Figure 2-5.) The level of gamma-G globulins (obtained from the mother) declines until about the fourth month, when it begins to rise, due to production by the infant. Care should be taken to protect the infant from exposure to serious illnesses during this time.

REFERENCES

1 L. L. Langley, Ira R. Telford, and John B. Christensen, *Dynamic Anatomy and Physiology,* McGraw-Hill, New York, 1969, p. 784.

2 Ibid. p. 734.

3 Louis M. Hellman, "The Birth Process," in Robert E. Cooke (ed.), *The Biologic Basis of Pediatric Practice,* McGraw-Hill, New York, 1968, pp. 1431–1432.

4 Geoffrey S. Dawes, *Foetal and Neonatal Physiology,* Year Book, Chicago, 1968, pp. 117–119.

5 Sheldon B. Korones, *High-Risk Newborn Infants: The Basis for Intensive Nursing Care,* Mosby, St. Louis, 1972, p. 13.

6 Karyn Smith Kaufman, "Complications during Labor and Delivery," in Joy Princeton Clausen, Margaret Hemp Flock, Bonnie Ford, Marilyn A. Green, and Elsa S. Popiel (eds.), *Maternity Nursing Today,* McGraw-Hill, New York, 1973, p. 785.

7 Sumner J. Yaffee and Charlotte S. Catz, "Pharmacology of the Perinatal Period," *Clinical Obstetrics and Gynecology,* September 1971, pp. 725–726.

8 Mary Lou Moore, *The Newborn and the Nurse,* Saunders, Philadelphia, 1972, p. 71.
9 Yaffee and Catz, op. cit., p. 730.
10 Ibid., p. 737.
11 Ibid., p. 732.
12 Hellman, op. cit., p. 1447.
13 Sol M. Shnider and Frank Moya, "Effects of Meperidine on the Newborn Infant," *American Journal of Obstetrics and Gynecology,* Aug. 15, 1964, pp. 1011–1012.
14 Hellman, loc. cit.
15 Robert O. Bauer, "Obstetrical Analgesia and Anesthesia and Resuscitation of Neonates," *International Anesthesia Clinics,* vol. 9, 1971, p. 77.
16 Moore, op. cit., pp. 68–69.
17 Bauer, op. cit., p. 75.
18 Ibid., p. 77.
19 Ibid., p. 78.
20 Moore, loc. cit.
21 Bauer, op. cit., p. 81.
22 Frank C. Greiss, "Obstetric Anesthesia," in Mary H. Browning and Edith P. Lewis (comps.), *Maternal and Newborn Care: Nursing Interventions,* American Journal of Nursing, New York, 1973, p. 78.
23 Moore, loc. cit.
24 Greiss, op. cit., p. 77.
25 Ibid.
26 Dawes, op. cit., p. 31.
27 Hellman, op. cit., p. 1433.
28 Arnold J. Rudolph, "Anticipation, Recognition, and Transitional Care of the High-Risk Infant," in Marshall H. Klaus and Avroy A. Fanaroff (eds.), *Care of the High-Risk Neonate,* Saunders, Philadelphia, 1973, p. 29.
29 Ibid., p. 30.
30 Petter Karlberg, "Developmental Anatomy and Physiology of the Lungs," in Cooke (ed.), op. cit., pp. 283–284.
31 Ibid., p. 284.
32 Dawes, op. cit., pp. 129–136.
33 Korones, op. cit., p. 122.
34 Dawes, op. cit., p. 138.
35 Karlberg, loc. cit.
36 Dawes, op. cit., p. 125.
37 Ibid., p. 126.
38 Ibid., p. 138.
39 M. Eugene Lahey, "The Erythrocyte: Physiologic Considerations," in Cooke (ed.), op. cit., p. 425.
40 Ibid., p. 424.
41 Ibid., p. 425.
42 Dawes, op. cit., pp. 92–93.
43 Ibid., p. 165.
44 Ibid., p. 166.

45 Ibid., p. 172.
46 Sue Rodwell Williams, *Nutrition and Diet Therapy,* Mosby, St. Louis, 1969, p. 67.
47 Michael K. Wald, "Problems in Chemical Adaptation," in Klaus and Fanaroff (eds.), op. cit., p. 29.
48 Peter A. J. Adam, "Control of Glucose Metabolism in the Human Fetus and Newborn Infant," *Advances in Metabolic Disorders,* vol. 5, 1971, p. 218.
49 Ibid.
50 Tibor Heim, "Thermogenesis in the Newborn Infant," *Clinical Obstetrics and Gynecology,* vol. 14, 1971, p. 792.
51 Ibid., p. 795.
52 Marshall Klaus and Avroy Fanaroff, "The Physical Environment," in Klaus and Fanaroff (eds.), op. cit., p. 61.
53 Heim, op. cit., p. 802.
54 Dawes, op. cit., p. 199.
55 Heim, op. cit., p. 798.
56 Ibid.
57 Ibid.
58 Ibid., p. 801.
59 Klaus and Fanaroff, op. cit., pp. 64–65.
60 Wallace W. McCrory, "Anatomic and Physiologic Considerations," in Cooke (ed.), op. cit., p. 999.
61 Alexander J. Schaffer and Mary Ellen Avery, *Diseases of the Newborn,* Saunders, Philadelphia, 1971, p. 376.
62 McCrory, op. cit., p. 1000.
63 Ibid., p. 1001.
64 William L. Nyhan, "Pharmacology," in Cooke (ed.), op. cit., p. 1464.
65 American Academy of Pediatrics, Committee on the Fetus and the Newborn, *Standards and Recommendations for Hospital Care of Newborn Infants,* American Academy of Pediatrics, Evanston, Ill., 1971, p. 104.
66 Janet Hardy, "Medical Care of the Newborn," in Cooke (ed.), op. cit., p. 1472.
67 Avroy Fanaroff and Marshall Klaus, "Neonatal Infections," in Klaus and Fanaroff, (eds.), op. cit., p. 208.
68 Richard T. Smith and John B. Robbins, "General Physiology," in Robert E. Cooke (ed.), op. cit., p. 522.
69 Ibid., p. 529.

BIBLIOGRAPHY

Adam, Peter A. J.: "Control of Glucose Metabolism in the Human Fetus and Newborn Infant," *Advances in Metabolic Disorders,* vol. 5, 1971, pp. 183–275.

American Academy of Pediatrics, Committee on the Fetus and the Newborn: *Standards and Recommendations for Hospital Care of Newborn Infants,* American Academy of Pediatrics, Evanston, Ill., 1971.

Bauer, Robert O.: "Obstetrical Analgesia and Anesthesia and Resuscitation of Neonates," *International Anesthesia Clinics,* vol. 9, 1971, pp. 63–93.

Clausen, Joy: "The Fourth Stage of Labor," in Joy Princeton Clausen, Margaret

Hemp Flock, Bonnie Ford, Marilyn A. Green, and Elsa S. Popiel (eds.), *Maternity Nursing Today,* McGraw-Hill, New York, 1973. pp. 527–552.

Dawes, Geoffrey S.: *Foetal and Neonatal Physiology,* Year Book, Chicago, 1968.

Fanaroff, Avroy, and Marshall Klaus: "Neonatal Infections," in Marshall H. Klaus and Avroy A. Fanaroff (eds.), *Care of the High-Risk Neonate,* Saunders, Philadelphia, 1973, pp. 205–227.

Greiss, Frank C.: "Obstetric Anesthesia," in Mary H. Browning and Edith P. Lewis (comps.), *Maternal and Newborn Care: Nursing Interventions,* American Journal of Nursing, New York. 1973, pp. 75–81.

Hardy, Janet: "Medical Care of the Newborn," in Robert E. Cooke (ed.), *The Biologic Basis of Pediatric Practice,* McGraw-Hill, New York, 1968, pp. 1467–1490.

Heim, Tibor: "Thermogenesis in the Newborn Infant," *Clinical Obstetrics and Gynecology,* vol. 14, 1971, pp. 790–820.

Helmrath, Thomas A.: "Energy Balance in the Newborn Baby: Aspects of Care of the Community Hospital," *Michigan Medicine,* December 1971, pp. 1121–1123.

Hon, Edward H.: *An Introduction to Fetal Heart Rate Monitoring,* University of Southern California School of Medicine, Post Graduate Division, Los Angeles, 1973.

Karlberg, Petter: "Developmental Anatomy and Physiology of the Lungs," in Robert E. Cooke (ed.), *The Biologic Basis of Pediatric Practice,* McGraw-Hill, New York, 1968, pp. 283–295.

Kaufman, Karyn Smith: "Complications during Labor and Delivery," in Joy Princeton Clausen, Margaret Hemp Flock, Bonnie Ford, Marilyn A. Green, and Elsa S. Popiel (eds.), *Maternity Nursing Today,* McGraw-Hill, New York, 1973, pp. 764–791.

Klaus, Marshall, and Avroy Fanaroff: "The Physical Environment," in Marshal H. Klaus and Avroy A. Fanaroff (eds.), *Care of the High-Risk Neonate,* Saunders, Philadelphia, 1973, pp. 58–76.

Korones, Sheldon B.: *High-Risk Newborn Infants: The Basis for Intensive Nursing Care,* Mosby, St. Louis, 1972.

Lahey, M. Eugene: "The Erythrocyte: Physiologic Considerations," in Robert E. Cooke (ed.), *The Biologic Basis of Pediatric Practice,* McGraw-Hill, New York, 1968, pp. 421–426.

Langley, L. L., Ira R. Telford, and John B. Christensen: *Dynamic Anatomy and Physiology,* McGraw-Hill, New York, 1969.

LeRoux, Rose S., and Shirley Stratton Yee: "The Physiological Basis of Neonatal Nursing," in Joy Princeton Clausen, Margaret Hemp Flock, Bonnie Ford, Marilyn A. Green, and Elsa S. Popiel (eds.), *Maternity Nursing Today,* McGraw-Hill, New York, 1973, pp. 638–686.

Littlefield, Vivian: "The Third Stage of Labor," in Joy Princeton Clausen, Margaret Hemp Flock, Bonnie Ford, Marilyn A. Green, and Elsa S. Popiel (eds.), *Maternity Nursing Today,* McGraw-Hill, New York, 1973, pp. 500–526.

Lutz, Linda, and Paul H. Perlstein: "Temperature Control in Newborn Babies," *Nursing Clinics of North America,* March 1971, pp. 15–23.

McCrory, Wallace W.: "Anatomic and Physiologic Considerations," in Robert E.

Cooke (ed.), *The Biologic Basis of Pediatric Practice,* McGraw-Hill, New York, 1968, pp. 989–1002.

Moore, Mary Lou: *The Newborn and the Nurse,* Saunders, Philadelphia, 1972.

Nyham, William L.: "Pharmacology," in Robert E. Cooke (ed.), *The Biologic Basis of Pediatric Practice,* McGraw-Hill, New York, 1968, pp. 1460–1467.

Patten, Bradley M.: *Human Embryology,* McGraw-Hill, New York, 1968.

Robbins, John B., and Richard T. Smith: "The Specific Immune Response," in Robert E. Cooke (ed.), *The Biologic Basis of Pediatric Practice,* McGraw-Hill, New York, 1968, pp. 507–521.

Rudolph, Arnold J.: "Anticipation, Recognition, and Transitional Care of the High-Risk Infant," in Marshall H. Klaus and Avroy A. Fanaroff (eds.), *Care of the High-Risk Neonate,* Saunders, Philadelphia, 1973, pp. 23–35.

Schaffer, Alexander J., and Mary Ellen Avery: *Diseases of the Newborn,* Saunders, Philadelphia, 1971.

Shnider, Sol M., and Frank Moya: "Effects of Meperidine on the Newborn Infant," *American Journal of Obstetrics and Gynecology,* Aug. 15, 1964, pp. 1009–1015.

Smith, Richard T., and John B. Robbins: "Developmental Aspects of Immunity," in Robert E. Cooke (ed.), *The Biologic Basis of Pediatric Practice,* McGraw-Hill, New York, 1968, pp. 521–536.

——— and ———: "General Physiology," in Robert E. Cooke (ed.), *The Biologic Basis of Pediatric Practice,* McGraw-Hill, New York, 1968, pp. 495–507.

Sturrock, Elizabeth W., and Sally Ann Yeomans: "The First Stage of Labor," in Joy Princeton Clausen, Margaret Hemp Flock, Bonnie Ford, Marilyn A. Green, and Elsa S. Popiel (eds.), *Maternity Nursing Today,* McGraw-Hill, New York, 1973, pp. 433–485.

Wald, Michael K.: "Problems in Chemical Adaptation," in Marshall H. Klaus and Avroy A. Fanaroff (eds.), *Care of the High-Risk Neonate,* Saunders, Philadelphia, 1973, pp. 168–182.

White, Mary, and William J. Keenan: "Recognition and Management of Hypoglycemia in the Newborn Infant," *Nursing Clinics of North America,* March 1971, pp. 67–79.

Wilkerson, Betty L.: "The Second Stage of Labor," in Joy Princeton Clausen, Margaret Hemp Flock, Bonnie Ford, Marilyn A. Green, and Elsa S. Popiel (eds.), *Maternity Nursing Today,* McGraw-Hill, New York, 1973, pp. 486–499.

Williams, Sue Rodwell: *Nutrition and Diet Therapy,* Mosby, St. Louis, 1969.

Yaffee, Sumner J., and Charlotte S. Catz: "Pharmacology of the Perinatal Period," *Clinical Obstetrics and Gynecology,* September 1971, pp. 722–744.

Zweymuller, E.: "Heat Loss in the Newborn Infant," *Indian Journal of Pediatrics,* March 1971, pp. 101–105.

Chapter 3

Labor and Delivery Room Care of the Term Infant

Although the welfare of the infant is influenced by the general level of health of the parents at the time of conception and, indeed, before then, the neonatal nurse becomes directly involved most often when the mother enters the hospital in labor. The total care the mother receives during her labor has an effect on the infant; however, this discussion will focus upon nursing care that is directly related to the welfare of the infant, beginning with assessment of fetal status during labor.

FETAL MONITORING

The usual way to determine fetal responses to labor is to monitor the fetal heart rate (FHR) and to evaluate it in relationship to uterine contractions. Traditionally, this has been done by palpation of the abdomen to feel the contractions and by auscultation of the FHR through the abdominal wall with a fetuscope, a modified stethoscope.

To palpate the abdomen for uterine contractions, the hand of the nurse should be in direct contact with the skin of the patient's abdomen. The fingers may be cupped lightly over the fundus of the uterus, with the palm of the hand resting lightly against the skin of the abdomen. As the uterus contracts, the nurse will feel a tightening of the fundus, and the uterus will rise slightly away from the spine of the patient. The nurse should indent the fundus slightly at the height of the contraction to determine its strength. Pressure on the uterus is uncomfortable for the patient, however, and unnecessary "kneading" of the abdomen should be avoided. The nurse's hand should be kept in place for several contractions so that the length of the contractions, the length of the rest period between contractions, and the degree of relaxation of the uterus during the rest period can be evaluated. The length of the contractions should be measured from the time the first tightening of the fundus is felt until the uterus is totally relaxed again. Any activity of the fetus between contractions should be noted, also, especially unusual agitation. Any contraction lasting longer than 90 seconds or incomplete relaxation of the uterus during the rest period should be reported immediately.

In order to hear fetal heartbeats with a fetuscope, it is necessary to determine the position of the fetus. Palpating the abdomen between contractions will enable the experienced examiner to determine the position of the fetus. The inexperienced student can best learn the skill from an experienced clinician. The fetal heart tones can be heard most clearly directly over the back of the fetus, as the fetus is in a flexed position, placing the back directly against the wall of the uterus. If the baby is in the vertex presentation, the heart tones usually can be heard in the lower quadrant of the mother's abdomen. Other, less frequent positions of the infant will place the audible fetal heart tones in the upper quadrants of the mother's abdomen or at the level of her umbilicus.

Traditionally, the fetal heart tones are auscultated between contractions and counted for 15 to 60 seconds. This does give some information about the condition of the fetus, but it has been found that by the time fetal distress is reflected in changes in rate of the fetal heart during uterine relaxation, considerable fetal asphyxia is likely to have occurred. For this reason pioneers in fetal monitoring have recommended that the FHR be counted for at least 20 consecutive 15-second periods with a 5-second rest between each of the counting periods.[1] These counting periods should start before a contraction begins and continue through the period of uterine contraction and for at least 2 minutes into the following period of uterine relaxation. Obviously, this kind of fetal heart monitoring takes considerable practice and skill, but it provides data much more useful in determining the status of the fetus than the less complex traditional method (though it is less satisfactory than electronic monitoring and may be very uncomfortable for the mother). Any time the FHR is taken with a fetuscope, the mother's pulse rate should be felt simultaneously to be sure that the audible beats are not those of the mother's blood pulsing through the placenta (uterine souffle) nor pulsations of her aorta.

Specific changes in FHR during the contraction will be discussed in detail in the section on electronic monitoring, but persistent rates of less than 120 beats/minute or more than 160 beats/minute usually indicate fetal distress and should be brought to the doctor's attention without delay.

Reed et al. recommend listening for the FHR at hourly intervals during early labor, increasing the frequency of auscultations to every 10 minutes during the second stage of labor and to every 5 minutes while the mother is on the delivery table.[2] When the mother is on the delivery table, her own vital signs should be taken every 5 minutes, also, because of the risk of maternal hypotension as a result of the anesthesia being used or because of supine hypotension syndrome. The FHR should be assessed when the amnionic membranes rupture if this occurs spontaneously and just before and immediately afterward if they are ruptured artificially. There is a chance that the cord may fall below the level of the presenting part if the part is not well engaged at the time the membranes are ruptured. Such an occurrence would lead to compression of the cord between the presenting part and the bony pelvis, an obstetric emergency. The presence of meconium in the amnionic fluid should be considered to be a sign of fetal distress until proved otherwise. (It is normal in breech presentations and may not be significant in some other situations.) Meconium in the amnionic fluid can be recognized by the greenish color of the fluid.

At best, auscultation of the FHR gives only partial data regarding what is happening to the fetus during labor. For this reason, electronic monitoring is widely used for both high-risk and "normal" patients.

ELECTRONIC MONITORING

Electronic devices now available make possible both the recognition of early fetal distress and the identification of impending distress. These instruments benefit the patient only when they are used with understanding and care, however. This is true whether the equipment is used for fetal monitoring or for monitoring the high-risk infant. Never can a nurse assume that equipment is functioning properly without checking it at frequent intervals. For instance, it is possible for the sensor devices to become detached from the patient or to be moved from their proper placement. If this happens and is not discovered, the information produced by the machine will be erroneous and may thus constitute a hazard to the patient.

When recordings from monitoring equipment are interpreted, the nurse should compare these interpretations with personal observations of the patient. If at any time the two do not seem to corroborate each other, the equipment should be checked for proper functioning. *There is no substitute for direct observation by a knowledgeable observer.*

The patient's comfort, psychological and physical, should also be kept in mind when monitoring equipment is in use. Anything that increases a mother's anxiety may constitute an extra stress for her and her infant since increased anxiety usually increases the need for medication. Most people are apprehensive about being attached to electrical equipment. Its use and function should be explained to the patient and to any family members who are present. Most patients assume when such devices are being used that something is dreadfully wrong. They need to be honestly reassured on this point. Since monitoring equipment is now being used in some hospitals "routinely," it is becoming more acceptable to patients.

A problem frequently encountered in using monitoring devices is that the patient is afraid to move. In their zeal to maintain proper functioning of the equipment nurses may forget that frequent position changes are necessary for the comfort and safety of the patient, especially in labor. No patient in labor should be required to remain on her back for long periods of time because of the danger of supine hypotension syndrome. The patient's moving will frequently dislodge external monitoring devices which are held in place by an elastic band. The patient should be told that the repositioning of these electrodes is an expected part of care, not an inconvenience to the nurse.

Another problem in the use of monitoring equipment is that the nurse may be tempted to focus attention on the machine rather than on the patient. This is especially true when readout equipment is located at the nurses' station, away from the patient's bedside. The equipment is to *augment* nursing care, not to replace it!

Available Equipment

For external monitoring of uterine contractions, a pressure transducer called a *tokodynamometer* is used. A transducer is an instrument that changes one form of energy to another. In this instance, a pressure transducer changes physical pressure into electrical signals and records them on graph paper. A large disk containing the transducer is held in place on the mother's abdomen with an elastic belt. During contractions, as the uterus rises in the abdomen and raises the abdominal wall, pressure is exerted against the transducer, which then emits electrical signals that are recorded graphically. Only the frequency and duration of contractions are recorded, not the intrauterine pressure. An internal monitor must be used to record actual pressure. For the external monitor to work, the sensing disk must be placed on the abdomen over the fundus, where the greatest displacement occurs. It may not work at all for obese patients or those who are especially restless during their contractions. Its use need not require the patient to lie prefectly still, however, and it should be remembered that frequent positional changes are necessary. Patients who are using abdominal breathing with their contractions may find the abdominal band rather uncomfortable. In addition, the pressure changes noted by the transducer may be less intense than would be registered on a patient who is not breathing abdominally.

FHRs may be monitored externally by a small microphone placed against the mother's abdomen. This method is not entirely satisfactory, however, since movement by the mother or the fetus may interfere with accurate recordings. Another instrument, using continuously emitted ultrasonic signals bounced off the fetal heart, may also record the FHR. The ultrasonic transducer must be placed where it can best bounce its signals off the fetal heart. The exact position should be determined by finding the fetal heart tones with a fetuscope and then placing the transducer where the loudest tones are heard. Since the ultrasonic transducer may pick up erroneous signals from the mother's uterine or aortic circulation, its placement must be checked by comparing the recorded rate with the mother's pulse.

Internal Monitoring

Internal monitoring is more accurate than external monitoring, but it can be used only after the cervix is partially dilated and the membranes have been ruptured. An internal device is often more comfortable for the patient than an external device, but, of course, its use carries with it danger of introducing infection into the vagina or uterus. The devices are always inserted under sterile conditions.

To monitor uterine contractions internally, a sterile catheter is filled with sterile water and inserted vaginally into the uterus behind the presenting part. It is important that the catheter be filled with fluid before inserting, because forcing air into the uterus may cause an air embolus to enter an open blood vessel which may be present if there has been any separation of the placenta from the wall of the uterus. If the presenting part is lying too low in the pelvis, insertion of the catheter may be impossible. Gentle upward pressure on the presenting part may move it enough to make the insertion, however. Whether or not this should be a nursing maneuver is debatable. Any bleeding or other indication of low-lying placenta prohibits the use of an internal monitor because of the possibility of premature separation of the placenta and subsequent hemorrhage. The catheter is connected to a transducer which converts pressure changes and records them graphically. An internal monitor has the advantage of being able to record changes quantitatively and of being an effective monitor for patients who cannot be monitored satisfactorily by external means. Patients often feel that they have more freedom of movement when monitored internally.

Internal monitoring of FHRs is done by means of an electrode attached to the presenting part which detects and transmits the actual fetal ECG. The electrode can be attached to any presenting part except the face, which is not used because of the danger of damaging the eyes mechanically. The electrode may become detached during labor if insufficient care is used in its application. Occasionally a sterile abscess forms at the site of attachment. Internal FHR monitoring has the major advantage of recording all variations in the baseline rate. This quality greatly increases the value of the recordings for identification of fetal stress which could lead to fetal distress. Hon and others are also developing means to determine the electromechanical interval, that time lapse between the electrical conduction reaching the heart and the actual opening of the atrial valves in the contracting phase.[3] They feel that this is a much better indication of actual fetal cardiac function than is currently available by the use of ECGs.

INTERPRETATION OF DATA

Electronic monitoring provides the patient with a degree of safety not achieved by even the most careful palpation of uterine changes and asucultation of FHR. Because the instruments receive and record even the very subtle changes in uterine contractions and FHR, not only can distress be identified as soon as it occurs, but indeed, signs of impending distress can be readily recognized. This enables the medical team to intervene before the infant suffers damage rather than afterward, as is often the case in nonelectronic monitoring. In interpreting data obtained from electronic monitors, procedures and definitions vary from institution to institution. What is presented below is a general discussion of data interpretation intended to give the student the basic concepts. Both knowledge of specific instrumentation and clinical experience are necessary for adequate use of monitors in a specific institution.

Evaluating Uterine Contractions

In examining the graphs produced by the monitors, consider first the data obtained by sensors of uterine contractions. Figure 3-1 shows a tracing of intrauterine pressure. Note that the pressure rises during contractions,

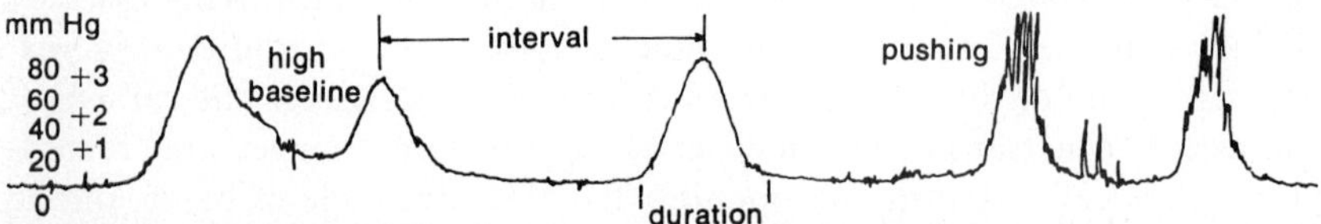

Figure 3-1 Intrauterine pressure during labor. *From "Electronic Monitoring of the Fetus," American Journal of Nursing, p. 1296, July 1974, by permission.)*

peaks, and then falls again to the original level, identified as the *baseline* and indicating a relaxed uterus. Intrauterine pressures normally reach 40 to 50 mmHg during contractions. The interval between contractions is measured from peak to peak, and the duration of the contraction is measured from the place where the line begins to rise to the point where it again reaches the baseline level. The area designated "high baseline" in the figure indicates that the uterus did not completely relax after the first contraction. If the uterus does not fully relax between contractions, the circulation of blood through the placenta is compromised, as was discussed in the last chapter. An occasional episode of incomplete relaxation is not significant, but frequent or prolonged tension in the uterus between contractions is very important. The contractions labeled "pushing" illustrate those toward the end of labor when the mother is contracting her abdominal muscles and "bearing down" to assist in the second stage of labor.

Evaluating the FHR

In evaluating the FHR, the baseline, the *predominant* rate per minute, should be assessed. The FHR graph in Figure 3-2 is typical in that the FHR is not a straight line; there is constant fluctuation. A steady baseline with no fluctuations usually indicates that the fetus has sustained enough damage to prevent the central nervous system (CNS) from reacting normally to stimuli. The normal baseline shows fluctuations of 5 to 15 beats/minute within the normal range of 120 to 160 beats/minute. An evaluation of the baseline may reveal tachycardia or bradycardia, but for either of those to be diagnosed, the increased or decreased rates must remain constant for a designated period of time. (Current usage seems to be 10 minutes to establish a baseline.)

Tachycardia By one definition, tachycardia is any baseline rate (sustained) above 160 beats/minute.[4] Moderate tachycardia is a rate of 160 to 179 beats/minute, and marked or severe tachycardia is over 180 beats/minute. Tachycardia may also be defined as an increase in the baseline rate of 20 to 30 beats/minute.[5]

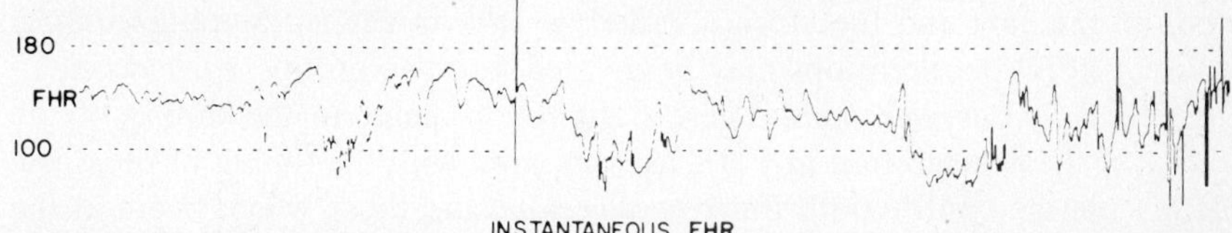

Figure 3-2 The fetal heart rate exhibits a constant fluctuation during labor. *(From Edward H. Hon, An Introduction to Fetal Heart Rate Monitoring, copyright Edward H. Hon, 1973, p. 19, by permission.)*

The clinical significance of tachycardia is somewhat open to interpretation. Russin et al. and Hon state that fetal hypoxia is one condition often associated with it.[6,7] Hon also cites fetal immaturity and maternal hyperthermia as frequently associated conditions. Tachycardia is often associated with FHR pattern changes which will be discussed later. This combination of rate and pattern changes may be very ominous for the infant.

Bradycardia Bradycardia is defined differently by different authors. For our purposes, Hon's definitions of *moderate bradycardia* as 119 to 100 beats/minute and *marked bradycardia* as less than 100 beats/minute will be used.[8] Hon states that bradycardia is not common but that when it does occur, it can lead to fetal acidosis because of the decreased flow of fetal blood through the placenta and the subsequent decrease in CO_2 exchange between mother and child. A frequent cause of bradycardia during labor is the use of oxytocin for the induction of labor.

Another cause of bradycardia may be maternal hypotension, precipitated usually by maternal position (supine) or by the use of regional anesthetics (caudal, spinal, or epidural). When bradycardia is noted for several weeks prior to the onset of labor, the most common cause is the presence of congenital heart defects.

Changes in FHR Patterns Besides evaluating the baseline FHR, it is important to note patterns of change in the rate. Hon identifies three types of FHR decelerations, which he calls periodic changes.[9] Other authors, notably Russin et al.,[10] have subdivided these types further, but for simplicity, Hon's definitions will be used here. Hon classifies the periodic changes according to two criteria: (1) the *shape* of the FHR wave on the graph as compared with the wave made by the sensors which measure uterine contraction and (2) the correlation in *timing* between the fetal deceleration and the uterine contraction.

When the FHR wave is closely correlated with the uterine contraction, it is consistently the same from one contraction to another and is therefore called *uniform* in shape. When there is no correlation between the FHR wave and the uterine contraction, it is not consistently the same from one time to the next and therefore is called *variable* in shape. (See Figure 3-3.)

Uniform decelerations may be divided into two groups, *early decelerations* and *late decelerations.* These designations refer to the timing of the onset of the deceleration in FHR as compared with the timing of the onset of the uterine contraction. *Early decelerations* are those which begin at the onset of the uterine contraction. *Late decelerations* are those which begin some time after the beginning of the contraction. Typically, early decelerations end and the rate returns to the baseline at the end of the contraction.

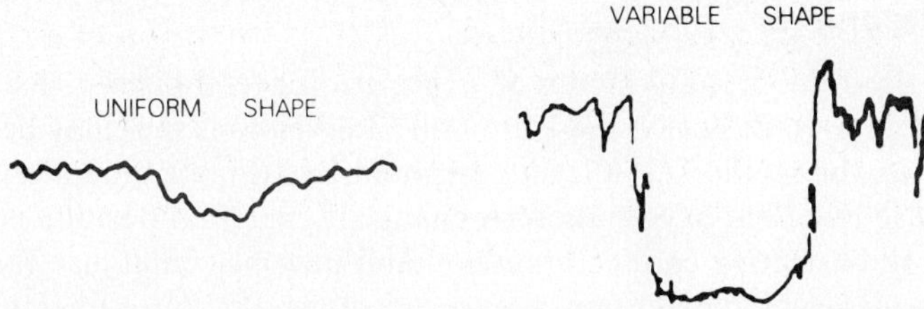

Figure 3-3 Fetal heart rate deceleration patterns may be classified as either uniform or variable. *(From Edward H. Hon, An Introduction to Fetal Heart Rate Monitoring, copyright Edward H. Hon, 1973, p. 24, by permission.)*

In late decelerations, the period of deceleration extends beyond the end of the contraction.

Clinical Significance of Deceleration Patterns

According to Hon, deceleration of the FHR is not a *normal* accompaniment of uterine contractions, though it is a frequent occurrence.[11] Hon sees all decelerations as an indication of *stress* in the fetus. Early deceleration patterns are the most common and the most innocuous. These are thought to be due to head compression by the uterine contraction, causing a vagal reflex that temporarily decelerates the FHR.

Late deceleration indicates some degree of uteroplacental insufficiency, such as premature separation of the placenta, or insufficient perfusion of the placenta, as might be caused by maternal hypotension or tetanic uterine contractions. Late deceleration is an indication of fetal *distress.* Often accompanying this pattern of deceleration is a baseline tachycardia. If it is accompanied by a smooth FHR baseline, it is particularly ominous, as this indicates inability of the fetal CNS to adapt to the stress.

Variable decelerations are caused by umbilical cord compression. Any appearance of cord compression is considered to be a warning sign of actual or impending fetal distress.

Identification of Fetal Distress

Hon delineates moderate tachycardia in the baseline (over 160 beats/minute) and mild variable decelerations in FHR as warning signs of *impending* fetal distress.[12]

Variable decelerations lasting more than 1 minute, decreases in FHR to less than 60 beats/minute, increasing numbers of variable decelerations over a short period of time, or the presence of late decelerations are indicators of *current* fetal distress. Late decelerations associated with a smooth baseline, indicate that the fetal CNS has already experienced great stress and is not reacting normally to stimuli.

Treatment of Fetal Distress

Hon has summarized the primary modes of treatment for fetal distress in a diagram (see Figure 3-4). Basically, there are four interventions that may be used: (1) reposition the mother, (2) alleviate hypotension, (3) relax the uterus, and (4) increase maternal oxygenation. A change in maternal position is especially useful in correcting cord compression and uteroplacental insufficiency caused by maternal hypotension. Figure 3-5 shows a monitor tracing for a patient who was experiencing marked variable deceleration. She was turned first to the right side and then to the left without alleviation of the FHR deceleration, but when she was placed in Trendelenburg's position, the variable deceleration stopped. (No woman who has received spinal anesthesia should be placed in Trendelenburg's position, however, as this causes upward progression of the anesthesia and may endanger the respiratory function.)

If a positional change alone does not correct the abnormal FHR pattern, it may be necessary to use other measures. (Doctor's orders are of course needed for most of these.) Elevation of the mother's legs and the administration of intravenous fluids may be needed to correct maternal

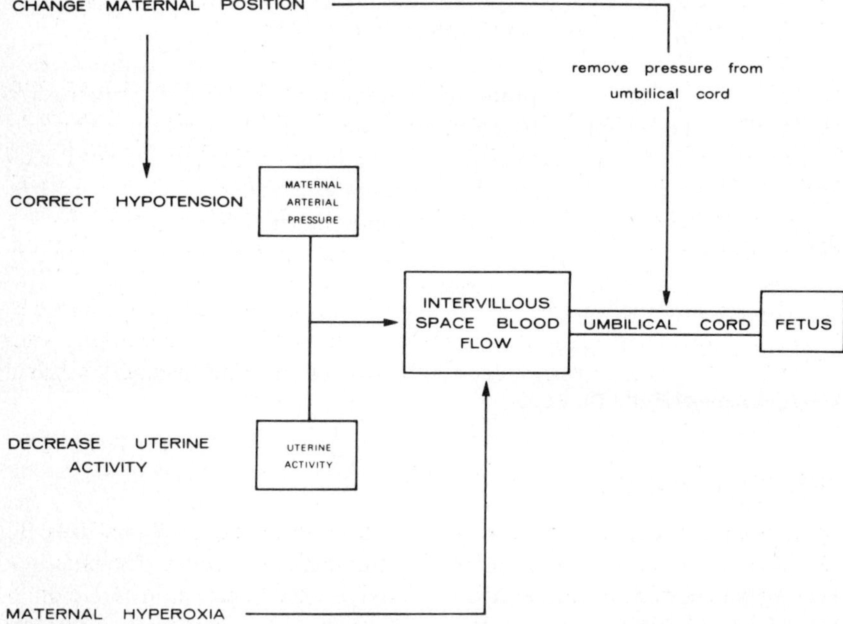

Figure 3-4 Fetal distress may be treated by changing the position of the mother, by correcting low blood pressure, by relaxing the uterus, and by increasing oxygenation of maternal tissues. *(From Edward H. Hon, An Introduction to Fetal Heart Rate Monitoring, copyright Edward H. Hon, 1973, p. 53, by permission.)*

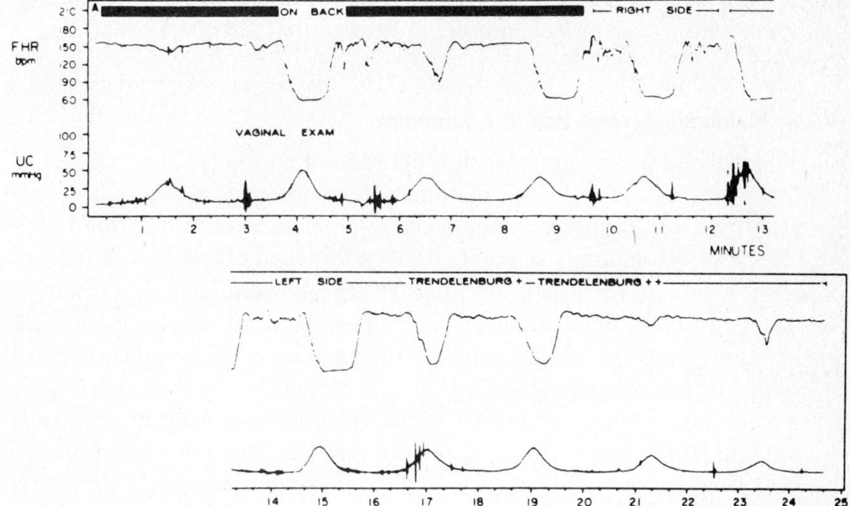

Figure 3-5 A patient showed marked variable deceleration of FHR while she was on her back for a vaginal examination. She was turned to the right side and then to the left and finally was put into a Trendelenburg's position. The variable deceleration was relieved in the Trendelenburg's position. *(From Edward H. Hon, An Introduction to Fetal Heart Rate Monitoring, copyright Edward H. Hon, 1973, p. 55, by permission.)*

hypotension. If uterine activity is greater than the fetus can withstand, and especially if oxytocics are being administered, measures should be taken to reduce the uterine activity. The discontinuation of oxytocics should be the first measure in the case of prolonged uterine contractions (more than 90 seconds in length or with incomplete relaxation between contractions). In addition, narcotics or diazepam (Valium) may be administered to relax the uterus.

The mother may also be given oxygen. Oxygen is usually administered by mask at relatively high rates (6 to 7 liters/minute).[13] It is important, also, to identify the cause for the fetal distress, since in some instances surgical intervention is necessary.

ELECTRICAL HAZARDS

Before leaving our discussion of electronic monitoring, it is important to mention the possibility of electrical hazard to the patient or the nurse. In electrical equipment, there may be a "leak" of some current from the operating parts of the machine to the metal case. If the machine is properly grounded, the excess current is carried away from the machine safely, and there is no danger of shock. If, however, the machine is not grounded correctly, a person touching the machine while touching a grounded object or standing on a damp floor can receive a shock; therefore, it is essential that those who use electrical equipment be sure that adequate grounding is provided.

Proper Maintenance and Use of Equipment

All electrical equipment must be stored and used correctly. The first step is to familiarize oneself with the manufacturers' instructions, both for safe operation and for proper maintenance. Equipment should be stored in a dry place away from areas where it could be knocked off shelves or banged about. It is an unsafe practice to use electrical equipment as a shelf or counter on which to place other objects, especially if the objects might leak or spill liquids onto the equipment. Any time a piece of electrical equipment is dropped or has something spilled on it, it should be checked thoroughly by an electrician before being used in patient care. The AAP recommends checking all equipment for grounding and leaks at least once a month.[14]

Any time an electrical device is to be used for patient care, it should be inspected for frayed or loose wires and broken plugs. When unplugging equipment, the entire plug should be grasped, not just the cord. Pulling on the cord often loosens the wires and breaks the plugs. All equipment should have a three-pronged plug; the round prong is a grounding prong. Adapters which allow three-pronged plugs to fit into two-hole outlets should not be used, as these negate the function of the grounding prong. If a fuse is blown, all the electrical equipment on the affected circuit should be checked for malfunction.

If the nurse notices a tingling sensation when touching the patient, if the patient responds with signs of pain when electrodes are attached, or if the patient reacts at recurring intervals corresponding to regular cycles in the functioning of the machine, the equipment should be disconnected and an electrician notified. If the equipment in use is life-support equipment, such as a respirator, then it should not be disconnected, but the doctor should be notified and a second machine readied for immediate use.

Occurrences of electrical shock are rare, but the nurse is the person most likely to be present when an equipment malfunction occurs; hence, the need for awareness of the potential hazards.

BLOOD GAS MONITORING

Fetal blood gases may be monitored if there are any indications of fetal distress. To obtain a sample of fetal blood, the membranes are ruptured, if they have not been ruptured, and the presenting part is visualized. A tiny incision is made in the presenting part (usually the scalp), and samples of blood are withdrawn. The blood is analyzed immediately for oxygen and carbon dioxide content and pH. The site for the blood collection is observed during at least one contraction to check for excessive bleeding. This is not usually a problem, however.

DELIVERY OF THE INFANT

Delivery of a newborn infant is one of the most exciting events in nursing. Even in normal pregnancies, there is always an element of suspense during the wait to see if the mother and baby will be all right and what the baby's sex will be. Nurses' responsibilities in relation to deliveries are varied. In some hospitals, nurses deliver some of the babies; in others, a doctor is always present to handle the deliveries. Usually, nurses are responsible for seeing that needed delivery room equipment is in working order and that all emergency supplies are readily available. (When the doctor is trying to resuscitate an apneic baby is no time to discover that the batteries in the lyringoscope are dead!) Nurses may also assist in giving anesthetics. In the administration of spinal anesthetics, the nurse is usually the person who times the injection so that the doctor can place the patient in a supine position after a specific number of seconds. In addition, taking vital signs of both the fetus and the mother are nursing responsibilities. The nurses in labor and delivery also need to keep the nursery staff informed of impending deliveries so that preparations may be made to receive the baby in the nursery. This is especially important if a high-risk infant is expected.

Establishment of Respiration

The primary concern immediately after birth is the establishment of respiration. Initially, the healthy infant will gasp and cry within a few seconds after the head is delivered. Often the first cry occurs even before the body is delivered. For this reason, as soon as the head is accessible, the person managing the delivery will suction the mouth first and then the nasal passages with a bulb syringe to prevent the infant from aspirating mucus or amnionic fluid in the first gasp. The suctioning itself may also assist in stimulating the first respiratory effort. After the body is delivered, the infant is held in a slight Trendelenburg's position while suctioning of the mouth and pharynx is completed. The infant is then usually placed on the sterile drapes on the mother's abdomen, and the cord is clamped in two places and then cut between the clamps (see Figure 3-6). The infant is then given to another person, usually a nurse, who is responsible for the infant's well-being while the placenta is delivered and the mother is prepared for transfer to the recovery room. It is vitally important that the infant be protected from heat losses immediately. This will be discussed in detail later. The infant should be placed in a slight Trendelenburg's position with the head turned to one side to facilitate drainage of fluid from the mouth.

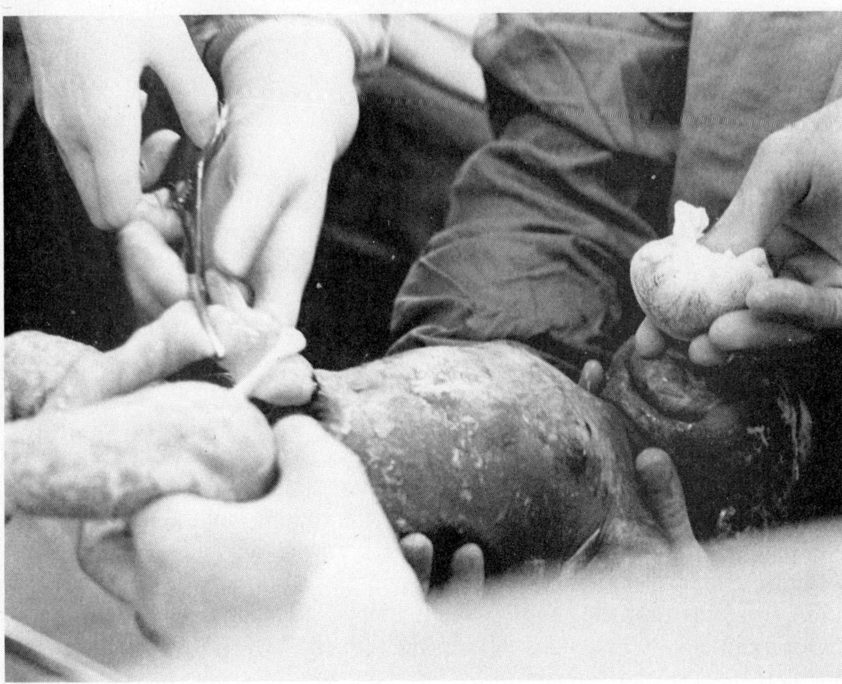

Figure 3-6 Clamping the umbilical cord after delivery. Note the shiny appearance of the umbilical cord and the presence of vernix on the skin. Note also that the infant is being suctioned orally while the cord is being clamped. *(Photo: Penelope Ann Peirce.)*

Table 3-1 Apgar Scoring

Sign	Score		
	0	1	2
Heart rate	Absent	Below 100 beats/minute	Over 100 beats/minute
Respiratory effort	Absent	Slow	Good
Muscle tone	Limp	Some flexion of extremities	Active
Reflex irritability (response to skin stimulation of feet)	None	Some motion	Cry
Color	Blue or pale	Blue extremities only	Pink

From Robert E. Cooke (ed.), *The Biologic Basis of Pediatric Practice*, McGraw-Hill, New York, 1968, p. 1451.

Apgar Scoring

Apgar scoring is a method of quick infant evaluation which has proved to be of great value both in assessing the immediate status of the infant and in predicting the later development of the child. It is usually done at 1 and 5 minutes after delivery. The 5-minute score correlates particularly well with future neurologic development.[15] Five parameters are checked: heart rate, respiratory effort, muscle tone, reflex irritability, and color (ranked according to importance). The child is given a score of 0, 1, or 2 points for each of the parameters examined, making the highest possible score 10. Table 3-1 summarizes the scoring system.

The heart rate should be taken apically for 30 seconds with a stethoscope. Any rate below 100 beats/minute should be reported to the doctor immediately. Respiratory effort, muscle tone, and color can be evaluated in a few seconds. Cyanosis of the hands and feet (acroncyanosis) is the rule for most babies, being present in approximately 85 percent of otherwise normal newborns.[16] As was mentioned in Chapter 2, this phenomenon may be an adaptive mechanism to preserve body heat. Reflex irritability can be checked by slapping the baby's foot lightly, by suctioning the oral cavity, or by inserting a suction catheter into the nares. The normal infant will respond by grimacing, crying, or trying to move away from the stimulus.

Apgar scores of 8 to 10 indicate that the infant is adapting to extrauterine life well; scores of 5 to 7 indicate moderate depression and the necessity for some intervention to assist early adaptive efforts; scores of less than 5 indicate severe depression and the need for vigorous resuscitative and supportive measures.[17] (Resuscitation techniques will be discussed in Chapter 9.)

Prior to the introduction of the Apgar scoring system (developed by Dr. Virginia Apgar in 1952), there was no systematic evaluation of newborns immediately after birth. As a result, many who were having difficulty adapting to extrauterine life were not identified immediately. Early identification of distressed babies has greatly increased their chances for survival and decreased the occurrence of neurological handicaps.

Prevention of Heat Loss

Prevention of heat loss is of great importance to all newborns; it may be of vital importance to preterm or distressed babies. The most important avenue of heat loss immediately after delivery is evaporation, since the infant is wet when born. The nurse should begin drying the infant with a soft flannel blanket as soon as the infant is laid on the mother's abdomen, even before the cord is cut. Then the infant is wrapped in another blanket and placed in a warmer.

Heat is also lost by convection, conduction, and radiation. Most delivery rooms are air-conditioned for the comfort of the staff. Drafts can be eliminated, however, thus decreasing heat losses due to convection. All surfaces on which the baby is laid should be warmed to prevent heat loss by conduction. Moore states that such surfaces should be 29 to 32°C (85 to 90°F).[18] It is important to remember, however, that warming a cold infant too rapidly may cause periods of apnea.

Poor conductors such as cotton mattresses are used in incubators to prevent heat losses due to conduction. Placing an infant in a warmed incubator is commonly practiced, though the walls of the incubator make resuscitative procedures difficult to perform. A radiant heat bed is a more convenient piece of equipment for assisting a distressed infant. It consists of a bed with low sides over which a radiant heater is suspended. Some of these heaters may not be approved for use in delivery rooms where certain anesthetic gases are present.[19] A room adjacent to the delivery room may be established for resuscitation of the infant, in such cases. The doctor or nurse who is caring for the infant in a radiant heater has free access to the infant without interfering with the heat source.

Two special covers for newborns have been described in the literature. One of these, developed in England, is the "silver swaddler," which is a plastic "blanket" laminated with a thin layer of aluminum.[20] One obvious problem with the swaddler is that the infant's respiratory efforts and heart rate cannot be checked unless the swaddler is wrapped around the baby's limbs, exposing the chest and abdomen, which of course decreases its efficiency.

A second device is a double-layered plastic bag and hood, containing air pockets.[21] One advantage of the clear plastic bag is that it is transparent, making observation of the infant more feasible. In addition, it can be torn and resealed for such procedures as clamping the cord and placing identification bands on the infant. In using either type of bag described, one must be aware of the possibility of overheating the infant and of suffocation should the infant's face become covered by the material.

Immediate Physical Examination of the Infant

There is disagreement as to when a physical examination of the newborn should take place; however, the AAP suggests that it is best for at least a brief examination to occur in the delivery room after the infant's condition has stabilized.[22] Of course, several observations have been made in obtaining the Apgar scores. In addition to those observations, the AAP recommends passing a soft catheter into the stomach to rule out obstruction of the esophagus. To insert the tube properly, first measure the distance from the mouth to the ear lobe and down to the ensiform cartilage at the tip of the sternum. The tube is marked and then carefully inserted through the mouth into the stomach. (Inserting the tube through the nares can cause mucosal swelling.) Placement of the tube in the stomach can be determined by withdrawing gastric contents through the catheter with a syringe, or by injecting a little air, ½cm³ (or cc), into the stomach while listening to a stethoscope placed over the stomach. (A swish will be heard.) Only a little air should be injected, and it should be withdrawn afterward. If, during the insertion of the tube, the infant becomes cyanotic or shows any other signs of respiratory distress, the tube probably has entered the trachea and should be removed immediately. It is recommended that the entire stomach contents be withdrawn at this time and measured to determine the quantity of fluid present.[23] A quantity of more than 20 ml indicates the possibility of an upper intestinal obstruction.

The AAP also recommends observing whether or not the infant can breathe with the mouth closed to rule out the possibility of choanal atresia (obstruction of the posterior opening of the nares).[24] The infant should be observed for the passage of meconium stool which would indicate a patent anus. If none is passed spontaneously, the AAP recommends passing a soft catheter into the rectum to check for patency.[25] Some authors state that it is preferable to wait 24 hours before passing the catheter into the rectum. It might be best to wait until after the second period of reactivity is over, as meconium is usually passed at that time.

The umbilical cord should be observed carefully. One thing that should be checked is the correct number of vessels (two arteries and one vein), since the presence of a single umbilical artery is highly correlated with serveral internal congenital malformations.

The arteries are smaller in diameter than the vein, and they have thicker muscular walls. Surrounding the vessels is a white gelatinous substance called Wharton's jelly. The relative amount of Wharton's jelly present may be helpful in determining the gestational age of the infant. The cord should also be observed for meconium staining, which can be recognized by a yellowish-green discoloration.

Any obvious abnormalities of the placenta should also be noted on the newborn record. The AAP also recommends weighing the infant in the delivery room and computing the precentile weight for gestational age.[26] This procedure seems to be more often done on admission to the nursery, and it will be discussed in that context.

Gonorrheal Prophylaxis

It has been required by law for several years that all newborns receive preventive treatment against gonorrheal infection of the eyes, which can cause blindness. The first treatment used was a 1 percent silver nitrate solution. This solution caused conjunctivitis in a large number of babies, resulting in a change to the use of antibiotic ointments. The development of antibiotic-resistant strains of gonorrhea, however, has resulted in the recommendation by the AAP that the use of 1 percent silver nitrate is again preferable.[27] To prevent conjunctivitis, it is recommended that the silver nitrate be rinsed from the eyes with sterile normal saline after it has been in contact with the conjunctival surface for at least 15 seconds.

Instilling drops into the newborn's eyes is not so easy as it might seem, since most newborns resist forceful opening of the lids. To perform this task correctly, it is helpful for the nurse to place a sterile gauze pad on each eyelid to prevent slipping of the fingers. Then the eyelids should be gently pulled open and one or two drops of medication instilled, with care taken to see that the tip of the dropper does not touch anything. It is best to turn the head slightly to one side and instill the drops in the inner canthus of the eye in the inferior position. Any solution which runs out of that eye will run down the side of the face away from the other eye, preventing the spread of infection if any should be present. Rinsing the eyes is done by the same procedure, using 1 to 2 ml of sterile normal saline for each eye. It is even more important during the rinsing to turn the head to one side to prevent the larger amount of fluid from flowing from one eye to the other.

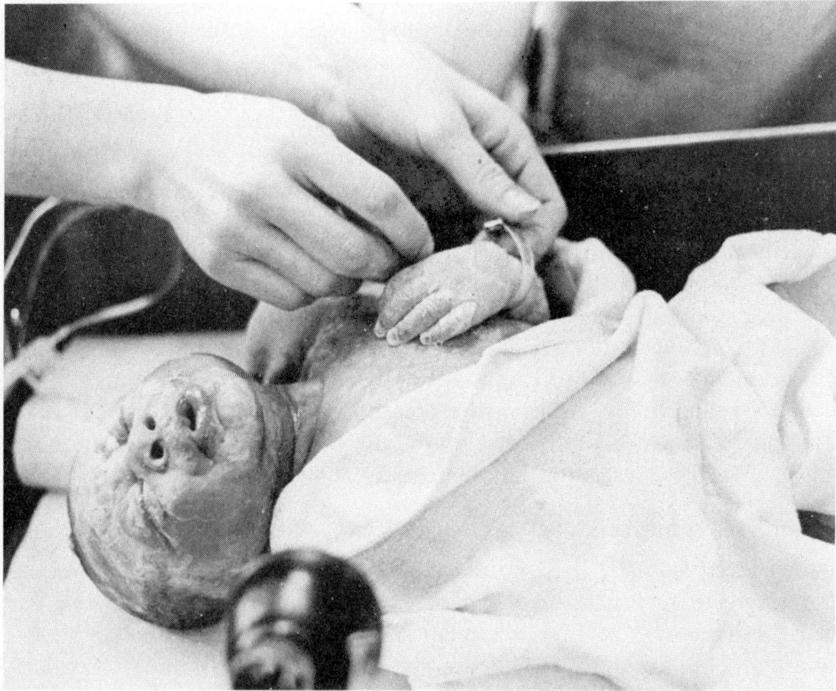

Figure 3-7 Identical identification bands are placed on the infant and the mother before either leaves the delivery room. Note flaring of the nares and pursing of the lips as the infant experiences the first period of reactivity. *(Photo: Penelope Ann Peirce.)*

Identification of the Infant

After the infant's condition has stabilized but before either the mother or the infant is allowed to leave the delivery room, the infant should receive proper identification. Usually, this is done by placing on the mother and the infant identical identification bands carrying code numbers and information (see Figure 3-7). A single band is usually placed on the mother's wrist, and the code number is recorded on her delivery record. Two bands are placed on the infant, either on both ankles or on one ankle and one wrist. The wrist bands tend to fall off when the baby moves around, so at least one ankle band should be used. The information on the bands contains the mother's full name and admission number, the date and time of delivery of the infant, and the infant's sex. In addition, in some hospitals footprints of the infant are taken along with a fingerprint of the mother. Care must be taken in obtaining these prints to be sure that they are clear; otherwise, they will be of no value. In placing the arm and leg bands, it is important that they be tight enough to prevent their falling off, but loose enough to allow for normal circulation. Correct identification of an infant is a serious nursing responsibility having both moral and legal ramifications.

Showing the Infant to the Mother

If the infant's condition is good and the mother is awake, she should be given an opportunity to see and, if possible, hold her infant. (See Figure 3-8.) It is best not to unwrap the baby at this time, as this would negate all

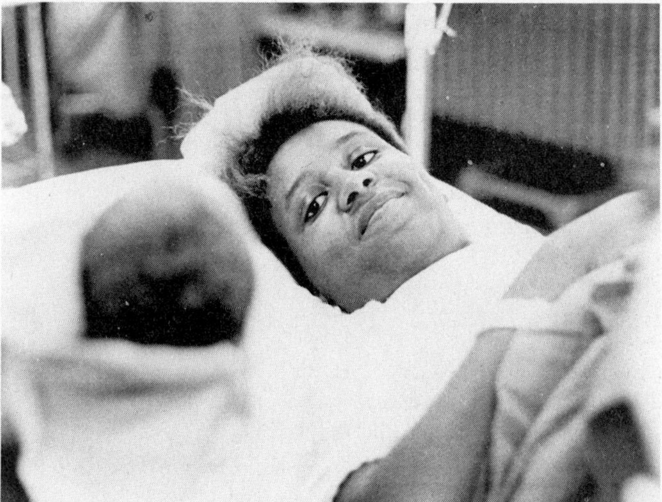

Figure 3-8 A mother sees her infant before leaving the delivery room. Note the mother's look of satisfaction. The infant is wrapped in a blanket to prevent heat loss. *(Photo: Penelope Ann Peirce.)*

the efforts that have been made to conserve body heat. Philips reports, however, no significant increase in heat loss when the mother holds a dried and well-wrapped infant after birth.[28] If the mother holds her infant, the nurse should stand by her side, as it is possible for the infant to fall from the mother's arms if she is very sleepy. Holding a newly delivered infant is one of life's special moments, however, and no mother should be denied this privilege unless the safety of her infant is clearly in jeopardy. If the father is in the delivery room, he, too, should be included in the initial contact with the infant. Some mothers may wish to nurse their infants at this time. This procedure is physiologically valid because it stimulates contraction of the uterus, thus aiding in preventing blood loss after delivery. It may help in preventing hyperbilirubinemia in the infant, also (see Chapter 9, The Infant with Hyperbilirubinemia, Resorption from the Gastrointestinal Tract). Most babies are wide-awake and are making sucking motions during the first period of reactivity for several minutes after birth.

REFERENCES

1 Erna Ziegal and Carolyn Van Blarcom, *Obstetric Nursing,* 6th ed., Macmillan, New York, 1972, p. 360.

2 Barbara Reed, Janet Sutorius, and Ronald Coen, "Management of the Infant during Labor, Delivery and in the Immediate Neonatal Period," *Nursing Clinics of North America,* March 1971, p. 5.

3 Edward H. Hon, personal communication, Nashville, Tenn., Mar. 21, 1975.

4 Edward H. Hon, *An Introduction to Fetal Heart Rate Monitoring,* Post Graduate Division, University of Southern California School of Medicine, Los Angeles, 1973, p. 40.

5 Ziegal, op. cit., p. 355.

6 Ann Woolbert Russin, Joan E. O'Gureck, and Jacques F. Roux, "Electronic Monitoring of the Fetus," *American Journal of Nursing,* July 1974, p. 1297.

7 Hon, op. cit., p. 45.

8 Ibid, p. 80.

9 Hon, op. cit.

10 Russin et al., op. cit.

11 Hon, op. cit., p. 7.

12 Ibid., p. 51.

13 Ibid., p. 60.

14 American Academy of Pediatrics, Committee on the Fetus and the Newborn, *Standards and Recommendations for Hospital Care of Newborn Infants,* American Academy of Pediatrics, Evanston, Ill., 1971, p. 60.

15 Barry S. Schifrin and Laureen Dame, "Fetal Heart Rate Patterns," *Journal of the American Medical Association,* Mar. 6, 1972, p. 1323.

16 Rose S. LeRoux and Shirley Stratton Yee, "The Physiological Basis of Neonatal Nursing," in Joy Princeton Clausen, Margaret Hemp Flock, Bonnie Ford, Marilyn A. Green, and Elsa S. Popiel (eds.), *Maternity Nursing Today,* McGraw-Hill, New York, 1973, p. 647.

17 Ibid.
18 Mary Lou Moore, *The Newborn and the Nurse,* Saunders, Philadelphia, 1972, p. 20.
19 Peter A. M. Auld, "Resuscitation of the Newborn Infant," *American Journal of Nursing,* January 1974, pp. 68–70.
20 J. W. Scopes, "A Simple Means of Reducing Heat Loss in Babies," *Triangle,* vol. 9, 1970, pp. 186–188.
21 Nicholas J. Besch, Paul H. Perlstein, Neil K. Edwards, William J. Keenan, and James M. Sutherland, "The Transparent Baby Bag," *New England Journal of Medicine,* January 1971, pp. 121–124.
22 AAP Committee on Fetus and Newborn, op. cit., p. 102.
23 Ibid., p. 103.
24 Ibid.
25 Ibid.
26 Ibid.
27 Ibid.
28 Celeste R. Nagel Philipps, "Neonatal Heat Loss in Heated Cribs vs. Mothers' Arms," *Journal of Obstetric, Gynecologic and Neonatal Nursing,* November–December 1974, p. 14.

BIBLIOGRAPHY

American Academy of Pediatrics, Committee on the Fetus and the Newborn: *Standards and Recommendations for Hospital Care of Newborn Infants,* American Academy of Pediatrics, Evanston, Ill., 1971.

Auld, Peter A. M.: "Resuscitation of the Newborn Infant," *American Journal of Nursing,* January 1974, pp. 68–70.

Beard, R. W., and E. G. Simons: "Diagnosis of Foetal Asphyxia in Labour," *British Journal of Anesthesia,* September 1971, pp. 874–885.

Besch, Nicholas, J., Paul H. Perlstein, Neil K. Edwards, William J. Keenan, and James M. Sutherland: "The Transparent Baby Bag," *New England Journal of Medicine,* Janaury 1971, pp. 121–124.

Cahill, Betty: "The Neonatal Nurse Specialist—New Techniques for the Asymptomatic Newborn," *Journal of Obstetric, Gynecologic and Neonatal Nursing,* January–February 1974, pp. 34–38.

Clark, Linda: "Introducing Mother and Baby," *American Journal of Nursing,* August 1974, pp. 1483–1484.

Clausen, Joy: "The Fourth Stage of Labor," in Joy Princeton Clausen, Margaret Hemp Flock, Bonnie Ford, Marilyn A. Green, Elsa S. Popiel (eds.), *Maternity Nursing Today,* McGraw-Hill, New York, 1973, pp. 527–552.

Dawes, Geoffrey S.: *Foetal and Neonatal Physiology,* Year Book, Chicago, 1968.

Edwards, Neil K., and Doris S. Edwards: "Are Babies Dying of Electrocution?" *Nursing Clinics of North America,* March 1971, pp. 81–91.

Hellman, Louis M.: "The Birth Process," in Robert E. Cooke (ed.), *The Biologic Basis of Pediatric Practice,* McGraw-Hill, New York, 1968, pp. 1429–1440.

Hon, Edward H.: *An Introduction to Fetal Heart Rate Monitoring,* Post Graduate Division, University of California School of Medicine, Los Angeles, 1973.

Littlefield, Vivian: "The Third Stage of Labor," in Joy Princeton Clausen, Margaret Hemp Flock, Bonnie Ford, Marilyn A. Green, and Elsa S. Popiel (eds.), *Maternity Nursing Today,* McGraw-Hill, New York, 1973, pp. 500–526.

Moore, Mary Lou: *The Newborn and the Nurse,* Saunders, Philadelphia, 1972.

Mueller-Heubach, Eberhard, and Karlis Adamsons: "Surveillance of the Fetus during the Intrapartum Period," *Mount Sinai Journal of Medicine,* September–October 1971, pp. 427–439.

Phillips, Celeste R. Nagel: "Neonatal Heat Loss in Heated Cribs vs. Mothers' Arms," *Journal of Obstetric, Gynecologic and Neonatal Nursing,* November–December 1974, pp. 11–15.

Reed, Barbara, Janet Sutorius, and Ronald Coen: "Management of the Infant during Labor, Delivery and in the Immediate Neonatal Period," *Nursing Clinics of North America,* March 1971, pp. 3–14.

Rice, Gail Taylor: "Recognition and Treatment of Intrapartal Fetal Distress," *Journal of Obstetric, Gynecologic and Neonatal Nursing,* July–August 1972, pp. 15–22.

Roberts, Joyce: "Suctioning the Newborn," *American Journal of Nursing,* January 1973, pp. 63–65.

Russin, Ann Woolbert, Joan E. O'Gureck, and Jacques F. Roux: "Electronic Monitoring of the Fetus," *American Journal of Nursing,* July 1974, pp. 1294–1299.

Schifrin, Barry S., and Laureen Dame: "Fetal Heart Rate Patterns," *Journal of the American Medical Association,* Mar. 6, 1972, pp. 1322–1325.

Scopes, J. W.: "A Simple Means of Reducing Heat Loss in Babies," *Triangle,* vol. 9, 1970, pp. 186–188.

Sturrock, Elizabeth W., and Sally Ann Yeomans: "The First Stage of Labor," in Joy Princeton Clausen, Margaret Hemp Flock, Bonnie Ford, Marilyn A. Green, and Elsa S. Popiel (eds.), *Maternity Nursing Today,* McGraw-Hill, New York, 1973, pp. 433–485.

Wilkerson, Betty L.: "The Second Stage of Labor," in Joy Princeton Clausen, Margaret Hemp Flock, Bonnie Ford, Marilyn A. Green, and Elsa S. Popiel (eds.), *Maternity Nursing Today,* McGraw-Hill, New York, 1973, pp. 486–499.

Ziegel, Erna, and Carolyn Van Blarcom: *Obstetric Nursing,* 6th ed., Macmillan, New York, 1972.

Chapter 4

Nursery Care of the Term Infant

When the infant is transferred to the nursery, all precautions should be taken to protect against heat loss, trauma, and exposure to hostile organisms. The cord should be checked immediately before and immediately after transfer to be sure there is no bleeding. A bulb syringe should be carried with the infant in case of respiratory distress. In some hospitals the infant may be transferred to the nursery in an incubator rather than being carried by the nurse. Public halls or elevators should be avoided. The infant may be shown to the father during the transfer procedure, depending upon the physical layout of the hospital; the infant should, however, not be unwrapped.

ADMISSION TO THE NEWBORN NURSERY

When a newborn is admitted to the nursery, the delivery room nurse is met at the door of the nursery by a nursery nurse, who receives the infant. This procedure prevents the carrying of organisms into the nursery from the outside. At the time of the transfer, the delivery room nurse should tell the nursery nurse of any complications of labor or delivery and of any resuscitative measures needed for the infant. These data should also be recorded on the infant's record, which accompanies the infant to the nursery. Usually, a carbon copy of the mother's record is attached to the infant's record, and it provides valuable information for the nursery nurse. The infant's identification bands should be checked with the number recorded on the carbon copy of the mother's record, the sex should be verified, and both nurses should sign the records. After the identity and general condition are noted, the infant is placed in a warmed environment (usually an incubator) to stabilize body temperature. Vitamin K prophylaxis is usually administered under standard orders if this has not been done in the delivery room. Usually an injection of 0.5 to 1.0 mg or an oral dose of 1.0 to 2.0 mg of vitamin K_1 is given to prevent blood loss due to normal vitamin K deficiency and its accompanying hypoprothrombinemia.[1] Injections are usually given in the thigh, to avoid the sciatic nerve. (See Chapter 8, Preventing Hemorrhage.)

Before discussing other specific care of the infant in the nursery, it is important to digress briefly to consider the physical layout of the nursery and aseptic technique to be used in giving care.

Physical Layout of the Nursery

The AAP now recommends an observation room for initial observations of newly delivered infants for the first 8 to 24 hours after delivery.[2] This area should be as close as possible to the labor and delivery suite. In most hospitals it is a part of the larger full-term nursery. This observation or transition room is usually next to the nurse's station, and it should have constant attendance by experienced personnel. The remainder of the nursery is usually divided into small rooms each housing 6 to 12 babies. It is important to be sure that there is adequate space between bassinets to allow for individual care of the infants and to prevent cross-infection. The floor may even be marked with bassinet stations to ensure adequate spacing. (Spacing requirements vary from state to state. Check with state health department.) Usually, each room is a self-contained unit, with all the necessary equipment for care of the infants. Supplies needed for individual infants are housed in the bassinet stands, and materials and equipment used by all the babies, such as scales, are located in a work area in the room. Hand-washing facilities are readily available throughout the nursery.

The nursery is completed with a nursing station, formula room, storage closets, treatment room, teaching room, utility room, conference room, and staff lounge and dressing area.

Aseptic Technique

In considering nursery aseptic technique, one can hope only to convey principles and an attitude which will enable the nurse to provide the protection needed in caring for infants. As has been emphasized in an article by Herrmann and Light, placing the infant in a sterile environment is neither possible nor even desirable.[3] Exposure to nonpathogenic organisms stimulates immunological responses (see Chapter 2, Specific Immune Responses), and it has been shown recently that the presence of certain strains of *Staphylococcus aureus* protects the infant from infection by other, more dangerous strains. In some places, babies are purposely being colonized by the nonpathogenic strains to prevent epidemics. This relatively new idea is called "bacterial interference."[4]

The goal then is not to provide a sterile environment, but to provide a medically clean environment, that is, one in which pathogenic organisms are absent. Specific techniques for reaching this goal change with time and place, and they must be modified as new equipment is introduced. Much of the complex equipment used in nurseries increases the possible loci for infectious organisms to grow. Nurses are in key positions, however, to ensure a safe environment. Indeed, it is primarily their responsibility to see that the environment is kept safe.

A Safe Zone It might help to imagine a zone of approximately 3 feet in all directions around a baby. Anything which enters this zone should be at least free from pathogens, if not sterile. Anything leaving the zone is considered to be "dirty" and must not be taken to a clean area or into another baby's safety zone. If this concept can be kept in mind, nursery aseptic technique is relatively simple.

Items that can be effectively sterilized, such as bed linens, clothing, and formula, are provided in individual packs for each baby. These are stored in a central "clean" area. Dirty objects (such as unwashed hands) must not enter such clean areas. An infant may be taken to some clean areas, such as a treatment room or the scales for weighing, but surfaces must be protected from direct contact with the baby by pads, or they must be disinfected before another baby is placed on them. Babies should never be taken to dirty areas, such as utility rooms where dirty equipment is stored. A nurse may handle clean objects and then handle a baby, but clean objects must not be touched after handling a baby, until hands have been washed. Nor should a baby be touched after handling dirty equipment, until hands are washed.

Aseptic technique associated with specific procedures will be discussed later in this chapter. There are, however, some general techniques that should be followed by anyone entering the nursery. Often it is the nurse who must see that all personnel follow these techniques. Such enforcement of rules is often a touchy business requiring tact and maturity and the support of other department heads. Most often tactful explanation of the rules and the reasons for them is sufficient to maintain adequate technique, but constant vigilance is a must.

Hand Washing By far, the most important single technique in protecting infants from infection is careful hand washing. Anyone entering the nursery to give patient care should follow specified hand washing procedures. Usually the persons who enter the nursery for a protracted period of time (such as nursing staff) change from uniforms to hospital-supplied scrub clothes. It is after changing clothes that they perform the initial scrub. Those who are entering the nursery for short periods of time, such as doctors or laboratory technicians, usually scrub first and put on short- or long-sleeved gowns over their clothing. Regardless of the timing, the technique is essentially the same.

Rings and watches should be removed and pinned to the clothing, taking care that they not be lost or discarded with the scrub clothes at the end of the day. The hands and arms are then scrubbed for a full 2 minutes (timed by the clock). Frequently soft brushes are provided for this purpose, though care should be taken not to abrade the skin, as this may increase the chances of a skin infection. Iodine preparations are especially favored currently for these scrubs because they are more widely effective against organisms than the hexachlorophenes which were widely used until recently. All aspects of the fingers, hands, and arms up to 2 inches above the elbows should be washed, and the fingernails should be cleaned with orange sticks or a similar device. The hands and arms should be dried with paper towels that are then discarded. Any time a baby or a dirty object is handled, the hands and arms should be washed again with a hexachlorophene or iodine solution, as provided for by nursery policy. A 15- to 30-second wash is generally considered sufficient for these secondary scrubs, depending upon the degree of contamination. Obviously, the important point is to remove the contamination, not just to go through a procedure. It is very easy to fall into the habit of following a ritual without thought to the results of the procedure. It is more helpful to be concerned with the end result and let the situation and knowledge of basic principles dictate the procedure.

Use of Nursery Gowns It is generally accepted practice that personnel entering the nursery either cover their clothes with a clean long- or short-sleeved gown or change into clean scrub clothes, taking their outer clothing off. The gowns worn by personnel coming from outside the nursery are discarded after use because they are likely to be contaminated with pathogens from other parts of the hospital. Except for doctors, laboratory personnel, and x-ray personnel, personnel generally are not allowed to work in the nursery if they are also working in what are considered to be contaminated areas (primarily other patient areas). Housekeeping personnel, for instance, usually are assigned only to the nursery areas, or possibly to labor and delivery and the nursery. The equipment they use, such as buckets and mops, should never be brought from contaminated areas into the nursery.

The potential for spread of infection via mops is phenomenal! Ideally, the nursery should have its own housekeeping staff, and they should be included in at least some staff conferences and made to feel the vital part they play in preventing nursery epidemics.

Parents are not usually allowed in the full-term nursery, but if they do enter for special reasons, they should be taught the same techniques used by other persons. Experience in intensive-care nurseries indicates that the presence of parents does not increase the risk of infection.[5]

Caps and masks were once a standard part of nursery apparel. In some hospitals caps still are worn, though most have discarded masks because they constitute a hazard when misused. The general feeling about caps seems to be that while they are not hazardous, they are unnecessary.

The scrub clothes donned by nursing staff are considered to be clean. In some hospitals, blankets are kept between the infant and the scrub clothes if the baby is picked up. These blankets are discarded when the baby is returned to the bassinet. In other nurseries, so long as only healthy babies are handled, the scrub clothes are not protected from contact with the babies, except by a plastic-backed pad under the diaper. Hands and arms should always be washed after contact with one baby before another one is handled.

CARE IN THE TRANSITIONAL NURSERY

How long the infant remains in the transitional nursery will depend upon hospital policy, population of the nursery at a particular time, and how the infant seems to be adjusting to extrauterine life. Most babies will go from the transition nursery to the normal newborn nursery. A few may be transferred to the intensive-care facility because of difficulty which develops or becomes apparent. The nurse is the key figure in the care of the newborn during this critical first day of life. Since the babies cannot talk, constant vigilance is essential, and the nurse needs to use all senses in observing infants. The nurse's role might for convenience be divided into the following functions:

1. Maintaining and supporting normal physiological adaptations
2. Collecting pertinent baseline data
3. Identifying risk factors
4. Recognizing and reporting symptoms of maladaption or illness
5. Protecting the infant from trauma and infection

While many of these functions are interrelated, they may be easier for the student to learn if they are discussed separately.

MAINTAINING AND SUPPORTING NORMAL PHYSIOLOGIC ADAPTATIONS

Respiration

The first concern is to maintain respiratory function. The newborn normally has an irregular respiratory rhythm, but the rate should be between 30 and 60 respirations/minute. Transient variations in the rate are not significant, but sustained tachypnea (over 60 respirations/minute), progressive tachypnea (rate that is steadily rising), a grunting sound in the expiratory phase, flaring of the nares, generalized cyanosis, or the presence of retractions are signs of inadequate adaptation.

Retractions are characteristic signs caused by the use of the accessory muscles of respiration. They can be recognized by the indentations of the tissue around the fixed structures of the chest wall on inhalation (see Figure 4-1). Especially common are sternal retractions. The lower tip of the sternum, the xiphoid process, is pulled in on inspiration. There may be similar indentations in the tissue above the clavicle and between the ribs. A deep indentation or groove below the lowest rib is commonly seen in severe retractions. The pulling in of tissues around the bones is thought to be due

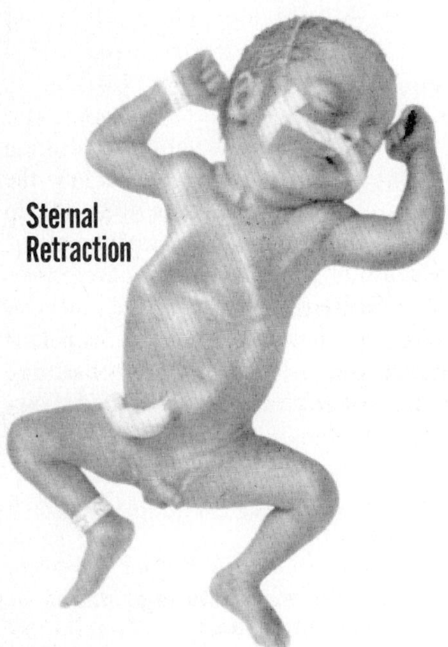

Figure 4-1 The soft tissues of the chest are sucked in during retractions. *(From The Premature Infant, Ross Clinical Education Aid #5, Ross Laboratories, Columbus, Ohio, by permission.)*

to increased negative pressure in the thorax which is produced as the diaphragm descends but the lungs do not expand as they should. Retractions are often accompanied by the grunting expiratory sound.

Brief pauses between respirations followed by one or two deep breaths are not unusual during the first and second periods of reactivity; however, periods of apnea lasting for more than a few seconds or those that are persistent or accompanied by any other signs of respiratory distress are highly significant.

At the onset of respiratory distress, nursing measures should be instituted as follows: (1) clear the airway of obstruction, (2) position the infant to facilitate respiratory efforts, (3) administer oxygen if policy permits, and (4) notify the responsible physician (not necessarily in sequential order).

Indications for needed suctioning include cyanosis, retractions, and an increased respiratory rate. Excessive oral mucus may be recognized by the infants' sticking out their tongues, "blowing bubbles" of saliva, and gagging or vomiting. To clear the upper airway, a bulb syringe should be used, suctioning the mouth first and then the nose. Suctioning the nose causes reflex gasping in which the infant is likely to aspirate oral secretions. The bulb syringe should be compressed before insertion to avoid forcing material from the upper to the lower respiratory tract. The bulb syringe should not be used for pharyngeal suctioning because it is too short, and tissue trauma is likely to result from attempts to use it for this purpose. A DeLee mucus trap or a catheter attached to a suction machine is appropriate for pharyngeal suctioning. The catheter should be lubricated with sterile water. The equipment can be checked at this time for patency by withdrawing a little water from its container. The catheter should then be introduced into the pharynx gently through the mouth or nose (preferably the mouth) with no suction being exerted by the catheter. The suction is then activated and the catheter is withdrawn slowly, rotating it gently to prevent the mucous membrane from being pulled into the eye of the catheter. Such suctioning should be limited to 10 seconds or less because prolonged suctioning of the throat may cause laryngospasm and because oxygen is removed from the airway along with mucus. Since passage of the catheter may stimulate the vagus nerve and cause bradycardia or cardiac arrhythmias, as well as unavoidably traumatizing the tissues to some extent, it is important to avoid unnecessary suctioning. A negative pressure of 3 to 5 inHg from a portable suction or 40 to 60 mmHg from wall suction is recommended.[6]

When performing any kind of suctioning, the positioning of the infant is important. Since gravity is an important adjunct to clearing the airway, the infant's head should be slightly lower than the body, with the head turned to one side. The infant can easily be positioned with one arm, leaving the nurse's other hand and arm free to manipulate the catheter and control the suction. Extreme positioning such as holding the infant upside down by the ankles is to be avoided, however, because it increases the risk of cerebral hemorrhage. In suctioning the lower airway, a small rolled towel placed under the infant's shoulders will slightly hyperextend the neck and prevent closure of the airway by the tongue.

Positioning of infants after suctioning will be determined by their responses to clearing the oral and nasal passages. If the problem does seem to be one of excessive mucus only, infants can be positioned on their abdomens so that mucus will drain better. If excessive mucus does not seem to be the problem, tilting the mattress of the incubator to place the infant in a slight semi-Fowler's position with the rolled towel under the shoulders may be helpful.

There should be standing orders in all nurseries regarding the administration of oxygen temporarily until a physician can be reached. Usually this is done via a mask or a hood which fits into the incubator. It is important to be sure that the oxygen is properly moisturized before it reaches the infant. If a hood is used, the oxygen must also be warmed (31 to 34°C or 87 to 93°F) to prevent cold stress, since the face is especially responsive to cold. During apneic episodes, respiratory efforts can be stimualted by gentle tactile stimualtion by gently lifting the abdominal musculature.

Roughness in handling or stimulating an infant should be avoided because of the damage that can be caused by traumatizing the skin and underlying tissues. Blood vessels are especially fragile in the preterm or distressed infant.

Body Temperature

Often associated with respiratory distress are the effects of cold stress. As has been emphasized in Chapter 2, maintaining body temperature is an obligatory function in the neonate, and to do so in a cold environment requires large amounts of oxygen. Cold stress may precipitate respiratory distress or it may simply accompany it, but it never helps it. Before considering specific nursing measures to prevent cold stress, let us first consider the concept of a thermoneutral environment.

Thermoneutral Environment Heim defines a thermoneutral environment as one in which minimal oxygen consumption (basal metabolism) is sufficient to maintain body temperature.[7] In terms of an incubator, a thermoneutral environment has been defined very precisely by him as 32 to 34°C (89 to 93°F) air temperature with the inner-wall temperatures of the incubator the same and the relative humidity inside the incubator at 50 percent. (Remember that heat is lost by radiation to solid masses near the infant.) Some incubators are equipped to regulate their own temperatures in response to the skin temperature of the infant as measured by sensors attached to the abdomen. These incubators are called "servocontrolled" incubators, and they are very useful so long as the temperature probes are functioning properly and so long as cold infants are not warmed too rapidly. (Rapid warming seems to cause apnea.) If they are used, they should be set to keep the abdominal skin temperature at 36 to 37°C (97 to 99°F).[8] However, these units are not accurate when infants are lying on their abdomens, if the probe is attached to the abdomen at that time. Placement of the incubator in areas away from air-conditioning vents or drafts is essential to prevent losses of heat due to convection and radiation. Simply placing the incubator next to a cold wall will increase the losses of heat due to radiation.

Body Temperature Normal newborns will probably be able to stabilize their body temperatures within 2 to 4 hours after delivery. After the temperature has remained stable for 2 to 4 hours and if there are no signs of respiratory distress, the complete physical exam and bath may be given. A brief physical exam should have been done earlier, however, and careful observations made during the intervening time.

In evaluating the infant's temperature, Lutz and Perlstein suggest taking concurrent readings of the infant's skin and rectal temperatures and the air temperature inside the warmer.[9]

Care should be taken always to note the air temperature inside the incubator before the incubator is opened. Incubator temperatures should be recorded hourly for normal babies and more often for sick ones, so that overheating is prevented.

A satisfactory rectal temperature is generally 36 to 37°C (97 to 99°F). If the skin temperature is the same or only slightly lower than the rectal temperature, the infant is probably in a thermoneutral environment. If the skin temperature is higher than the rectal temperature, the newborn may be in an environment that is too warm (this too can cause increased metabolic activity). If the air temperature in the incubator is more than 2 to 3°C (2.6 to 5.4°F) lower than the skin temperature, the infant is probably in too cold an environment. (This is true for full-term infants only until their temperatures have stabilized within the normal range. After that they can be kept at room temperature unless there is difficulty maintaining normal body temperature.) If a baby must be warmed after delivery to obtain a normal temperature reading, it is very important that this be done very slowly, since it has been observed that babies who have experienced cold stress and then are warmed rapidly develop apenic episodes.[10,11] The reason for this phenomenon is not known. Babies in unheated bassinets can be kept adequately warmed by the use of flannel blankets. The AAP recommends that nursery room temperature be kept at 28 to 30°C (82.4 to 86°F).[12] (Many nurseries are maintained at lower temperatures, however.)

In taking temperatures, a rectal thermometer should be lubricated and then inserted not more than ½ inch to avoid perforating the rectum. The thermometer should be held throughout the procedure and the infant's legs restrained to prevent kicking (see Figure 4-2). The rectal temperature may be taken without removing the diaper (just unpin one side) to prevent unnecessary heat loss. Axillary temperatures should be taken for 3 minutes (AAP recommendation[13]) or as dictated by nursery policy. They should be taken before unwrapping or undressing the infant.

Newer electronic devices are now available that permit the taking of accurate temperatures in seconds. These instruments are convenient if they are available.

Nutrition

The infant may be fed when fully awake, especially if signs of hunger are shown, unless nursery policy dictates a standard waiting period before the first feeding. The first feeding (or feedings, depending on policy) should always be of sterile water, and the nurse should give it. Both milk and glucose water can cause great lung irritation if aspirated. It is important at the time of the first feeding to evaluate the infant's sucking reflex and ability to swallow without choking and to rule out the possibility of tracheoesophageal fistula (an opening between the esophagus and the trachea

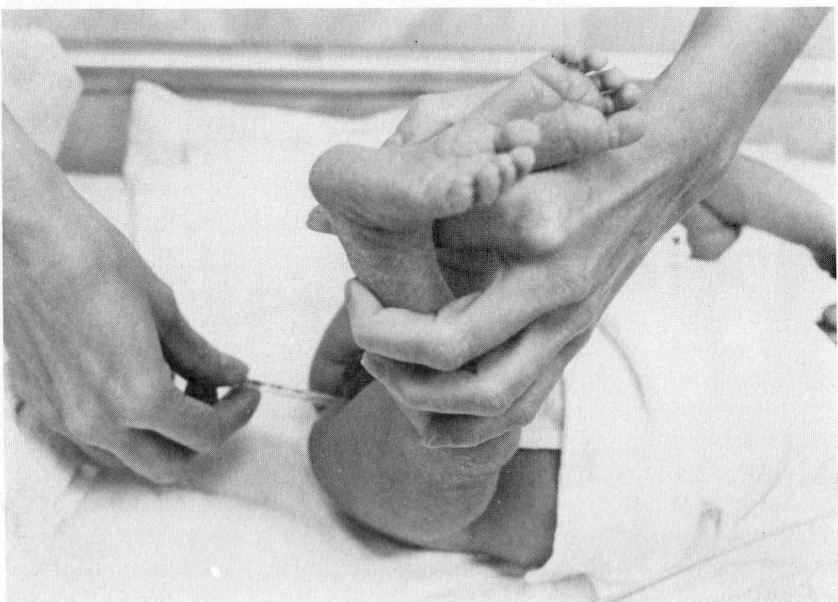

Figure 4-2 When taking a rectal temperature, restrain the infant's legs to prevent kicking of the thermometer and injuring the rectum. *(Photo: Penelope Ann Peirce.)*

which would cause the fluid ingested to run into the lungs). Any baby who has excessive oral mucus or drooling should have the patency of the esophagus checked before feeding (by inserting a feeding tube to the stomach). If the mother has had excessive amnionic fluid (polyhydramnios), the patency of the esophagus should be checked before feeding because excessive amnionic fluid often is caused by some blockage of the gastrointestinal tract. (The fetus normally swallows and digests some amnionic fluid in utero.) If the baby chokes when being fed, or swallows once or twice and then the fluid overflows the mouth, the feeding should be stopped and the infant's oral pharynx suctioned to prevent further aspiration. The patency of the esophagus should then be checked if this has not already been done. If the esophagus is patent, excessive mucus in the oral pharynx may be the cause for the regurgitation. Careful suctioning before attempting to feed will usually take care of the problem. The feeding may be attempted again after a few minutes rest, with care taken to be sure that the passages are clear of excessive mucus before beginning. If the esophagus is not patent or if there is strong suspicion that there is a fistula, the infant should be placed in a semi-Fowler's position and the physician notified immediately. The infant should be observed for circumoral cyanosis (blueness around the mouth) during the feeding, as this may indicate the need for rest periods during the feeding.

One often overlooked cause of choking in early feedings is a nipple with too large a hole. Nipples should be checked before every feeding. This can be done by holding the bottle upside down. The water or milk should flow out in distinct drops, about one per second. Water flowing faster than that is likely to choke the infant. A nipple through which no fluid drips may be all right or it may be clogged. Clogging can be checked by watching for bubbles to rise in the water when the infant sucks on the bottle. (This is true only for non-vacuum-type bottles.) If no air bubbles rise in the water or if the infant tires rather quickly and does not seem to decrease the amount of fluid in the bottle, it is likely that the nipple is clogged. It may be opened by inserting a sterile injection needle in the hole, taking care not to touch the nipple with the nurse's fingers. The infant should be burped after each ounce taken.

Students and parents should be helped to realize that newborns need time to learn to coordinate the reflexes required for sucking and swallowing. Patience is necessary during the early feedings.

IDENTIFICATION OF RISK FACTORS

While the infant is sleeping during the quiet period between the first and second periods of reactivity (see Chapter 2, Adaptation to Extrauterine Life), the nurse should study carefully the records that came to the nursery with the infant. (It should be noted that the nurse does not leave the room to do this reading of the records.) The records, though brief, will include pertinent data for identifying the high-risk infant, the infant likely to need special care. For convenience, this discussion will consider only prenatal risk factors and labor and delivery risk factors. Postnatal risk factors will be discussed in Chapter 7.

Prenatal Risk Factors

In studying the mother's record, it is especially important to note the expected date of confinement (EDC) and the mother's age and parity. Parity refers to the number of times the mother has delivered a baby at the age of viability (usually about 28 weeks). The date of delivery should be compared with the EDC. A discrepancy of more than 2 or 3 weeks should alert the nurse to the possibility of the birth of a preterm or postterm infant. (Criteria for evaluating the age and development of the infant from direct observations will be presented later.) Mothers over 35 years of age are especially likely to produce children with Down's syndrome (Mongolism) or to have prolonged or difficult labors. Anyone who has had a spontaneous abortion or stillbirth should be considered to be a high-risk mother. Early neonatal deaths noted on the record are of particular importance, also.

The mother's general health and nutritional status should be noted. Chronic diseases, especially diabetes, thyroid disorders, and cardiac and renal conditions, are of particular importance. A noted infection of the mother, especially in the first trimester of pregnancy, is frequently associated with congenital abnormalities. In addition, a number of drugs taken by the mother, again especially in the first trimester, are associated with numerous congenital anomalies. Korones gives a detailed list of maternal infections and drugs and their consequences for the newborn.[14] Bleeding during the third trimester or complications of pregnancy such as toxemia are also significant. It is important to note when the membranes were ruptured. If they ruptured as long as 24 hours before delivery, neonatal infection is likely. The mother's blood group and type should also be noted because of the likelihood of blood incompatibilities and subsequent jaundice in infants of couples who have either Rh or A, B, or O incompatibilities. (See Chapter 9, Hemolytic Disease of the Newborn.)

Labor and Delivery Risk Factors

It is important to note from the labor and delivery record, the length of each stage of labor, the type of analgesic or anesthetic used, the occurrence of maternal hypotension, the dosage and timing of drugs administered, the intrauterine presentation of the baby, the condition of the infant at birth, the use of resuscitative measures, and the results of the physical examination of the infant, if one was given in the delivery room.

Precipitous labors, lasting less than 3 hours total, may result in trauma to the head. Prolonged labors (longer than 24 hours) after the onset of regular contractions may result in excessive molding of the head, trauma to the head, and asphyxia.[15]

The presentation of the baby in utero will be noted on the record. If the baby's head is down as is usual, the presentation will be noted as vertex. Abnormal presentations may result in prolonged labors, central nervous system trauma, or asphyxia. A prolapsed cord or cord around the neck should alert the nurse to the likelihood of intrauterine asphyxia.

In considering the drugs given during labor, it should be remembered that narcotics are readily transferred to the fetus via the placenta. Doses of narcotics given 2 to 3 hours before delivery seem especially likely to result in a depressed infant. Regional anesthetics may be inadvertently absorbed by the mother and passed on to the fetus. Spinal anesthetics are especially likely to cause sudden drops in maternal blood pressure, resulting in fetal asphyxia. General anesthetics are the most likely to result in a depressed infant at birth.

Any indication of fetal distress during labor, as determined by fetal monitoring, or the presence of meconium in the amnionic fluid (except in breech presentations) should be noted. Examination of the placenta and cord may reveal further risk factors. Infarctions in the placenta may indicate the possibility of low glucose stores and asphyxia. The absence of one of the umbilical arteries is often associated with renal abnormalities.

The condition of the infant at birth can best be determined by noting the 5-minute Apgar score. In addition, the use of resuscitative measures should be noted. It is important to look closely at the physical examination given after birth. It is especially important to note any abnormalities and to note exactly what examinations were done (such as testing patency of the nares, the esophagus, and the anus) so that these will not be repeated in the nursery. Whether or not the infant voided or passed a stool should also be noted.

The careful perusal of the records will enable the nurse to anticipate problems and to make a more knowledgeable physical examination in the nursery. It should help determine placement of the infant when transferred from the observation nursery either to the normal newborn nursery or to the high-risk nursery.

COLLECTING PERTINENT BASELINE DATA

Collection of baseline data should receive top priority because of its importance in evaluating the infant's current status and adaptation to extrauterine life. Vital signs, including heart rate and respiratory rate, should be taken every 30 to 60 minutes until they are stable. Just what constitutes stability may be debatable. For our purposes, if the heart rate does not vary more than 10 beats/minute and the respiratory rate does not vary more than 5 respirations/minute for comparable activity states, the vital signs are stable. When recording the vital signs, the level of activity of the infant (awake, crying, asleep) should be noted since the activity level may greatly alter the vital signs. Respiratory rates should be taken before the infant is disturbed, followed by pulse rates and then temperature. After the vital signs have stabilized, they may be taken at increasing intervals, but they probably should be taken at least every 2 hours during the infant's stay in the observation nursery and at least once every shift thereafter. Such matters, of course, must be determined to some extent by nursery policy.

The infant's temperature should be taken on admission to the nursery and once every hour until it reaches normal levels. In some hospitals, after the temperature has been normal for 2 to 4 hours, the infant is given an admission bath and physical examination. In others, the infant is not bathed completely but merely sponged off to remove excess blood from the delivery. The most recent recommendation by the AAP Committee on the Fetus and the Newborn is that only blood from the delivery be washed off, with the vernix left undisturbed.[16] Recommendations regarding daily care suggest that only the buttocks and perianal region be washed routinely and that this be done with sterile water only, or with a mild, nonmedicated soap that is rinsed off thoroughly. The complete physical examination may be delayed for several hours, depending upon the baby's condition and the nursery policy. After being bathed or sponged off, the infant is dressed and either returned to the warmed incubator or placed in an unheated bassinet. Close check should be maintained for another 2 to 4 hours to determine the infant's ability to maintain a constant temperature under room temperature conditions. This should be one criterion for transferring the infant to the full-term nursery from the observation nursery.

Dextrostix determinations of blood glucose levels should be done within the first hours after birth and at appropriate intervals thereafter. (See Chapter 8, Preventing Hypoglycemia and Hypocalcemia.)

The general behavior of the infant should also be observed to determine levels of activity (lethargy, jitteriness, etc.), the effects of trauma (failure to move an extremity, for instance), and responses to stimuli.

Determining Gestational Age

Determining gestational age is a relatively new concept which aids in predicting the infant's ability to adjust to extrauterine life. It can be important in anticipating problems, and it may be one criterion for placing the infant in full-term or intensive-care nurseries after leaving the observation nursery. Obviously immature or distressed babies will in most instances be taken directly to the intensive-care nursery from the delivery room. While it is highly unlikely that very immature infants would be placed in the observation nursery, it is possible that an occasional infant who is really a preterm baby will be large enough to be mistaken for a full-term infant. It is possible, for instance, that a baby of a diabetic or prediabetic mother will be assumed to be a normal full-term infant when in fact the infant is an immature one grown to an unusually large size for the gestational period. This infant needs special care not needed by a full-term infant. Equally needful is the postterm infant, born more than 42 weeks after the beginning of gestation. The special care needed by these infants will be discussed later in the book, but for now the important point is to differentiate the preterm and postterm infant from the term infant.

Definitions First, the AAP has defined three categories in terms of length of gestation from the first day of the last completed normal menstrual period.[17] The *term infant* is one born between 38 and 42 completed weeks of gestation. *Preterm babies* are those who have completed less than 38 weeks of gestation, and *postterm babies* are those born after 42 weeks.

At one time gestational age was determined entirely by weight at birth. It was found, however, that this criterion did not result in an accurate determination of gestational age. Numerous factors, such as genetic inheritance, social and economic circumstances of the mother, and nationality, influence the weight of babies born after a full 40 weeks of gestation, so that in some cultural conditions a 5½-lb baby is the rule rather than the exception. No exact method of determining gestational age has been developed. There are too many factors that cannot be determined, such as the exact date of conception. The calculated age of the infant is measured from the first day of the last menstrual period, as the mother can remember it. This, as you might guess, is frequently a rather inaccurate date.

To make estimation of gestational age as accurate as possible, certain easily observable signs have been defined and their time of appearance in fetal development determined from examination of fetuses and babies whose dates were reliable. These external signs then can be used to determine estimated age of infants within a 3-week range on either side of the age which would be calculated if the menstrual dates were known. There are several systems that have been proposed for this purpose. These shall be explored in some depth in Chapter 8 (Classification of the Preterm Infant). Here, however, physical findings which can be observed in a brief examination by the nurse are presented so that a preterm or postterm infant can be readily distinguished from the term infant. (See Table 4-1.) The doctor should be notified when either a preterm or postterm infant is identified.

PHYSICAL EXAMINATION

Besides estimating gestational age, it is helpful for the nurse to perform a physical examination of the infant. Hospital policy differs widely as to the

Table 4-1 External Signs for Estimating Gestational Age

Characteristics	Late Preterm (34–38 weeks)	Term (38–42 weeks)	Postterm (42 weeks)
Vernix	Covers most of body	Covers part of body	None
Breast	1–2 mm in diameter (palpated)	More than 4 mm	Undetermined
Nipples	Good definition, areola flat	Good definition, with areola raised	Same
Sole creases	Less than two-thirds of anterior sole has creases; none on heel	Creases involving at least two-thirds of anterior sole progressing to include the heel as well	Creases cover entire bottom of foot
Ear cartilage	Thin cartilage; external ear returns to original shape slowly after being folded over	Thin to firm cartilage; ear springs back when folded over	Ear retains erect position away from head
Hair (on head)	Fine, woolly; individual strands hard to identify	Well-defined individual strands	Same
Lanugo	A little lanugo on shoulders	None	None
Skin texture	Smooth	Smooth	Desquamation
Skin color and opacity	Pink to red; some large vessels seen over abdomen	Pink; few to no vessels seen	Pale pink; no vessels visible
Posture at resting	Knees flexed; hips relaxed; minimal elbow flexion	Total flexion of arms and legs	Total flexion
Recoil (extend and then release)	None in arms; good in legs	Slow recoil in arms, to good recoil in arms; good in legs	Good recoil in arms and legs

*(Adapted from Lula O. Lubchenco, ''Assessment of Gestational Age and Development at Birth,'' *Pediatric Clinics of North America,* February 17:125-45, 1970, pp. 125–145.)

ultimate responsibility of the nurse for this type of examination. There is no reason, however, why it cannot be done for obtaining nursing data regardless of hospital policy, so long as it is done after the infant's condition has stabilized. Doing a systematic physical examination will sharpen considerably the nurse's powers of observation which are so necessary in caring for infants. Perhaps the most important point to remember is that specific observations need to be made and a written form completed to be sure all points have been checked. The examiner will probably develop a system for determining the order in which the observations will be made. This order may vary a little from time to time depending upon such factors as the wakefulness of the infant. There is really no reason why the determination of gestational age and the physical examination cannot be combined if checklists are available so that none of the needed observations is forgotten.

For a nurse to become a competent examiner, many babies need to be examined alongside a skilled practitioner who can confirm or correct findings as they are made. Audiovisual materials may help the student learn what to observe for, but clinical skills of this sort must be learned in clinical settings. However, an attempt shall be made here to provide a guide for the beginner in making an examination meaningful. It will be helpful for the beginning examiner to have an assistant to record findings as the examination is done. Emphasis will be placed on normal findings and nonpathologic variations in these findings. Pathologic findings most common will also be mentioned with an attempt made to describe how these pathologic signs can be identified. For those desiring a more detailed account of a physical examination, an excellent chapter has been written by Anne Noordenbos Smith in *Maternity Nursing Today* (see reference list).

Basically, the examiner is looking for *normality of appearance, indication of normal function,* and *presence of pathology.* In considering appearance, one should consider color and texture, symmetry, relative size, completeness, alignment, and assumed position. In determining evidence of normal function, characteristics such as spontaneous and evoked movements, sounds, range of motion, and response to stimulation will be considered. In detecting pathology, one must be alert to evidence of trauma and infection, the presence of abnormal masses, anomalous structures, and abnormal behavior, such as seizures. Abnormalities should be reported to a physician as soon as possible.

Initial Observations

Before a detailed examination of the infant is begun, one should simply observe the infant lying in the crib. The infant should be uncovered but otherwise left undisturbed at first.

Color Color should be noted. Usually it will be either pink or, perhaps, ruddy. Blueness of the hands and feet is normal for several hours after birth. Generalized blueness or grayishness are signs of inadequate oxygenation of the tissues, however. Paleness may indicate anemia; extreme pallor may be very serious.

The presence of jaundice is abnormal in the first 24 hours. Its appearance in the second or third day is normal, but the degree of jaundice needs to be observed. Kramer reports a very interesting and potentially useful system for evaluating the level of serum bilirubin by observing the location of jaundice in the skin.[18] Kramer has defined five zones of dermal icterus as listed in Table 4-2. Study has indicated that for the full-term infant, when jaundice is present only in zone 1, the indirect serum bilirubin level is between 4 and 8 mg/100 ml. Progression of dermal icterus to the second zone indicates a level of 5 to 12 mg/100 ml; the third zone corresponds to 8 to 16 mg/100 ml; zone 4 indicates a level of 11 to 18 mg/100 ml; and finally, when zone 5 is involved, the level is 15 mg/100 ml or higher. There were no infants in the study with levels above 18 mg/100 ml whose palms and soles were not jaundiced. Kramer points out that there may be some overlapping in zones and that preterm babies may progress through the zones at lower bilirubin levels than do term babies, but that generally, the skin observations do correlate well with blood values. When the bilirubin level becomes stationary, the skin signs also remain stable. When the bilirubin levels decrease, the skin signs fade uniformly all over the body, rather than regressing toward the head. However, if the level rises a second time, the progression in the skin signs is repeated. Kramer emphasizes that the observations he describes are not meant to replace blood studies, but that they could be used adjunctively. (Other observations are helpful in evaluating bilirubin levels, also. See Chapter 9, Moderate Hyperbilirubinemia, Early Recognition.)

Table 4-2 Dermal Icterus Zones

Zone	Location	Bilirubin level
1	Face and neck	4–8 mg/100 ml
2	Trunk from neck to umbilicus	5–12 mg/100 ml
3	Umbilicus to upper thighs	8–16 mg/100 ml
4	Elbows to wrists and knees to ankles	11–18 mg/100 ml
5	Feet and hands	15 mg/100 ml or above

Adapted from Lloyd I. Kramer, "Advancement of Dermal Icterus in the Jaundiced Newborn," *American Journal of Diseases of Children,* September 1969, pp. 454–458.

Symmetry Any obvious discrepancies in the symmetry of appearance or movement of any part of the body should be noted. Symmetry of facial movement and of movement of the extremities should be observed when infants are quiet and when they are crying.

Relative Size Infants' heads will appear to be quite large in proportion to their bodies. (Measurements will be taken later.) The presence of obvious swelling or bulging on the head should be noted. General body edema may be present with or without pitting, or may be localized in the presenting part. Localized edema in the presenting part is not unusual. According to Korones, some generalized edema may also be present for a few days after birth without undue concern, but severe edema is highly abnormal.[19] With some experience, one can learn to evaluate the infant's relative state of nutrition and hydration from observing the size of the extremities. Well-nourished full-term infants have layers of subcutaneous fat which give them a rounded "filled-out" appearance. Preterm or malnourished infants appear frail and thin by comparison. The skin of an infant who is dehydrated or who has lost weight in utero due to intrauterine growth retardation appears to be too big for the body. It is obvious that the infant has lost subcutaneous fat or fluid. If a fold of skin is picked up in the abdominal region, it does not spring back to its normal tightness, but rather only slowly returns.

Texture The normal infant's skin will be smooth in the first 24 hours after birth. It may dry and become flaky the second or third day. The presence of flakiness at birth is a common finding in postterm infants. The skin may be covered with a cheesy white material, *vernix caseosa.* The amount of this material should be noted, as this will help determine the gestational age of the infant. After the first day, most of the vernix either has been washed off or has dried and disappeared. Small white papules called *milia* may be present, especially on the nose. The papules are common findings caused by blockage of sebaceous glands. They disappear in a few days or weeks, and should be left alone (mothers need to be told not to squeeze them). The presence of fine hair, *lanugo,* on the face and body should be noted. It, too, helps determine the maturity of the infant. Some term infants with dark hair on their heads, may, however, have some dark body hair that is not indicative of gestational age.

There is one common skin lesion that appears to be very pathologic when seen for the first time. *Erythema toxicum* presents as a pink papular rash with vesicles interspersed. The vesicles, which may appear to be purulent, often look like insect bites. (It is sometimes called "flea-bite" rash, though it has no relationship to fleas.) The cause for the rash is not known, but it does not seem to be related to any known pathology. It appears in the first few days of life and disappears spontaneously. Petechiae on the head and shoulders due to pressure during delivery are common.

Completeness In the initial observation of the infant one should note any obvious missing parts, such as fingers, toes, and the like.

Alignment and Posturing Most newborns will assume the position they held during their intrauterine existence. Usually, this includes flexion of the neck, with chin resting on the chest; flexion of the elbows, with the hands and upper arms crossed in front of the chest; and flexion of the hips and knees, with the legs drawn up on the abdomen and the ankles close to each other or crossed. It is quite common for the ankles and feet to be adducted and rotated medially so that they may appear to be deformed. Most often, this is simply a matter of the intrauterine position and no cause for alarm. (More precise examination of the feet will be discussed later.) The degree of flexion of the arms and legs should be noted, as this will be helpful in determining gestational age. Unusual intrauterine positions are the most common reason for deviations from these described postures. For instance, the infant may have a hyperextended neck if the face rather than the back of the head was the presenting part in the delivery. Injuries of the nerves, however, must also be considered in unusual posturing. These will be described later.

Evidence of Normal Functioning In the initial appraisal, the infant's color can give information about both the circulatory and respiratory systems and the liver (presence of jaundice.) Further evidence of respiratory function can be obtained by observing closely the movements of the chest and abdomen as the infant breathes. It is best to do this before the infant is disturbed. One should observe rate and character of respiration. Irregular rates are the rule, but prolonged apneic periods should be noted with great care. The presence of retractions should also be noted, as should grunting sounds during exhalation and flaring of the nares. The chest and abdomen should rise and fall at the same time. Alternate motions resulting in a "see-saw" appearance are usually a sign of respiratory distress. The chest should be observed for symmetry of expansion also. A visible heart beat should be noted.

Spontaneous motor movements of the infant should be observed. It is normal for the extremities to jerk as the infant moves them about, but a repeated, regular, rhythmic jerking may be a clonic seizure indicating neurologic dysfunction. Failure to move an extremity may be an indication of trauma during the delivery. The presence of nystagmus in the eye movements should also be noted. A lack of coordination of eye movements, however, is normal until 3 months of age; hence, many newborns appear to have "crossed" eyes from time to time.

Pathology In the initial appraisal of the infant, only the grossest pathological signs, obvious deformities for instance, will be observed. These should be described as accurately as possible.

Birthmarks or nevi may be seen on the skin. There are several types, some requiring no medical intervention and some requiring eventual surgery. A common type called *telangiectatic nevi,* or commonly, "stork bites," are flat pink areas caused by capillary dilation. They are most often found on the eyelids or on the back of the neck. They are of no special significance and fade in a few months. A *nevus flammeus,* or "port wine stain," is a larger, darker area of mature capillaries which is flat and does not fade. It can be covered with cosmetic preparations when the child is older. *Nevus vasculosis,* or strawberry hemangioma, is a raised red lesion which may be seen immediately after birth, or may appear in the first or second week. It tends to enlarge in the first year of life, after which it slowly disappears. Most such lesions are totally absorbed by the time the child is 7 or 8 years old. They are usually untreated unless they interfere with function. *Cavernous hemangiomas* are large raised dark vascular areas which do not decrease in size. They are sometimes removed surgically because of possible bleeding if they are traumatized and for cosmetic reasons.

Birth trauma is sometimes evidenced by the presence of ecchymotic areas or erythematous forceps marks, especially on the face. Petechiae may also indicate increased intravascular pressures during the delivery, or they may be an indication of infection. Petechiae due to delivery pressures are usually observed on and near the presenting part, for instance on the face, neck, and upper chest in vertex deliveries. Extensive bruising or petechiae may indicate a greater than usual bleeding tendency, such as hemophilia. Large areas of bruising should alert the examiner to the possibility of later high bilirubin levels as the extravasated blood is resorbed.

Systematic Examination

After as much information as possible is learned from the simple observation of the infant, a systematic examination is done. The exact procedure through which this is accomplished may vary according to the examiner and according to the conditions at the time, but a checklist should be available to be sure that no observations are omitted. Smith suggests examining the extremities first as this is less upsetting to the infant.[20] It may be advantageous to begin with auscultation of the chest and abdomen, if possible, since these observations require the infant to be quiet. A pacifier may be used later, however, to quiet a crying infant if the examiner prefers.

Ascultation of the Chest and Abdomen A good stethoscope with a pediatric bell rather than a flat diaphragm is needed to hear the sounds well. The heart may be checked first. The rate should be counted and any abnormalities in rhythm noted. There are two distinct heart sounds representing the closing of the heart valves. The first sound is a little lower-pitched than the second, and it is caused by the closing of the mitral and triscupid valves. The second sound, which is higher-pitched, is the result of closure of the aortic and pulmonary valves. The resulting "toc-tic" rhythm should be distinct and sharp. Murmurs heard between the sharp sounds may be indications of pathology, though Korones states that most are benign.[21] The sounds of the individual valves can be detected by moving the stethoscope to different areas of the chest. The specific sounds to listen for have been described in detail by Alexander and Brown in their book *Pediatric Physical Diagnosis for Nurses.* The nurse who will be responsible for differentiating these sounds is referred to that reference (see reference list).

The functioning of the lungs should also be evaluated during auscultation of the chest. Evaluation of the breath sounds is difficult in the neonate because the small size of the chest makes it very difficult to localize sounds. One should listen for diminution of breath sounds from one side of the chest to the other and for the presence of rales and rhonchi, which are indications of fluid in the chest. Rales sound similar to the crackling produced by rubbing hair between two fingers close to the ear; rhonchi sound more like snoring.[22] (As in other aspects of the physical exam, there can be no substitute for guided clinical experience in learning to identify the sounds accurately.)

In auscultation of the abdomen, one is listening for evidence of peristalsis. These sounds are described as metallic tinkling occurring approximately 2 to 5 times/minute.[23]

Palpation of the Abdomen Following auscultation of the abdomen, and while the infant is still quiet, the abdomen is palpated to determine the presence of abnormal masses, tenderness, or rigidity and to determine the state of the abdominal muscle structure. Normally the lower edge of the liver can be palpated just below the lower border of the right ribs. The spleen may sometimes be palpated in the left upper quadrant. Korones states that each kidney should be palpated in the first 4 to 6 hours after birth to determine presence and appropriate size.[24] This can be done by placing one finger behind the flank of the infant. The other hand is then pressed into the abdomen from the front. A round oval mass should be palpable between them. If the kidneys are normal size, they should not extend below 1 or 2 cm above the umbilicus. Extension beyond this point leads to the suspicion of kidney enlargement. Next, the abdomen should be percussed. This is accomplished by placing one finger firmly against the abdominal wall and tapping it with the index finger of the other hand. Increased resonance especially in the presence of distension indicates the presence of gas in the abdomen.

Examination of the Head After completing auscultation and percussion of the abdomen, the examiner may then proceed with examination of the infant's head. First the entire scalp should be observed for swelling. Generalized edema called *caput succedaneum* is a result of pressure on the head during the delivery. It is a self-limiting condition and requires no treatment. In this condition, the swelling crosses suture lines. *Cephalhematoma,* in contrast, is a condition in which there is a smaller area of swelling which does not cross suture lines. It is caused by bleeding between the bone and the periosteum and usually does not require treatment, though it may remain evident for several weeks. The forehead should be observed in profile for any unusual protuberance which may indicate hydrocephalus. The head may have been molded by pressure during labor and delivery, resulting most often in a rather pointed appearance of the top or back of the head. This is of no major significance, as it will disappear in a few hours or days. It should be noted, however, that any unusual shape of the head may be of great concern to a new mother. The nurse should anticipate the need for parent teaching and reassurance.

The sutures and fontanels should be palpated (see Figure 4-3). The primary sutures are the *coronal suture,* which separates the frontal bones from the parietal bones, and the *sagittal suture,* which runs from back to

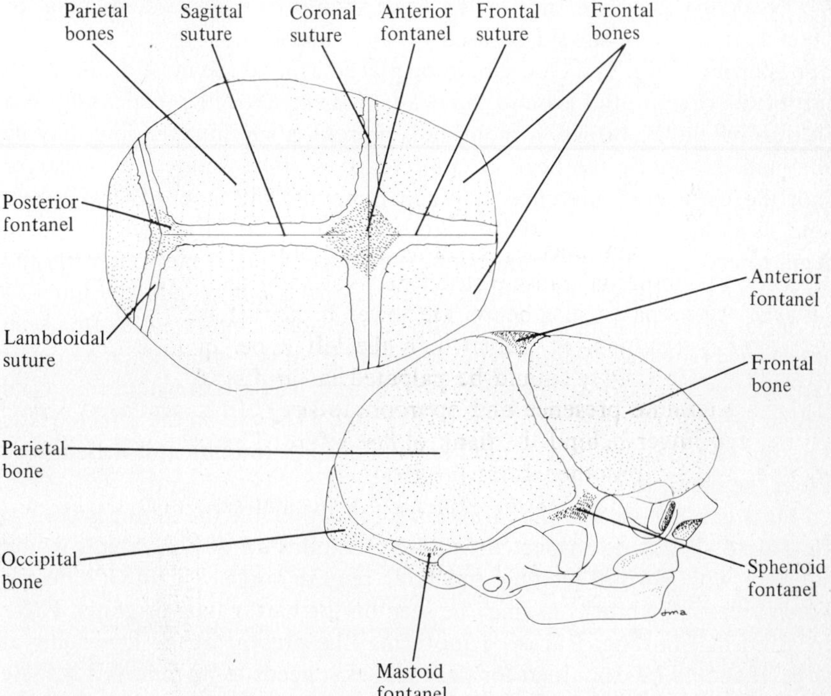

Figure 4-3 The sutures and fontanels should be palpated during a neonatal physical examination. *(From M. Alexander and M. Brown, Pediatric Physical Diagnosis for Nurses, McGraw-Hill, New York, 1974, p. 34, by permission.)*

front across the top of the head between the two parietal bones. The *lambdoid suture* separates the parietal bones from the occipital bone at the back of the head. The anterior fontanel is a diamond-shaped area at the juncture of the coronal and sagittal sutures. It is usually 1 to 5 cm in width at its widest point. The posterior fontanel is a triangular area at the juncture of the sagittal and lambdoid sutures. It is usually smaller than the anterior fontanel. In normal infants, the fontanels are flat when the baby is quiet, and they bulge when the baby is crying. Pulsations in the anterior fontanel are normal. In malnourished infants, the fontanels and sutures appear flat and soft; in infants with increased intracranial pressure, the fontanels are bulging and tight. If the infant is dehydrated, the fontanels may be sunken. The sutures and fontanels appear on palpation to be spaces between the cranial bones. It is important in palpating them to note their width and the level of tension present. A width of more than 1 cm in the sutures may indicate increased intracranial pressure. If molding of the head is present, there may appear to be ridges where sutures should be found. This is due to the overlapping of the cranial bones as they adapted to the shape of the mother's pelvis. Complete evaluation of the infant's head may have to be delayed until it assumes a more normal shape.

Next, the circumference of the head should be measured. A metal or paper tape measure should be used because it does not stretch, as a cloth tape is prone to do. The tape should be placed around the most protuberant part of the occiput and around the head, crossing above the ears and just a little above the eyebrows. If molding is present, a spurious reading may be obtained. Normally the head circumference is approximately 2 cm larger than the chest circumference.[25] (When removing the tape, lift the baby's head to avoid scratching or cutting the scalp.) As the infant will probably begin to cry during this examination, symmetry of facial movement should be observed during crying. Failure to move one side may indicate injury to the facial nerve. The mouth will droop on the side of injury, as is often seen in victims of a stroke. Spontaneous recovery from this condition may occur within a few weeks, or surgery may be required. The infant will need special care in feeding and may need special eye care if the eye on the affected side does not blink normally. The mother will need information and reassurance about the condition.

It is easy to observe the inside of the mouth while the infant is crying; the palate should be inspected for the possibility of a cleft which would interfere with normal feeding and later require surgery. Epstein's pearls, which are small white cysts, may be seen on the hard palate or gums. These are a normal finding. Rarely, a tooth may be present in the lower jaw at birth. It should be examined for tightness as it needs to be removed if there is any danger of its falling out and being aspirated. The relative size of the lower jaw should be evaluated. An abnormally small jaw may contribute to respiratory distress by allowing the tongue to fall back into the pharynx. Babies with this condition need special care to prevent occlusion of the airway. Patency of the nose should be observed since its occlusion can cause severe respiratory distress. Patency can be checked by inserting a very small catheter through each of the nares. (The newborn record should indicate whether this was done in the delivery room.)

Examination of the eyes may be difficult if the infant is crying and because babies tend to shut them when anyone tries to open them. For these reasons, it might be more convenient to observe the eyes during a quiet period. Gently rocking the head or placing the infant in an upright position may cause the eyes to open. When the eyes are open, the color of the sclera should be noted, especially if any yellow (representing jaundice) is present. It is not unusual to note small hemorrhages in the sclera due to pressure from labor and delivery. The eyelids may be swollen because of chemical irritation caused by the silver nitrate drops administered in the delivery room. In addition, a whitish discharge may be present. This should be cleaned from the eyes several times a day, but it usually disappears without further treatment. If a greenish-yellow discharge is present, an infection is likely, and it should be evaluated by a physician. Using the ophthalmoscope or a flashlight, light should be shone into each eye, to evaluate pupillary reaction and the blink reflex. Opacities of the cornea or lens will be observable at this time, also. The shape of the iris (round, oval, or irregular) should be noted. If an ophthalmoscope is being used, it should be set at 0 or -1 and the light directed into the pupil. A reddish-orange spot should be visible. This phenomenon, called the *red reflex,* is the result of light shining on the retina. It indicates that there are no opacities present in the structures between the cornea and the retina. The spacing and shape of the eyes should be noted. Excessively widely spaced eyes (hyperteliorism) or closely spaced eyes (hypoteliorism) are often associated with major syndromes involving extensive congenital defects. Eyes that slant up in the outer corners are often found in children with Down's syndrome. Eyes in which the sclera is visible above the iris ("setting sun" sign) are typical of children with hydrocephalus.

The ears should be examined primarily for position (see Figure 4-4). The top of the ear should be even with or slightly above a line drawn from the outer corner of the eye to the most prominent part of the occipital bone. (Again, this may be somewhat difficult to determine while excessive molding of the head is present.) Another imaginary line drawn from the point of insertion of the lobe to the point of insertion of the top of the pinna should be not more than 10° from a vertical line. Abnormal positioning of the ears is frequently associated with kidney abnormalities and extensive chromosomal abnormalities.

The infant's hearing should be tested by making four different noises

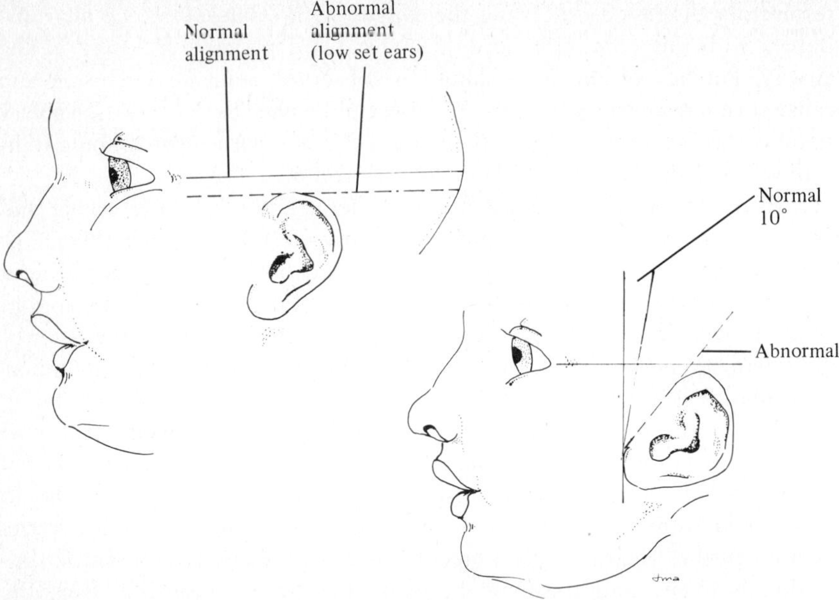

Figure 4-4 The ears should be observed for normal positioning. *(From M. Alexander and M. Brown, Pediatric Physical Diagnosis for Nurses, McGraw-Hill, New York, 1974, p. 72, by permission.)*

with rattles or bells near the infant's head but out of eyesight. Hearing the sound will cause infants to cease their activity, blink their eyes, or startle in response. It should be noted here that Daniel Ling of Canada has called to question the validity of screening newborns using only a single sound.[26] According to his study, an unacceptably high number of babies pass such hearing tests and later are found to have significant hearing losses. He states that the only safeguard against such false positive responses is to require the infants to pass three of four trials preferably with four different sounds. This procedure is not totally accurate, since many babies with normal hearing may fail to pass such a test in the newborn period. It seems, however, that it would be preferable to err on the side of suspecting hearing losses when they were not present than to pass infants who do indeed have hearing losses.

The head should be rotated to determine the range of motion of the neck. Any particular resistance to movement should be noted. With the head turned to the right, the left sternocleidomastoid muscle should be palpated for the presence of a mass. Similarly, the right muscle should be palpated.

Examination of the Chest Initially the chest is inspected for symmetry of shape and movement. Uneven expansion may indicate uneven lung expansion. The nipples are inspected to determine whether the areola are well defined and whether they are raised or flat. These observations are specific for determining gestational age. The breast tissue is palpated and its diameter is estimated, again as an adjunct to determining gestational age. It should be noted here that after the second or third day of life, engorgement of the breast is not unusual. This phenomenon is a result of the abrupt withdrawal of maternal hormones at delivery. Sometimes the engorged breasts secrete a fluid. Usually the engorgement will resolve itself in about 2 weeks. Mothers should be cautioned not to massage the breasts nor to try to remove the fluid, as this may cause breast abscesses.

The examiner should palpate the entire length of the clavicles to determine the presence of a mass which might indicate a fracture.

The circumference of the chest should be measured just above the nipple line. This measurement should be compared with the head measurement.

Examination of the Arms The arms should be examined for masses, for unusual posturing, and for range of motion of each joint. The fingers should be observed for color, clubbing, webbing, and the presence of extra digits. The shape of the fingers, especially the little finger, should be noted. Curving of the little finger is commonly present in Down's syndrome. The length of the fingernails should be noted. They are especially long in postterm babies. The *grasp reflex* can be elicited by pressing the examiner's finger into the palm of the infant's hand. The infant should grasp the finger and hold on tightly. Grasping with both hands simultaneously, the infant should have enough strength to be raised off the surface of the bed as the examiner pulls forward. It is very important to note failure to move one arm spontaneously, as this is indicative of injury to the fifth or sixth cervical nerves (brachial plexus palsy). The affected arm will require special positioning until the damage resolves spontaneously or until surgery is done. A broken clavicle also limits the movement of the arm. (This is the bone most frequently broken during delivery.)

Examination of the Feet and Legs Each joint of the legs is put through its range of motion. Of particular importance is the hip joint. With the infant in a supine position, the legs should be flexed on the abdomen and then abducted as the examiner pushes them laterally toward the bed. Uneven or limited abduction is often found in congenital dislocation of the hip. Unsymmetrical skin folds on the posterior aspect of the thigh also are common in dislocation of the hip. The toes should be counted and unusually wide spacing between the first and second toe or webbing of the toes noted.

The alignment of the feet and legs should be considered. Most newborns maintain an alignment of the feet reflecting the fetal position, with the feet turned inward and the soles of the feet touching each other. Other positions may be noted, depending upon the exact position of the infant in utero. The feet should be able to be brought into correct alignment by simple manipulation by the examiner without the use of force. If not, the infant should be evaluated for clubfeet.

Examination of the Spine With the diaper off and the infant in a prone position, the spine is observed for the presence of masses, dimples, and tufts of hair. Dimples and tufts of hair may indicate a spina bifida occulta which rarely requires treatment if nerve function is unimpaired. The anus should be inspected for any redness or excoriation. The presence and character of stools should be noted, and the patency of the anus should be determined if this has not been done. At this time, the presence of Oriental spots, bluish discoloration of the skin of the buttocks, may be noted. They are normal findings, especially in infants of Oriental or Negro parentage.

Examination of the Genitalia The infant is then turned over, and the external genitalia are examined. For the female, the presence of the labia majora, labia minora, clitoris, and vaginal orifice are determined. The relative sizes of the labia minora and labia majora should be noted, as this may help in determining gestational age. An unusually large clitoris should also be noted, as it may indicate adrenogenital syndrome, a serious endocrine disorder. A white mucoid or blood-tinged discharge may be present as a physiological response to maternal hormones. It usually disappears in a few days.

The male should be examined for the presence of testes in each side of the scrotum. This is determined by palpation. The penis should be inspected for the presence of the urinary orifice in an abnormal position. The glans penis is usually covered by the prepuce, which in the newborn most often cannot be retracted. If the prepuce fully covers the glans, the meatus may be assumed to be in its normal position at the center of the glans. If, however, there is an area of the glans not covered by prepuce, the urinary orifice is probably located abnormally. The inguinal area should be palpated for the presence of hernias.

Neurological Examination Finally, in evaluating total function of the infant, it is important to assess neurologic function. One important observation to be made throughout the examination is that of muscle tone. A limp, "floppy" baby is a baby in trouble. Most normal term babies maintain a posture of flexion at rest. In addition, if their extremities are extended, they will return them to the flexed position. This characteristic is called *recoil.* The degree of recoil present is important in estimating gestational age. The infant's head control should also be observed. The infant is raised slowly from a supine to a sitting position and should be able to control the head well enough to prevent the chin from falling on the chest or to raise it to an upright position after an initial slump. In general, poor muscle tone and poor response to reflex stimulation is indicative either of immaturity or of previously suffered hypoxia.

There are several reflexes that can be checked. The *grasp* reflex has already been described. The *rooting* and *suck* reflexes are best tested when the infant is hungry. A sterile nipple is rubbed lightly on the cheek at the corner of the lips. Infants should turn their heads toward the nipple (see Figure 4-5). The suck reflex can be evaluated by allowing the infant to take the nipple into the mouth. Infants should suck vigorously if they are hungry. The *Moro* or *startle* reflex can be elicited by placing the baby on a blanket and suddenly pulling the blanket as though to pull it out from under the infant, or by holding the infant supine above the bassinet and allowing the head suddenly to fall back approximately 30°. The characteristic response is to throw the arms outward and then bring them back to the midline as though to embrace. The legs are usually flexed briefly during this time, also. Alexander and Brown state that the Moro reflex is the most important single reflex for evaluation of overall neurologic function in the neonate.[27] Its absence is indicative of CNS trauma or depression. If it is present and then disappears, it may indicate early kernicterus (staining of the gray matter of the brain caused by excessively high levels of bilirubin and often accompanied by neurological damage).

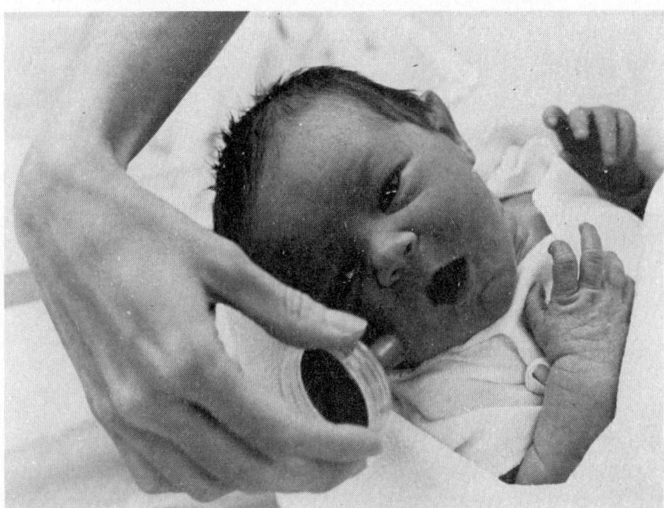

Figure 4-5 A hungry infant will turn his head toward an object that touches his cheek (rooting reflex). Note the open mouth in preparation for grasping the nipple and the eyes "looking" toward the nipple. *(Photo: Penelope Ann Peirce.)*

DAILY NURSERY CARE OF THE FULL-TERM INFANT

After moving from the transitional nursery to the full-term nursery, full-term infants receive daily care according to established nursery procedures. Usually they will be weighed daily, and will be taken to their mothers for at least daytime feedings. Daily baths are no longer being given in some nurseries because of possible toxicity of hexachlorophenes and in an attempt to promote colonization of infants with their own bacterial flora as a deterrent to growth of pathogenic organisms. Term babies receive most of their care from technicians or aides. This does *not*, however, relieve the head nurse or team leader of the responsibility for knowing an infant's condition and observing the infant frequently to be sure that no problems are developing. The nurse must also be sure that the persons who are caring for the infant are using good aseptic technique consistently.

Because students frequently begin their care of newborns in the full-term nursery, the following sections will provide a detailed account of suggested procedures to be used in the daily care of the infants. More experienced students or graduates may wish to use this section as a quick review.

Morning Care

Normally, morning care includes taking the vital signs and cleaning and weighing the infant. Feeding will be considered separately, as it is usually done by the mother. The student should be familiar enough with the procedures and the nursery to gather the needed materials before touching the infant. Exactly what is needed will vary from nursery to nursery, but in general, the student will need the following items:

For the taking of vital signs:

1. Thermometer (and lubricant if rectal temperatures are taken)
2. Stethoscope (preferably one with a pediatric bell)
3. Pen and paper
4. Watch with second hand or clock on wall

For the bath (if one is given):

1. Soap or soap substitute (if used)
2. Dry sterile cotton balls
3. Flannel blanket
4. Alcohol-soaked cotton balls for cord care if these are used
5. Fresh bed linen and clothing (usually prepared in sterile packs for each day)
6. Disinfectant-dampened paper towel for cleaning bassinet (not used in all nurseries)
7. Warm water, basin, blanket for drying

Vital Signs

The infant should be observed, first, before being disturbed. Color should be noted, as should any spontaneous movements. The nurse should be especially alert to repeated clonic movements indicating possible seizure activity. The respiratory and heart rates should be counted for a full minute if the infant is quiet. If the infant is crying, it may be preferable to count the respiratory rate at a later time. The heart rate should be counted apically with a stethoscope. The axilla is recommended as the site of choice for taking the temperature of newborn infants.[28] The AAP recommends holding the thermometer in place for 3 minutes with the infant's arm pressed gently but tightly against the side of the body. In some hospitals, rectal temperatures are preferred as a more accurate measure of "core" temperature. In taking the rectal temperature, the thermometer should be inserted into the rectum gently, not more than ½ inch (1.27 cm) and held in place for 3 minutes.[29] Care should be taken to be sure that movement of the baby does not cause the thermometer to injure the rectum. Rectal thermometers should always be lubricated before insertion. Temperatures should be taken before completely undressing the infant.

Manipulating the Infant

Many students find it difficult to pick up or turn over an infant if they are not used to handling newborns. There are any number of ways to do these maneuvers. The following descriptions are meant to serve only as a guide. Any way which is comfortable for the student and safe and comfortable for the infant is acceptable. It is important in moving the infant to be gentle but firm so that the infant feels secure. Smooth motions are much less upsetting than hesitant or jerky ones.

Turning the Infant Newborns should be kept in a prone or lateral position to prevent aspiration. It is easier to pick an infant up from a supine position, however, so the baby must be turned over, first. To do this, the nurse places one hand on the back of the infant's neck, supporting the head and neck. With the other hand, the pelvic region is gripped and the infant is gently turned toward the hand supporting the head and neck (see Figure 4-6).

Lifting the Infant The infant may be lifted from a supine position by raising his feet and legs slightly with the nurse's right hand while the left hand slides under his back to support the head and neck. When the left hand is in place under the head, the right hand is placed under the buttocks with a firm grip around one leg. The infant can then be lifted from the bed and held as shown in Figure 4-7*a*.

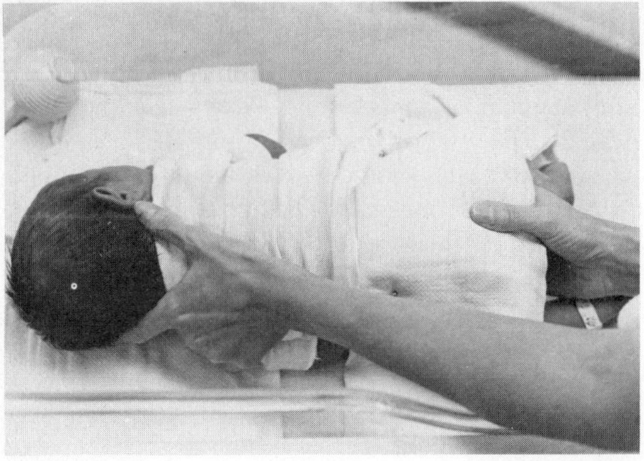

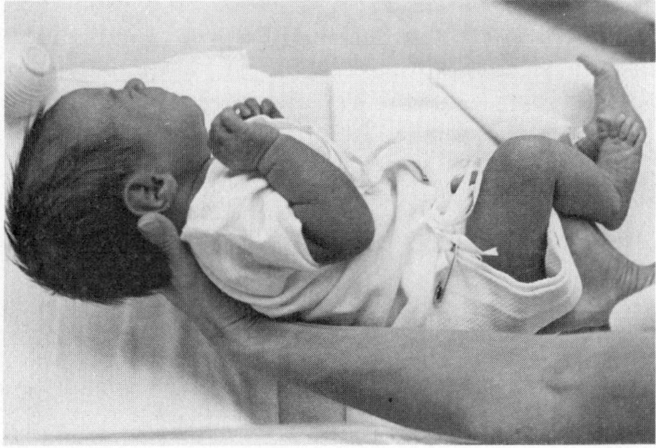

Figure 4-6 The head and pelvis are supported as the infant is turned from a prone to a supine position. Note the presence of the identification band on the ankle and the suction bulb in the upper left-hand corner of the bassinet. Extra diapers under the infant's head and pelvis provide pads that can be changed easily without changing all the linens. *(Photo: Penelope Ann Peirce.)*

Dressing and Undressing

Dressing and undressing an infant is awkward for some students. It is easier if the nurse grasps the infant's hands and gently pulls them through the sleeves of the shirt. Shirts that open in the front are much easier to use than those which must be pulled over the infant's head. (Expectant mothers who are preparing layettes need this information.)

The diaper should be put on snugly to prevent its slipping off. Lapping the back of the diaper over the front will prevent stools from falling out of the diaper. The nurse's fingers should be held between the diaper and the baby if diaper pins are used so that the pins do not prick the infant. Pins

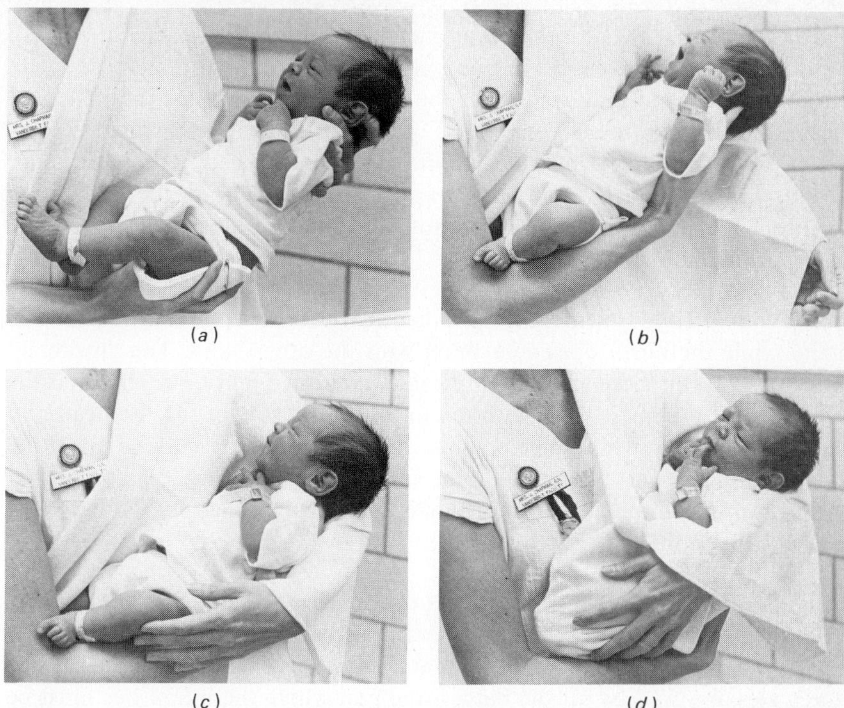

Figure 4-7a Swaddling the infant in preparation for taking him to the mother. Note the blanket on the nurse's shoulder and her hands supporting the infant's head and gripping the pelvic region. **b** The right hand and arm support both the head and body as the infant is positioned in the crook of the nurse's left arm. **c** The nurse's left arm now unfolds the infant, and she grasps the baby's left leg with her left hand. Note how the infant stops crying as he is enfolded. **d** With her left hand and arm supporting the weight of the infant, the nurse brings the blanket up under the infant and around the feet and legs. The blanket will lightly cover the head as the infant is carried to the mother. *(Photos: Penelope Ann Peirce.)*

should be pointed toward the infant's back so that they will not injure the abdomen if they come open. Disposable diapers are available now with tapes, however, so that pins are not used in most hospitals. No plastic protectors are used in the nursery other than those on the plastic-backed disposable diapers.

Swaddling After the infant is dressed, he may be swaddled, or wrapped in a blanket, to be taken to the mother for feeding. This is easiest to accomplish if a clean blanket is placed over the nurse's left shoulder, as illustrated in Figure 4-7*a*. The infant is then picked up with the nurse's left hand supporting the head and neck and the right hand supporting the buttocks. The right hand is slid along the back until it reaches the head. With the right hand supporting the entire weight of the infant, the nurse slides the left hand and arm under the infant's neck until the infant's head lies in the crook of the left arm (see Figure 4-7*b*). The infant is then enfolded by the nurse's left arm, and the infant's leg is grasped by the left hand, freeing the nurse's right hand to complete the wrapping of the infant (see Figure 4-7 *c* and *d*; in the figures, note how a crying infant is quieted by being enfolded in the nurse's arms).

Football Hold Sometimes it is necessary to hold the infant with one hand while the nurse does something with the other hand. The "football" hold is ideal for these situations. As illustrated in Figure 4-8, the infant is held against the nurse's hip with the nurse's hand supporting the head and neck of the infant while the elbow presses the hips of the infant against the nurse's hip. It is very important to be sure that the feet and legs are in such a position that the infant cannot brace them against the nurse's body and "push off" out of the nurse's grasp.

Weighing the Infant The infant can be weighed either before or after the bath. (It should be done before feeding, however.) It is perhaps better to weigh the baby before the bath, so that there is less chance of chilling. Since the scales are used by all the babies, the pan where the infant lies must be protected from contamination. Usually this is done by placing on the pan a

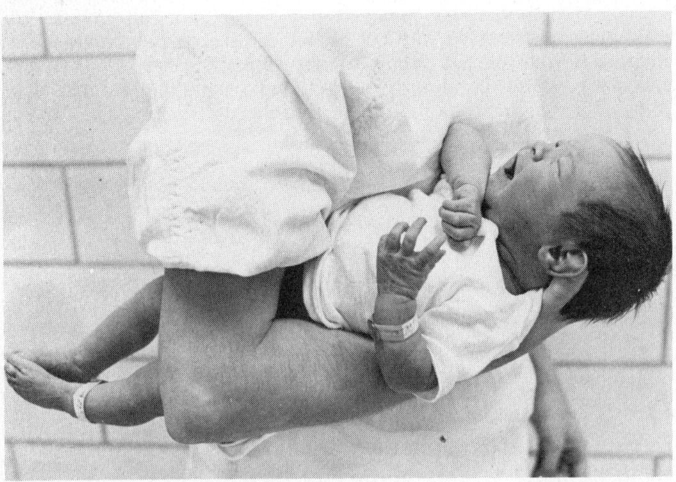

Figure 4-8 The "football hold" frees one of the nurse's hands to do other things, such as change the linens in the bassinet. Note that the infant's feet and legs are held away from the nurse so that he cannot "push off" against her hip. *(Photo: Penelope Ann Peirce.)*

paper or plastic-backed pad upon which the infant lies. The scales should be balanced with this pad in place. If the scale weights must be manipulated by hand to determine the infant's weight, then a paper towel or similar material should be used to protect the weights from the "contaminated" hands of the nurse. The scales should be totally prepared before undressing the infant.

The infant is weighed undressed, but may be covered with a blanket while being carried to the scales, to prevent chilling. It is a good idea also to hold a diaper in place while carrying the infant. The infant is laid in the pan of the scales, the blanket and diaper are removed, and the weight is read. It is important for the nurse to keep one hand over the infant as illustrated in Figure 4-9 to prevent his wiggling out of the weighing pan. After the weight is taken, the infant is covered with a clean blanket to prevent unnecessary chilling and replaced in the bassinet. The scales should be cleaned with a disinfectant if the infant voids or defecates on them. Otherwise, the used pad may simply be discarded and a fresh one placed on the pan. The weight should be recorded. If a common pen is used for recording the weight,

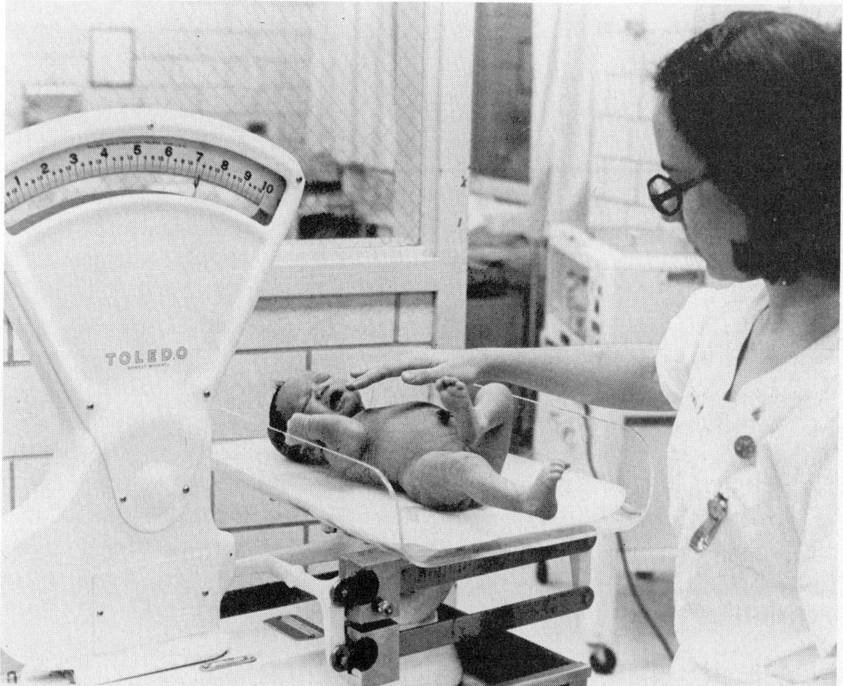

Figure 4-9 When the infant is weighed, the nurse's hand should be held just slightly above him to prevent his wiggling off the scales. *(Photo: Penelope Ann Peirce.)*

either the nurse's hand should be washed before handling the pen or else the pen should be manipulated with a paper towel to prevent its being a means of cross-infection.

Bathing the Infant

When an infant is bathed, how it is done, and whether it is done at all in the hospital nursery varies from one locality to another. The following is a suggested guide for giving a bath. Whether or not the nurse gives a bath in the nursery, establishing policy, supervising others, and/or teaching parents the basic principles and techniques involved are usually nursing responsibilities.

Cotton balls may be used in place of a washcloth because they are softer and less abrasive to the tender skin of the infant. (It is acceptable for the mother to use a soft cloth at home.) Hexachlorophene soap may or may not be used depending upon nursery policy. If it is used, it should be rinsed well to prevent absorption of the hexachlorophene through the skin. The AAP recommends the use of a nonmedicated soap, if any is used at all.[30]

Each eye should be bathed separately with clean water and a sterile cotton ball to prevent the spread of any infection from one eye to the other. There is frequently a heavy white discharge from the eyes as a result of irritation from the silver nitrate administered in the delivery room. This exudate should be wiped away carefully several times a day and always before taking the infant to the mother.

If a complete bath is given, no soap is put on the infant's hands, so that he will not put the soap in his mouth. Only a small part of the body is soaped, rinsed, and dried at a time with the rest of the infant covered with the blanket to prevent chilling. The diaper region should be cleaned last. It is a good idea, especially when bathing a boy baby, to keep the diaper in place until it is time to wash the diaper region. The cord should be kept dry during the bath to promote healing and prevent infection.

After bathing infants, wrap them in a blanket. Their hair may be washed. Clean water should be used for this part of the bath. In some nurseries, the hair is washed and dried immediately after washing the face so that the bath water need not be changed. It is usually easiest to wrap the blanket as a mummy restraint (see Figure 4-10) and then to hold the infant in a football hold with the head over the bath pan. Tipping the infant in a slight Trendelenburg's position will prevent water from running into the eyes. Each auditory meatus should be covered with the nurse's finger or thumb (of the hand supporting the head) to prevent water from running into the ears.

Cord Care There is some disagreement about what constitutes the best procedure in cord care. The AAP recommends that "some measure" be

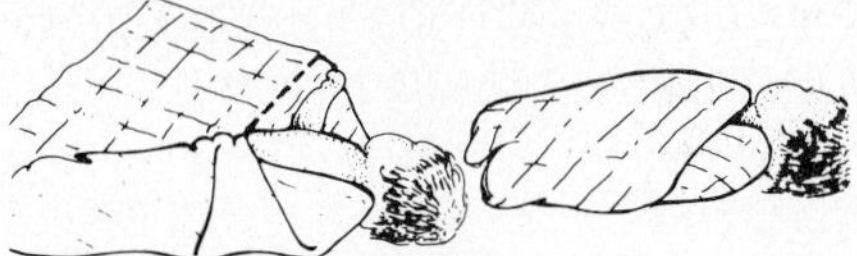

Figure 4-10 A mummy restraint holds the infant so that treatments or procedures may be done more safely. *(Adapted from G. Scipien et al., Comprehensive Pediatric Nursing, McGraw-Hill, 1975, p. 933, by permission.)*

used to prevent the colonization of the stump by bacteria.[31] A procedure commonly used is to wipe the stump of the cord with an alcohol-soaked cotton ball 1 to 3 times a day. (See Figure 4-11.) It is important to get the alcohol well around the base of the cord. The stump of the cord should be left above the edge of the diaper, never covered by it. Any redness around the stump, oozing of blood, or purulent discharge from the stump (all indicating an inflammatory process) should be reported.

The cord dries over a period of several days, turning first brown and then black. (This may worry some mothers.) By the end of the first week it has usually dropped off. At the time of the final separation between the cord stump and the umbilicus, some oozing of blood may occur, but this should be very slight (only a drop or two). Alcohol should be applied to the umbilicus for 2 to 3 days after the cord comes off so that it will dry thoroughly and heal without infection. Mothers frequently ask about coins

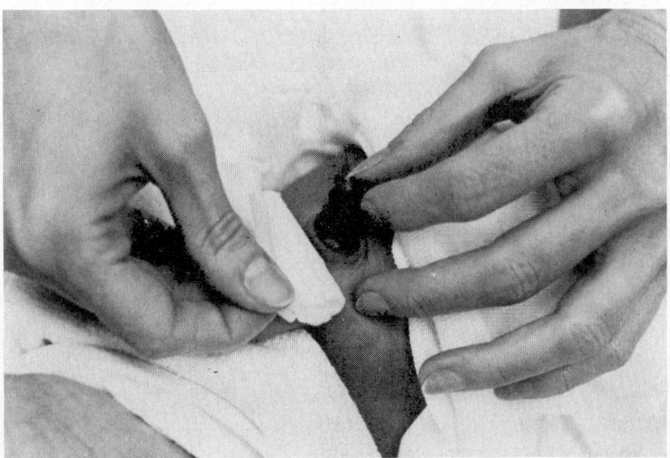

Figure 4-11 In giving cord care, it is important to wipe all aspects of the cord. Note how the cord has dried and turned black. Note, also, that the nurse's fingernails are short, clean, and free of polish. *(Photo: Penelope Ann Peirce.)*

tied on the umbilicus or bands tied around the abdomen to prevent a protuberant umbilicus. Such devices are of no value and frequently contribute to infection; hence, they should be discouraged. Umbilical hernias are fairly common. These are considered to be no threat to the child and are usually not treated. They tend to disappear as the child gets older.

Care of a Circumcision Circumcisions are most often done during the infant's stay in the nursery because of cultural pressures, although this practice is currently being questioned by the AAP.[32] An operative permit must be signed by a parent before the procedure is done. As for any such permit, the procedure and its risks should be fully explained. If a circumcision is done, it should not be done within an hour after a feeding because of the danger of aspiration. (The infant is restrained in a supine position.) An application of a petroleum jelly, usually in the form of impregnated gauze, is placed on the wound afterward to protect it from irritation. This dressing should not be allowed to dry out and adhere to the wound. A fresh dressing should be applied when necessary to keep it moist and clean and with each diaper change. The infant should not be positioned on his abdomen for several hours after the procedure is done. A lateral position is best.

The dressing should be inspected frequently for bleeding. If bleeding occurs, direct pressure should be applied to the dressing. If the bleeding is not stopped easily (within 3 to 5 minutes) the doctor should be notified.

The mother should be taught how to care for the infant after discharge. Prevention of irritation and infection and observing for bleeding are the main points. By the time the cord has dropped off and the umbilical stump has healed, the circumcision is usually healed enough to permit tub baths. For those who are interested, a detailed description of a circumcision procedure is given in the article by Melges (see reference list).

Observations to Be Made

Probably the most important aspect of the infant bath is the observations that can be made during the procedure. The infant should be observed for the development of an infection and for signs of other illness that may not have been apparent during the first few hours after birth. The infections most likely to be seen in the full-term nursery are thrush, skin lesions, and diarrhea. Other symptoms which may develop are jaundice, drug withdrawal symptoms, and seizure activity.

Thrush Thrush is an infection of the mouth by *Candidiasis (Monilia) albicans,* a fungus found frequently on mucous membranes of the mouth or vagina and in the intestinal tract. The organism may be present without symptoms. When growth becomes excessive, however, symptoms appear.

Thrush is seen as white patches on the tongue and the mucous membrane of the mouth. The tissue under the white patches becomes sore and the infant may refuse to eat. These white patches look like milk curds in the mouth. A small amount of sterile water may be given to the infant orally to differentiate the two. If the white patches are washed away by the water, they are milk curds. If not, thrush should be suspected, and the doctor notified. As with any diagnosed or suspected infection, care should be taken to protect other babies and personnel.

The infection is usually treated with an oral suspension of a fungicide such as nystatin (Mycostatin). Occasionally in some hospitals the lesions may be painted with a 1 percent solution of aqueous gentian violet. The gentian violet is irritating to the stomach if swallowed and should be used sparingly. The infant should be placed in a prone position after the treatment so that as the gentian violet becomes mixed with saliva, much of it will drain out of the infant's mouth. Stains on clothing or bedding that result from the use of this substance can be removed with a paste of sodium bicarbonate. If gentian violet is used, the mother should be informed of its purpose and the staining it will cause. (She should also be told how to remove the stains.) Tissue staining inside the infant's mouth disappears in a few days.

Impetigo A skin infection that is directly related to aseptic technique in the nursery is impetigo. The organism most often involved in *Staphylococcus aureus,* and spread of the infection is associated with either the presence of carriers in the nursery or poor aseptic technique. The characteristic skin lesions appear first in the diaper region. Vesicles filled with cloudy fluid appear, and then the vesicles burst, leaving behind a red, moist lesion devoid of skin. The lesions dry and heal by reepithelialization. Lesions in all stages of development may be present. The lesions may be treated with topical ointments or by being painted with 1 to 2 percent solutions of gentian violet. If more than one or two lesions appear, the infant is usually given systemic antibiotics.

An infant who has impetigo must be isolated immediately or removed from the nursery. It must be noted here that infants cannot be isolated simply by placing them inside incubators. An incubator has forced air flow that prevents organisms from entering, but it may actually disseminate organisms that are present inside the incubator. Incubators thus operate as *reverse* isolation only. Infected infants should be placed in a separate room and cared for with isolation precautions.

The AAP recommends that when an infant is diagnosed with impetigo, the organisms causing the outbreak should be identified by phage typing.[33] Then, all the infants in the nursery should have cord and nasal cultures to determine the extent of colonization. Personnel should also have nasal cultures. It is not uncommon to find persons with *S. aureus* strains in their nasal cultures different from the one causing the infection. It is accepted that carriers of strains different from the offending one need not be treated. In fact, the presence of the different strain is probably protecting the person from the pathogenic strain. In some nurseries, babies and personnel are purposely colonized with strains of staph different from the one causing an infection in an effort to control the infection.[34] Persons who are carrying the offending strain or who have skin lesions should be removed from the nursery and treated with antibiotics before being allowed to return to work. If the epidemic is widespread, the nursery may have to be closed for a time and new admissions made to a different location in the hospital. All the babies present in the nursery and those who have been recently discharged should be followed for possible later evidence of infection. After the nursery is emptied, all equipment must be thoroughly cleaned and sterilized where possible. The AAP recommends weekly surveillance cultures of the nursery and its occupants for at least 2 months after a serious outbreak of impetigo. An investigation of general aseptic technique should also be made and retraining instituted wherever indicated.

Diarrhea Epidemic diarrhea in the nursery is most often caused by certain strains of *Escherichia coli.* This organism, while not normally pathogenic to healthy adults, may be readily pathogenic to infants. Diarrhea must be defined for the neonate. The number of stools per day is not a sufficient criterion. Infants who are breast-fed may normally have as many as six liquid yellowish stools per day.[35] Other infants who have only one or two loose stools in a day may become rapidly acidotic and dehydrated. A sick infant will usually be identified by lethargy, refusal to eat, and temperature instability.[36] A dehydrated infant will have sunken fontanels and a loss of elasticity of skin. If a fold of abdominal skin is "pinched up," it will return to its former position only very slowly. The AAP recommends that when an *E. coli* epidemic is discovered, the sick infants be isolated and the nursery be closed to new admissions.[37] The AAP also recommends that all babies have stool cultures and be given prophylactic antibiotics for the duration of their nursery stay and for 48 hours after discharge. Stool cultures should also be taken from all personnel. Carriers of the offending organism should be removed from duty and treated appropriately. Thorough cleaning of the nursery and equipment and evaluation of general nursery aseptic techniques should be made prior to admitting any new babies to the nursery.

Jaundice The infant should be observed daily for the presence of jaundice. Jaundice in the newborn is caused by a combination of increased red blood cell destruction in the first days of life and liver immaturity. Poor oxygenation and low blood glucose levels compound the problem, as both oxygen and glucose are needed for metabolism of bilirubin in the liver. Excessive doses of vitamin K given to the mother during labor to prevent neonatal bleeding in the infant may also cause increased hyperbilirubinemia. Extravascular pools of blood formed by hematomas, extensive petechiae, or extensive bruising as a result of delivery may also contribute to excessive levels of bilirubin. (The blood in these pools is broken down, and large quantities of bilirubin may be resorbed in a short period of time.)

Physiologic jaundice occurs in over half of full-term babies. This is a relatively low level of hyperbilirubinemia (less than 12 mg/100 ml) which becomes evident after the first 24 hours of life and which does not reach levels high enough to cause neurologic damage. It should be noted here, however, that the bilirubin level that can cause neurologic damage for a specific infant is dependent upon many factors such as birth weight and serum albumin level. Thus, all jaundice deserves careful medical evaluation. Treatment for physiologic hyperbilirubinemia may include exposure to sunlight or a phototherapy light which converts bilirubin to less toxic metabolic products. The metabolism of bilirubin in this instance appears to occur in the skin.[38]

If phototherapy is used, the infant is undressed and exposed to the light of a daylight fluorescent bulb for several hours. It is very important that the infant's eyes be covered while under the light. The eye covers should not be too tight, and care must be taken that the eyes are closed when the covers are applied. The covers may need frequent readjustment for especially active infants. The covers should be removed daily to check the eyes for conjunctivitis. If the baby's condition permits, he or she may be dressed (with eye patches removed) and taken to the mother for feedings as usual.

The condition of the infant and the length of treatment can be determined only by blood studies, as skin color is no longer a valid means of determining serum bilirubin levels. The infant's temperature should be monitored closely, as overheating may occur. Loose stools which have a greenish color due to excreted bilirubin are a common side effect of the treatment. Extra fluids should be offered orally to compensate for fluid losses.

The light bulbs used for phototherapy lose their effectiveness after about 200 hours.[39] Therefore, a record of the length of time they have been used should be kept with the equipment.

As was mentioned in Chapter 2, phenobarbital may also be administered to increase hepatic metabolism of bilirubin.[40]

Drug Withdrawal With the recent increases in narcotic addiction, it has been more and more common to find newborns who are physically addicted to the drugs taken by their mothers. Early diagnosis and treatment is essential to their ultimate recovery. Withdrawal symptoms usually appear 1 to 5 days after birth. In preterm infants, nonspecific respiratory difficulty is usually the first symptom evident. Vomiting and diarrhea following the first feedings are characteristic. Otherwise, the infants are hyperactive. They cry for prolonged periods, and their cry has an unusually high pitch. They appear to be very hungry, sucking and chewing on their fists constantly, but feeding is followed by vomiting and diarrhea. If untreated, they may develop tremors and convulsions and finally slip into a coma and die. Treatment varies according to medical judgment and preference. Schaffer and Avery note that while the use of narcotics in treating the symptoms fell into disfavor for a while, the use of paragoric, which is an opium derivative, is once again recommended.[41] It is important to note here that the dosage of paragoric for infants is measured in *drops,* not in cubic centimeters, as most other medications are measured. Paragoric is a very potent drug and overdosages can cause respiratory arrest.

Mothers are sometimes advised to give paragoric for colic. Great care should be taken to be sure that the mother understands the correct dosage of the drug.

Seizure Activity Repeated clonic movements, tremors, or twitches are considered to be seizure activity in the neonate equivalent to generalized convulsions in older children and adults.[42] The tremulous movement of the extremities and the quivering of the lower jaw of the neonate when disturbed, however, is normal and should not be confused with seizures. Any suspected seizures should be recorded in detail and reported as soon as possible.

DISCHARGING THE INFANT HOME

Infants being discharged home are usually taken to the mother to be dressed. It is vitally important at that time to check the infant's identification bracelets and to compare them with those of the mother. One bracelet is usually removed and kept in the hospital with the record; the other should be left on until the baby is home. The mother usually will be asked to sign a release indicating that the baby has been adequately identified. These procedures should be taken very seriously, as the consequences of a mistake are grave.

Preparation for discharge should be unhurried. The mother should be assisted so that she does not tire herself in dressing the baby and packing. She will be understandably excited, but she should be encouraged to rest as much as possible after getting home and to try to conserve her energy for the care of the baby. If the discharge is near mealtime, her departure should be delayed until after she has eaten, if it is at all possible.

REFERENCES

1 American Academy of Pediatrics, Committee on the Fetus and the Newborn, *Standards and Recommendations for Hospital Care of Newborn Infants,* American Academy of Pediatrics, Evanston, Ill., 1971, p. 104.
2 Ibid., p. 67.
3 Judith Herrmann and Irwin J. Light, "Infection Control in the Newborn Nursery," *Nursing Clinics of North America,* March 1971, pp. 55–65.
4 Ibid., p. 55.
5 Sheldon B. Korones, *High-Risk Newborn Infants: The Basis for Intensive Nursing Care,* Mosby, St. Louis, 1972, p. 212.
6 Joyce E. Roberts, "Suctioning the Newborn," *American Journal of Nursing,* January 1973, p. 64.
7 Tibor Heim, "Thermogenesis in the Newborn Infant," *Clinical Obstetrics and Gynecology,* vol. 14, 1971, p. 790.
8 Korones, op. cit., p. 63.
9 Linda Lutz and Paul H. Perlstein, "Temperature Control in Newborn Babies," *Nursing Clinics of North America,* March 1971, p. 18.
10 Ibid., p. 16.
11 Korones, op. cit., p. 64.
12 American Academy of Pediatrics, Committee on the Fetus and the Newborn, *Standards and Recommendations,* p. 57.
13 Ibid., p. 89.
14 Korones, op. cit., pp. 38–42.
15 Erna Ziegel and Carolyn Van Blarcom, *Obstetric Nursing,* 6th ed., Macmillan, New York, 1972, p. 431.
16 American Academy of Pediatrics, Committee on the Fetus and the Newborn, "Skin Care of Newborns," *Pediatrics,* December 1974, p. 682.
17 Ibid., *Standards and Recommendations,* p. 19.
18 Lloyd I. Kramer, "Advancement of Dermal Icterus in the Jaundiced Newborn," *American Journal of Diseases of Children,* September 1969, pp. 454–458.
19 Korones, op. cit., p. 93.
20 Ann Noordenbos Smith, "Physical Examination of the Newborn," in Joy Princeton Clausen, Margaret Hemp Flock, Bonnie Ford, Marilyn A. Green, and Elsa S. Popiel (eds.), *Maternity Nursing Today,* McGraw-Hill, New York, 1973, p. 688.
21 Korones, op. cit., p. 102.
22 Ibid., p. 101.
23 Smith, op. cit., p. 693.
24 Korones, op. cit., p. 102.
25 Mary M. Alexander and Marie Scott Brown, *Pediatric Physical Diagnosis for Nurses,* McGraw-Hill, New York, 1974, p. 39.

26 Daniel Ling, "Response Validity in Auditory Tests of Newborn Infants," *The Laryngoscope,* March 1972, pp. 376–380.
27 Alexander and Brown, op. cit., p. 250.
28 American Academy of Pediatrics, Committee on the Fetus and the Newborn, *Standards and Recommendations,* p. 8.
29 Celeste R. Nagel Phillips, "Neonatal Heat Loss in Heated Cribs vs. Mothers' Arms," *Journal of Obstetric, Gynecologic and Neonatal Nursing,* November–December 1974, p. 13.
30 American Academy of Pediatrics, Committee on the Fetus and the Newborn, "Skin Care."
31 Ibid., *Standards and Recommendations,* p. 109.
32 Ibid., p. 110.
33 Ibid., pp. 45–46.
34 Ibid., p. 45.
35 Mary Lou Moore, *The Newborn and the Nurse,* Saunders, Philadelphia, 1972, p. 122.
36 Alexander J. Schaffer and Mary Ellen Avery, *Diseases of the Newborn,* Saunders, Philadelphia, 1971, pp. 271, 679.
37 American Academy of Pediatrics, Committee on the Fetus and the Newborn, *Standards and Recommendations,* p. 43.
38 Korones, op. cit., p. 74.
39 Jane M. Brightman and Stephanie Clatworthy, "Care of the High-Risk Infant and His Family," in Clausen, Flock, Ford, Green, and Popiel (eds.), op. cit., p. 845.
40 Schaffer and Avery, op. cit., p. 540.
41 Ibid., p. 848.
42 Korones, op. cit., p. 180.

BIBLIOGRAPHY

Alexander, Mary M., and Marie Scott Brown: *Pediatric Physical Diagnosis for Nurses,* McGraw-Hill, New York, 1974.

American Academy of Pediatrics, Committee on the Fetus and the Newborn: "Nomenclature for Duration of Gestation, Birth Weight, and Intra-uterine Growth," *Pediatrics,* June 1967, pp. 935–939.

———: "Skin Care of Newborns," *Pediatrics,* December 1974, pp. 682–683.

———: *Standards and Recommendations for Hospital Care of Newborn Infants,* American Academy of Pediatrics, Evanston, Ill., 1971.

Brightman, Jane M., and Stephanie Clatworthy: "Care of the High-Risk Infant and His Family," in Joy Princeton Clausen, Margaret Hemp Flock, Bonnie Ford, Marilyn A. Green, and Elsa S. Popiel (eds.), *Maternity Nursing Today,* McGraw-Hill, New York, 1973, pp. 820–867.

Farr, V., R. G. Mitchell, G. A. Neligan, and J. M. Parkin: "The Definition of Some External Characteristics Used in the Assessment of Gestational Age in the Newborn Infant," *Developmental Medicine and Child Neurology,* October 1966, pp. 507–511.

———, D. F. Kerridge, and R. G. Mitchell: "The Value of Some External Characteristics in the Assessment of Gestational Age at Birth," *Developmental Medicine and Child Neurology,* December 1966, pp. 657–660.

Finnstrom, Orvar: "Studies on Maturity in Newborn Infants, Part II, External Characteristics, and Part IV, Comparison between Different Methods for Maturity Estimation," *Acta Paediatrica Scandinavia,* January 1972, pp. 24–41.

Heim, Tibor: "Thermogenesis in the Newborn Infant," *Clinical Obstetrics and Gynecology,* vol. 14, 1971, pp. 790–820.

Herrmann, Judith, and Irwin J. Light: "Infection Control in the Newborn Nursery," *Nursing Clinics of North America,* March 1971, pp. 55–65.

Korones, Sheldon B.: *High-Risk Newborn Infants: The Basis for Intensive Nursing Care,* Mosby, St. Louis, 1972.

Kramer, Lloyd I.: "Advancement of Dermal Icterus in the Jaundiced Newborn," *American Journal of Diseases of Children,* September 1969, pp. 454–458.

Le Roux, Rose, and Shirley Stratton Yee: "The Physiological Basis of Neonatal Nursing," in Joy Princeton Clausen, Margaret Hemp Flock, Bonnie Ford, Marilyn A. Green, Elsa S. Popiel (eds.), *Maternity Nursing Today,* McGraw-Hill, New York, 1973, pp. 638–686.

Ling, Daniel: "Response Validity in Auditory Tests of Newborn Infants," *The Laryngoscope,* March 1972, pp. 376–380.

Lubchenco, Lula O.: "Assessment of Gestational Age and Development at Birth," *Pediatric Clinics of North America,* February 1970, pp. 125–145.

Lutz, Linda, and Paul H. Perlstein: "Temperature Control in Newborn Babies," *Nursing Clinics of North America,* March 1971, pp. 15–23.

Melges, Frederick J.: "Newborn Circumcision with a New Disposable Instrument," *Obstetrics and Gynecology,* March 1972, pp. 470–473.

Moore, Mary Lou: *The Newborn and the Nurse,* Saunders, Philadelphia, 1972.

Reed, Barbara, Janet Sutorius, and Ronald Coen: "Management of the Infant during Labor, Delivery, and in the Immediate Neonatal Period," *Nursing Clinics of North America,* March 1971, pp. 3–14.

Roberts, Joyce E.: "Suctioning the Newborn," *American Journal of Nursing,* January 1973, pp. 63–65.

Schaffer, Alexander J., and Mary Ellen Avery: *Diseases of the Newborn,* Saunders, Philadelphia, 1971.

Shimek, Mary Lynne: "Screening Newborns for Hearing Loss," *Nursing Outlook,* February 1971, p. 115.

Smith, Ann Noordenbos: "Physical Examination of the Newborn," in Joy Princeton Clausen, Margaret Hemp Flock, Bonnie Ford, Marilyn A. Green, and Elsa S. Popiel (eds.), *Maternity Nursing Today,* McGraw-Hill, New York, 1973, pp. 687–704.

Ziegel, Erna, and Carolyn Van Blarcom: *Obstetric Nursing,* 6th ed., Macmillan, New York, 1972.

Chapter 5

Infant Feeding and Postpartum Parent Education

Subject of much debate is the question of whether to bottle-feed or breast-feed infants. While arguments are presented with great fervor, very little objective evidence has been shown that clearly demonstrates differences in the development of children, either physical or emotional, that can be traced directly to the techniques of feeding used by their mothers.[1]

BREAST-FEEDING AND BOTTLE-FEEDING COMPARED

Comparing the two methods of feeding is really very difficult because of the involvement of such uncontrollable factors as differences in the basic personality structure of mothers who choose to breast-feed and those who choose to bottle-feed. In addition, the decision to breast-feed may be as much cultural as rational, as evidenced by distribution of breast-feeding mothers among specific cultural groups. For instance, mothers in middle and upper socioeconomic groups are more likely to breast-feed than are mothers in lower socioeconomic groups. Also, modern technology has negated many of the reasons why breast-feeding was so much better for children than bottle-feeding when artificial feeding was first introduced in the late nineteenth century.

As with most arguments where feelings are involved, the issues tend to be greatly oversimplified. Just the assumption that all bottle-feeding or all breast-feeding is the same is one such oversimplification. For instance, if the infant's family runs out of grocery money at the end of each month and the mother dilutes the baby's formula to make it last longer, the infant will have very different feeding experience from that of an infant whose mother provides a consistent formula in ample quantities. Similarly, the composition of breast milk may vary somewhat with the mother's diet.

Niles Newton has presented arguments that suggest that there is a great deal of difference between "unrestricted breast feeding," which is practiced in many societies and advocated by many people in this country and "token breast feeding," which Dr. Newton says is the predominantly *practiced* form of breast-feeding in this country.[2] The mother who has read about breast-feeding and who does not recognize the differences in practice may be very disappointed if she fails to have the satisfying experience cited in the literature. Not only are many of the advantages of breast-feeding not realized in token breast-feeding, but also new problems develop which seem to make the practice generally less desirable than bottle-feeding.

Although her findings have been questioned, Madeline Schmidtt states that nurses as a group are strongly biased in favor of breast-feeding.[3] Because of their contact with expectant and new mothers, nurses need to be aware of possible biases and avoid pressuring mothers, however subtly, to conform to their views. The major issues involved in evaluating the two methods of feeding with arguments for and against each method are presented here to provide a basis for understanding the choices mothers make and to assist them in making those choices.

Composition of Milk

Cow's milk is the usual substitute for human milk for infants. While cow's milk contains more protein than does human milk, the protein is less digestible and therefore of no more value to the infant. It does in fact increase the solute load on the kidneys and may in this way constitute a problem for the infant whose kidneys are especially immature or under stress. There is less carbohydrate proportionately in cow's milk; hence, most formulas using cow's milk have added sugar. The fat content is higher, but the fat is less digestible than that found in human milk. Both human and cow's milk seem to be deficient in vitamin D. Human milk is adequate in vitamin C if the mother's intake is adequate. Because of the processing it undergoes, cow's milk seems deficient in vitamin C by the time it reaches the infant. The B vitamins seem adequate in both kinds of milk. Iron is low in human milk and cow's milk.

This comparison is especially important for mothers in lower socioeconomic groups. These are the mothers most likely to bottle-feed their infants because of peer pressure and social norms. At the same time, they may not be able to afford the newer specially prepared formulas which compensate for many of the deficiencies of simple cow's milk. These mothers may also not understand the importance of preparing formulas exactly as directed and may not add the needed sugar, or they may dilute the milk with a greater proportion of water in order to decrease the cost.

Mothers in higher socioeconomic groups who bottle-feed turn almost exclusively now to the specially prepared infant formulas which have modified cow's milk and added vitamins and iron so that the resulting formula is very digestible and nourishing for infants.

It should be noted here that the composition of breast milk is influenced by the mother's diet and that there are some foods that mothers may need to avoid. Spicy foods, onions, and chocolate are examples of foods that may need to be eliminated from the mother's diet. Elimination of certain foods is not universally advised, but many new mothers are advised to follow some dietary restrictions. If elimination of certain foods requires significant deviation from the usual family eating habits, it may be difficult. Most drugs are transmitted to the baby via breast milk. One especially perplexing problem is faced by nursing mothers who have been advised by their doctors to take a laxative regularly during the last months of pregnancy. They may be faced in the postpartum period with a laxative dependence, while the pediatrician is advising against taking most laxatives because of their transmission to the infant. (Milk of magnesia is an acceptable laxative to take while nursing.[4]) While not of major importance from a medical point of view, such a situation may be seriously difficult for the new mother. Breast-feeding mothers may also be advised against taking oral contraceptives, which may add anxiety about the possibility of an unplanned pregnancy. The new mother who is breast-feeding should remind her doctor, whenever medications are prescribed for her, that she is nursing the baby. This is especially true if the mother is being treated by a variety of specialists rather than a family doctor.

An occasional mother's milk contains a progesterone metabolite which interferes with the infant's conjugation of bilirubin in the liver. The babies of these mothers may become jaundiced during the second week of life. The question of whether or not this condition is a contraindication to breast-feeding is not clearly resolved at this time, but it does represent a problem not faced by mothers who bottle-feed.

Protection from Infection

The transfer of immune globulins to the infant via mother's milk is one advantage to breast-feeding. Evidence indicates that this immunity is especially effective against enteric pathogens, such as *E. coli.*[5,6,7] More generalized protection against communicable diseases, as stressed by such groups as the La Leche League (an organization of mothers who have nursed their children) seems not to be supported by the available research.[8]

Allergies

Allergies to cow's milk may have serious consequences. Babies from families known to have allergic tendencies may need to be breast-fed in order to avoid the possibility of severe allergic reactions. However, it has been noted in such cases that restrictions must be made in the mother's diet. One study noted by Schmidtt seems to indicate that a formula prepared from soybean seemed to be more satisfactory for highly allergic babies than either cow's milk or breast milk.[9]

Economics

The economic advantages of breast-feeding have not been carefully documented. The increased food in the mother's diet required by breast-feeding may well negate the savings which might accrue from not having to buy milk for the infant. Other factors which need to be considered here, also, are the type of formula which would be substituted for breast milk, the form of the formula which is used (powdered formulas are much less expensive, for instance, than the same formula in liquid form), the source of the mother's food (home-grown vegetables are less expensive than highly prepared convenience foods, for instance), and the extent to which breast-feeding delays the introduction of solid foods to the infant.

Convenience

Breast-feeding is more convenient if one compares it with preparation of formula. The situation most often cited by proponents of breast-feeding is a middle-of-the-night feeding when the mother who is bottle-feeding her infant must take time to heat the bottle (and then cool it if it got too hot) while the nursing mother simply tucks the baby in bed with her and nurses as she calmly falls asleep again. The extremes in the situation are somewhat overdrawn. In the first place, most babies when they awaken must be changed before they can be fed. A bottle can be warmed if necessary while the baby is being changed. For mothers whose homes are essentially clean, many physicians are encouraging discontinuation of sterilization of bottles at a very early age. These mothers can use clean equipment and powdered formulas mixed with warm tap water to prepare individual bottles of formula as they are needed. If the dry powder is measured into a dry baby bottle when the mother goes to bed, final preparation of the formula requires only a few seconds.

Tucking the baby snugly in bed with the mother for its night feedings may sound simple, but here, too, there can be problems. There is the possibility (rare though it may be) of the baby's rolling out of bed or being rolled onto by the mother or father. Also, since many doctors advocate that no plastic pants be used in the first few months of the infant's life (because their use seems to contribute to the development of diaper rash), one has only to care for an infant for a short time to realize that a bed with a baby in it will soon be a very wet bed. It also seems possible that older infants might become accustomed to the cosiness of their parents' bed and prefer it to their own.

All this is not to say that breast-feeding is not more convenient than bottle-feeding. To a great extent, there is much less work involved and a quicker response to the needs of the infant. The issue is just not quite so simple as it is frequently presented.

Convenience must also be considered from other aspects. It is more convenient, at times, for someone other than the mother to feed the baby. This is true if older children in the family need her attention, and it is especially true when she is up for much of the night with the infant and unable to sleep during the day because of toddlers or preschoolers in the home who must be supervised. Most newborns do *not* awaken at neat 4-hour intervals and then quickly go back to sleep, especially when they are breast-fed.

Also, in spite of assurances that nursing a baby is a perfectly natural activity, many mothers and even more fathers are uneasy about an infant being nursed in a public place or even in the presence of friends. Many mothers find the necessity of providing a private place to nurse their infants a highly inconvenient aspect of breast-feeding.

Bacterial Contamination

Here the advocates of breast-feeding cannot be disputed. Except in the presence of a breast infection, breast milk does not become contaminated. (The nipple may become contaminated, but even this is unlikely.) Contamination of milk is one of the problems faced in bottle-feeding, especially when adequate sanitation and refrigeration are lacking.

Psychological Benefits

Schmidtt cites a number of studies which indicate that no specific psychological benefits from breast-feeding can be identified.[10] Closeness to mother is a needed quality in early infancy, but there is no evidence that such closeness cannot be obtained during bottle-feeding as well as breast-feeding. It is true that bottle-fed babies tend to be left to hold their own bottles as they get older, but there is no evidence that this in itself is psychologically damaging.

One aspect of psychological benefits not explored by Schmidtt is the mother's satisfaction in breast-feeding. Most mothers who breast-feed find it very satisfying, and it does tend to raise their self-esteem and enhance their self-concepts as mothers. It may in this way contribute significantly to the development of "motherliness."[11] Breast-feeding can also enhance and strengthen the bonds of attachment which are important in the early mother-child relationship, but there is no evidence that these bonds cannot be established when the infant is bottle-fed. On the other hand, not being able to breast-feed successfully or having to stop before she is psychologically ready to can be a devastating blow to a mother's self-esteem. One mother who was advised by her physician to cease breast-feeding put it this way, "I felt as though I had lost my baby."

One pitfall, psychologically, in breast-feeding is the tendency of the mother to become possessive in her relationship to the infant. The father may feel very left out of the relationship, and if his exclusion is complete enough, he may turn to the "absentee father" role and fail to establish a close relationship with the infant. One husband admitted to a nurse that he felt very jealous of his wife's ability to quiet their infant by nursing him when he was unable to do anything to help.

Ability to Succeed

It certainly would seem that modern women are no less able physically to nurse their infants than women of yesteryear. In practice, however, there may be a number of factors that interfere with successful breast-feeding. At the top of the list is the advice of well-meaning friends and even a few physicians that to breast-feed is too much trouble or that the mother does not have enough milk. The geographic separation of the nuclear family unit from supportive relatives may also be a factor. The new mother may not have enough household help to be able to rest sufficiently to produce enough milk, especially if there are older children in the family. The simple fact that breast-feeding is not the norm also mediates against its success, because mothers worry about their ability to succeed. Worry and tension definitely do affect the availability of milk for the infant. The inconvenience imposed by the predominant cultural attitudes (i.e., it is not nice to breast-feed in public) may also discourage the new mother in her early attempts. Even the mass media, with advertisements of clean, shiny floors and sparkling, white laundry may interfere with successful breast-feeding. New mothers are in subtle ways coerced into judging their worth according to such criteria and may in their zeal to be good mothers expend their energies on housekeeping tasks rather than resting and relaxing so that they can produce sufficient quantities of milk for their infants.

Token Breast-Feeding

Finally, in considering the issues presented by the breast-feeding–bottle-feeding question, some attention should be paid to an article by Niles Newton.[12] Dr. Newton describes unrestricted breast-feeding as that in which the infant receives only breast milk for food and is allowed unrestricted nursing priviledges for several months. Babies typically are fed as often as every 2 hours in the first few weeks of life; as late as the sixth to twelve month most are still receiving six feedings a day. There are no rules about when to feed the baby or how long to nurse at each feeding. Weaning occurs usually late in the second year, and even toddlers are allowed to nurse whenever they desire to do so.

In contrast, Dr. Newton describes breast-feeding as it is usually practiced in this country as "token breast feeding." There are many "rules and regulations" regarding how long the infant should nurse at a time and how long to wait between nursings. Solid foods are introduced early in the first year, and weaning to either the bottle or cup also occurs in the first year. Mothers who practice token breast-feeding also usually give bottles at least part of the time, concurrently.

Newton feels that mothers who practice token breast-feeding experience more difficulties with the actual feeding process itself than do those who feed without restriction. Their nipples, especially, are more prone to soreness and lesions when sucking is restricted. Engorgement is also likely to be a recurrent problem, or the supply of milk may not become established. If the baby does not seem to be satisfied by the breast or requires feeding as often as every 2 hours, the mother is usually advised by her physician to supplement the feedings with bottle-feedings, or she may do so because of her own need for sleep. Since formulas are usually sweeter than breast milk and because obtaining milk from the bottle is easier and requires less effort, the infant may soon show a preference for the bottle. The infant's rejection of the breast is very depressing to the mother and usually results in guilt feelings and lowering of her self-esteem.

According to Newton, infants also have a frustrating time when token breast-feeding is practiced. Use of two very different sucking techniques during feeding is required if the standard long rubber nipple is used. (Short ones that resemble the breast are also available.) Infants are also being offered very different tasting milk at different times. The timing rules often imposed (nurse for 10 minutes on each side and no more often than every 4 hours) may require the infant either to wait for feeding when he or she is hungry or to stop sucking before the need to suck has been satisfied. Breast engorgement is likely to occur with infrequent nursing. When engorgement occurs, the breast becomes hard and the nipple may be very difficult to grasp. If the mother has a strong let-down reflex at this time, the infant may be choked by the gush of milk that results.

Early weaning from the breast is one of the defining characteristics of token breast-feeding. Abrupt weaning at 3 months due to the mother's feeling tied down was noted in one study.[13] This is the age when object attachment to the breast is strong, and weaning at this time, especially abrupt weaning, may be very upsetting to the infant.

In all, it seems that token breast-feeding can be a very frustrating experience for both mother and child. Expectant mothers who are choosing their method of feeding need to know some of the pitfalls of token breast-feeding so that they can either avoid them by allowing unrestricted breast-feeding or at least approach them with some understanding.

BREAST-FEEDING

Physiology of Milk Production

The functional portion of the breast is composed of 15 to 25 lobes which are divided into lobules containing the milk-producing cells and collecting tubules called *lactiferous ducts.* Anteriorly, the lobes end with the nipple which contains the terminal orifices of these ducts. Under the areola of the nipple are enlargements of the ducts called *ampulae.* When the baby grasps the nipple correctly during nursing, his jaws squeeze the ampulae to eject milk into his mouth (see Figure 5-1). Posteriorly, the lactiferous ducts end in clusters of *acini* or *alveoli,* which contain milk-secreting cells. All the components of milk are secreted by these cells. As the milk is secreted, it is stored in the ducts and in the alveolar cells until the pressure of the milk present is sufficient to cause cessation of milk production.

The alveoli and the small ducts leading from them are surrounded by myoepithelial cells which contract when stimulated by oxytocin. When the baby nurses, nerve endings in the nipple are stimulated. The impulses travel to the hypothalamus, which in turn stimulates the anterior pituitary to secrete *prolactin,* a hormone that stimulates the production of milk in the alveoli. The posterior pituitary is also stimulated. It secretes *oxytocin,* which stimulates contraction of the myoepithelial cells surrounding the milk ducts.

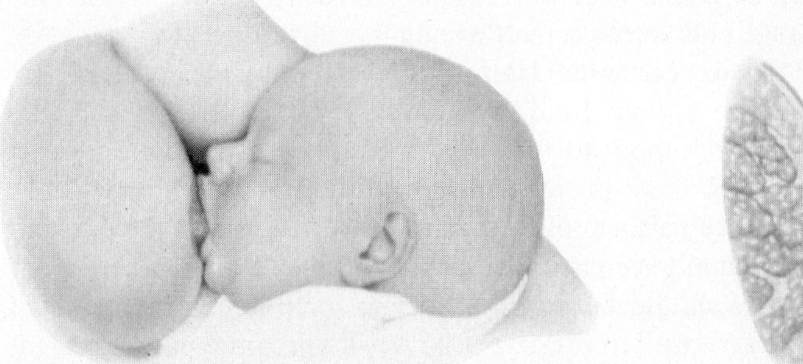

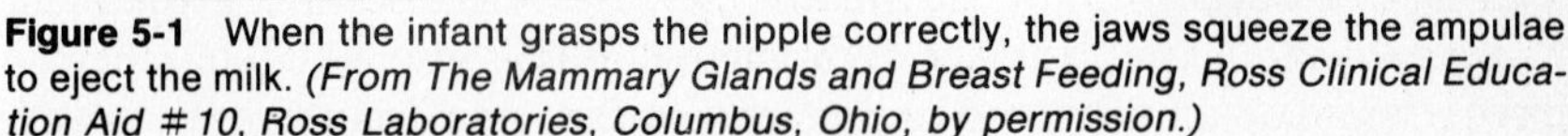

Figure 5-1 When the infant grasps the nipple correctly, the jaws squeeze the ampulae to eject the milk. *(From The Mammary Glands and Breast Feeding, Ross Clinical Education Aid # 10, Ross Laboratories, Columbus, Ohio, by permission.)*

The contraction of these cells moves the milk from the alveolar cells, through the ducts, to the ampulae, making it available to the infant. The movement of milk to the ampulae is called the *let-down reflex* or *milk-ejection reflex*. Until it functions, the milk present in the breast is not available to the baby. Emotional stress can interfere with its activation, as can physical tension and fatigue.

Emotional states also interfere with milk production and secretion by the cells of the alveoli. It is thought that an emotional upset stimulates the sympathetic nervous system, which decreases the blood flow through the mammary glands almost entirely.[14] Without blood supply, there can be no milk production.

Let-Down Reflex

The availability of the milk to the infant is dependent upon the let-down reflex, which develops in response to the crying of the infant. The mother experiences this reflex as a tingling sensation in the nipples and a "drawing" sensation in the breasts. She soon learns to recognize it. She may notice milk dripping from the nipple of the breast the infant is not nursing. If this occurs, putting pressure against that nipple with a clean cloth is usually sufficient to stop the flow. If she happens to be in a public place when she notices the tingling, she can unobtrusively cross her arms in front of her and stop the leaking. Most mothers find it necessary to wear pads inside their nursing bras in order to keep their clothing dry. Plastic-backed pads are available commercially, but a clean handkerchief is generally more satisfactory because it allows air to circulate to the nipple, and it is more absorbent than a commercial pad. Maceration of the tissues due to the lack of air circulation is more likely to occur when plastic-backed pads are used. The mother may need to check the wetness of the pad or cloth periodically, so that it does not become saturated and wet her clothing.

Engorgement

The most common physical discomfort experienced by nursing mothers is breast engorgement. This event occurs about the third day after delivery, when the milk begins to "come in." (Before then the baby is getting colostrum, a yellowish, high-protein fluid.) When the milk first comes in, the greatly increased blood supply to the breasts causes severe congestion. It can be very painful and needs prompt nursing attention. The mother needs to have either heat or ice packs applied to the breasts as soon as the swelling becomes apparent. Usually ice packs are used, and they do relieve much of the discomfort. There should be standing orders for this treatment for all nursing mothers in the hospital; if not, the nurse should anticipate the need, as a delay in applying the ice greatly increases the discomfort. Frequent nursing to empty the breasts of accumulated milk is also a help in relieving discomfort. The mother needs a nursing bra that supports the breasts well, and she may need to support the breasts with her hands, also, if she is up and about or as she turns in bed until the swelling subsides. The severe engorgement usually lasts only about 48 hours. It may be less severe and last a shorter period in mothers who have nursed children before. Mothers who are discharged after a short hospital stay should receive written instructions for the treatment of engorgement at home.

The mother may also notice some engorgement when there has been an unusually long period of time between feedings. This is a good indication that the milk supply is being produced in response to the baby's needs. At these times, as well as when the first engorgement occurs, it may be difficult for the baby to grasp the nipple. The mother may need to express a small amount of milk to soften the breast sufficiently for the baby to grasp the nipple and areolar area. When the breasts are engorged, the baby may also have difficulty breathing while nursing. The mother needs to hold the breast tissue away from the nursing infant's nose. It is also possible to shift the baby's position with the legs across the mother's abdomen so that the nose is not occluded by breast tissue. When engorgement is present, the mother may find that the milk gushes out of the breast too fast, causing the baby to choke. If this happens, manual expression of a little of the milk will also help.

Sore Nipples

If the mother's nipples become sore, they should be examined for cracks and fissures. Air drying the nipples after each feeding will help prevent and/or treat the problem. Plastic pads should be avoided. If the nipples are especially sore, the application of hot towels before nursing to stimulate the let-down reflex will help decrease trauma to the nipples as the baby nurses.

Sometimes an ointment is prescribed. It should be one that will not be harmful to the baby if a small amount is ingested during nursing. Usually, if it is rubbed thoroughly into the nipple after feeding, no cleansing of the nipple is needed before the next feeding. If the skin is broken, treatment with dry heat in the form of heat lamps should be instituted. The mother may sit about 18 inches from a gooseneck lamp with a 20-watt bulb in it for 5 to 10 minutes several times per day. She should be cautioned against using bulbs of higher wattage and to time the exposure carefully. Sometimes ultraviolet bulbs are recommended. If they are used, the exposure time is limited to 30 seconds the first day and should not extend beyond 2 minutes even after a tolerance is built up. This treatment should be done only once a day. The mother should be especially careful not to extend the exposure time inadvertently because sunburn is the inevitable result of prolonged exposure to ultraviolet rays. When an ultraviolet light is used, the mother should be seated no closer than 4 feet from it, and she should protect her eyes from the rays of the bulb.[15]

Fatigue

One of the least-discussed problems of the nursing mother is chronic fatigue. The baby will probably need to nurse about every 2 to 3 hours day and night. This pattern of feeding is not at all suited to the mother's pattern of sleeping. (For a lengthy discussion of fatigue and its effects, see Chapter 6, The First Weeks at Home, The Mother's Need for Sleep.) The overly tired mother may find that she is unable to relax and fall asleep easily when the baby does go to sleep. It would be helpful for nurses to teach the new mother relaxation techniques which will allow her to fall asleep quickly when the baby does. There are several relaxation exercises which might be used, but one which is easy to learn is for the mother to lie down on her back and relax her muscles systematically. If she has had preparation for childbirth, she may already be familiar with one or more systems for accomplishing this task. If not, have her imagine her feet in a tub of warm water. Have her think about the warmth of the water and how soft and comfortable it feels on her feet. When she indicates that she can feel the warmth of the "water" on her feet, ask her to allow the warmth to move upwards to include her ankles, then her calves, and so forth, until her body is warm and relaxed all over. Usually, she will fall asleep during the exercise. To end the period of relaxation, if she does not fall asleep, the mother may simply count slowly from 10 to 1 while thinking about "getting up." She should feel very refreshed and have a sense of renewed vigor after a period of deep relaxation. The nurse should help the mother practice the exercise several times during her postpartum stay in the hospital. It is important to note that when the mother is deeply relaxed she may be more than unusually susceptible to accepting uncritically comments heard in her environment. The nurse should avoid making any extraneous comments, especially those which might be misconstrued as critical or otherwise be damaging to the mother's self-esteem. The mother should know that she will be able to respond to any of her baby's needs while practicing this exercise just as she would if she were falling asleep "naturally." Practicing this exercise for 10 to 15 minutes when she does not have time to take a nap will improve her stamina and help her fight the chronic fatigue which accompanies the care of a newborn.

Hospital Routine With regard to the problem of fatigue, mothers should never be awakened at night in the hospital for extraneous procedures such as "routine" temperature taking. If temperatures need to be taken, they should be taken when the mother is awakened for the baby's feedings. Similarly, daytime visitors should be greatly restricted so that the mother may rest and nap as much as possible during the day. It will be several months before she will again enjoy an uninterrupted night's sleep, and she needs as much rest as she can possibly have. Similarly, I feel, and it is a personal opinion formed as a result of having nursed two children, that the nursing mother should have uninterrupted sleep the last night in the hospital before being discharged, leaving the baby in the nursery for at least the 2 A.M. feeding. Otherwise her fatigue, especially if she has other children at home, quickly becomes unbearable.

Combating Fatigue at Home If it is at all possible to have help at home, the nursing mother should take advantage of every opportunity to rest. She would profit from sleeping at least 6 hours without interruption for at least one night per week. This will probably require some one, the baby's father for instance, to feed the infant during the mother's sleeping time. An occasional bottle of milk will not interrupt the milk supply once it is established. If a bottle is used, it is best to use the type with short nipples so that the baby will not be confused by the change. The mother may even want to express breast milk ahead of time and refrigerate it or freeze it for later use. The nursing mother should plan to lie down and rest for at least an hour during the day, even if she is not able to sleep because of having to supervise toddlers. (For some reason, toddlers and newborns almost never take naps at the same time!) She should simplify her housekeeping routines so that she conserves as much of her energy as possible. If household help is available and within her means, it can be very valuable. Besides getting the work done, it also frees the mother for giving the all-important attention to older brothers or sisters of the infant. Visitors in the home should be greatly restricted in the first few weeks after the baby comes home both to protect the infant from exposure to infection and to conserve the mother's strength. The mother may need to see special friends, however, so that she does not feel isolated. The most helpful visitors are those who can socialize with the mother and also help with some of the household chores.

Techniques of Breast-Feeding

Most babies when presented with the breast grasp the nipple and begin nursing correctly without assistance, but because breast-feeding is not the "norm" and because most women have not observed other women nursing their babies, it has become a technique that must be learned. The nurse in the hospital plays a very important role in assisting the new mother to become comfortable nursing her baby. The nurse should be knowledgeable about breast-feeding and should work to establish a warm, supportive relationship with the mother.

Preparation for Nursing The mother should wash her hands before taking the baby from the nurse. In many hospitals, mothers are notified a few minutes before the babies are brought to them so that they can be ready. Hospital policy differs as to the necessity of washing the nipples before nursing the infant. The AAP recommends only that the mother take a daily shower and wash her hands prior to feeding.[16] No drying solutions should be used on the nipples at any time, as such solutions tend to make the nipples more susceptible to cracking and fissuring.

The mother should be assisted to a position which will allow her to nurse the infant without any muscle strain. It may be more comfortable at first to nurse the infant lying down (see Figure 5-2). Some mothers find a sitting position more comfortable, and it is much easier in this position to move the baby from one breast to the other. If the mother chooses to nurse in the sitting position, her back and arms should be well supported with pillows to prevent fatigue (see Figure 5-3).

Helping the Infant to Nurse The sucking behavior of newborns has been described and classified by Dr. Anton Lethin as follows:[17]

1 "Baracudas"—infants who nurse very vigorously immediately when put to breast. They do not usually need any assistance, but they may on occasion hurt the nipple.

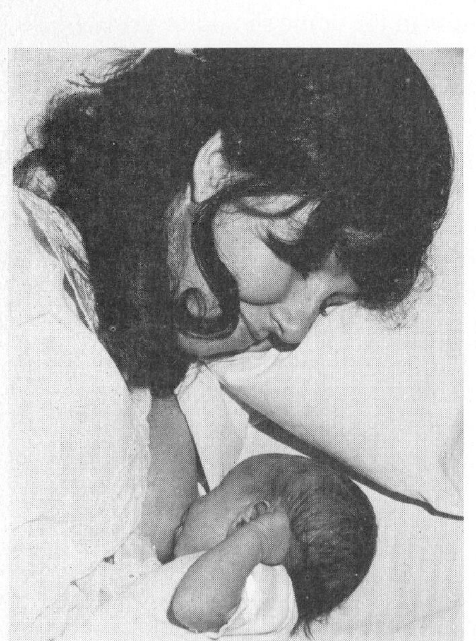

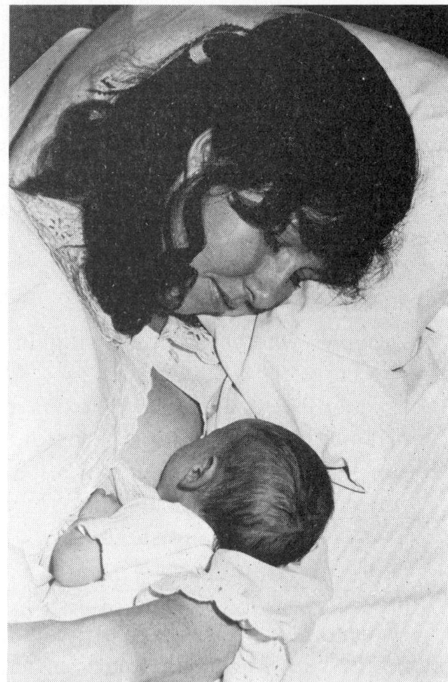

Figure 5-2 Some mothers find it more comfortable at first to nurse their babies lying down. *(From J. Clausen et al., Maternity Nursing Today, McGraw-Hill, 1973, p. 583, by permission.)*

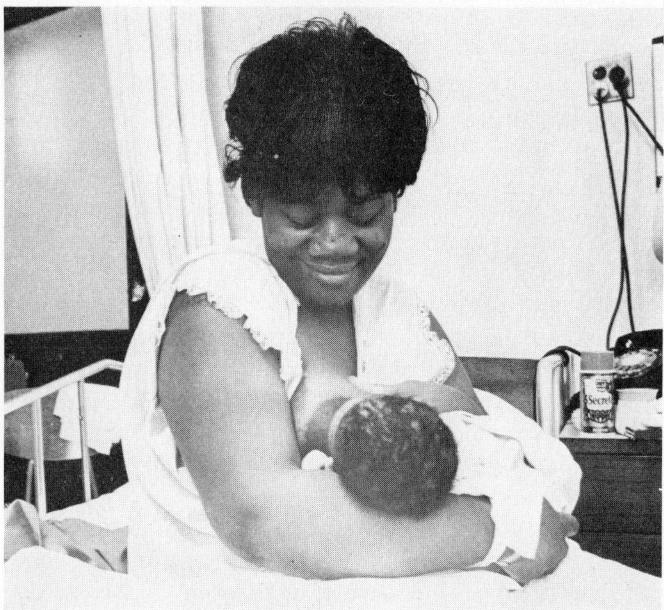

Figure 5-3 Some mothers prefer to sit up to nurse their infants. (Although this mother seems very comfortable with her baby, she would probably be more comfortable with a little more back support.) *(Photo: Penelope Ann Peirce.)*

2 "Excited Ineffectives"—babies who grasp and lose the nipple repeatedly in their excitement to nurse. They usually become very agitated and cry and need to be quieted before proceeding.

3 "Procrastinators"—infants who do not show any interest in nursing until the milk comes in. They should not be rushed, as they usually do well once they get started.

4 "Gourmets" or "Mouthers"—babies who taste a little milk and smack their lips a few times before settling down to steady nursing. They become quite upset if rushed, but do well when left alone.

5 "Resters"—infants who nurse awhile and then rest awhile. There is no hurrying them, but they nurse well if given plenty of time.

In assisting mothers and babies in early breast-feeding experiences, these differences should be kept in mind and perhaps explained to the mother.

In helping the infant to grasp the breast, initially, it may be necessary first for the mother to quiet the infant by holding him close in her arms. If the infant is hungry, stroking the corner of the mouth closest to the breast will cause him to turn his head toward the breast. Mothers commonly try to turn a baby's head toward the breast by pushing it from the side farthest away from the breast. This causes the infant to turn his face away from the breast rather than toward it, as he roots in an attempt to find the nipple. If the infant is having difficulty finding the nipple, the mother may grasp the breast and make the nipple more prominent. When the infant grasps the nipple, it is important to grasp as much of the areola as possible. If the infant is held close to the breast, this will be more likely. The correct placement of the nipple and areola in the infant's mouth can be checked by listening for a soft clicking sound during swallowing and by checking to be sure that the areola is drawn into the baby's mouth as sucking proceeds. Loud sucking noises indicate most often that the nipple is grasped improperly. Grasping only the nipple causes pain and may lead to cracking and fissuring which may necessitate temporary discontinuation of nursing. The appearance of small blisters, often filled with blood, on the nipples usually indicates that the baby is not grasping enough of the areola. The presence of the blisters is not a contraindication for nursing, however. Even if they burst during the nursing, no harm is done unless they subsequently become infected.

When the mother wants to take the baby off the breast, she should first insert her finger into the corner of the baby's mouth to release the suction.

As the baby begins vigorous sucking, the mother may feel some discomfort in her nipples and breasts. In addition, the sucking stimulates uterine contractions which may be quite painful, especially in multiparas. (Uterine contractions are caused by the oxytocin released from the pituitary.) The mother needs to know that both these kinds of pain will disappear in a few days. For severe discomfort, pain medication may be administered a few minutes prior to nursing. Some of the initial nipple pain ceases when the infant begins sucking in long rhythmic strokes because the milk begins flowing and the baby swallows, breaking the negative pressure. This kind of sucking indicates an ample flow of milk.

Alternate Massage The mother can help in establishment of the let-down reflex by performing alternate breast massage during the feedings during the first few days after birth.[17] To do this, the mother observes the infant's suck pattern. When short, choppy strokes are observed, the mother should massage an area of the breast with her fingers until the tissues become soft. For convenience, the breast may be divided into three or four sections, each section extending from the areola to the outer margins of breast tissue. The mother massages one section at a time. When the infant's suck changes back to the long strokes, massage is stopped so that the milk does not flow too fast. An attempt is made to massage all sections of the breast during the establishment of breast-feeding. After the let-down reflex becomes well established, the massage is stopped.

Time for Nursing There is some difference of opinion as to the length of time the baby should be nursed. Newton seems to indicate that the nursing period should be unrestricted.[18] The La Leche League recommends nursing on one side for 10 minutes and then switching sides and allowing the infant to nurse until satisfied on the other side.[19] Another recommendation is to allow the baby to nurse 3 to 5 minutes on each side the first day and then to increase the time gradually until the nipples can tolerate the baby's nursing 10 minutes on the first side and 20 minutes on the second.[20]

It is generally recommended that the baby nurse both breasts at each feeding, especially while the milk supply is being established. According to Joseph and Peck, the baby gets about 90 percent of the milk present in the first breast in the first 5 to 10 minutes of vigorous nursing.[21] Because the infant nurses less vigorously on the second side, it may not empty so completely; therefore, the mother needs to alternate the side that is nursed first. One way for the mother to remember is to pin a safety pin to her bra on the side nursed last so that she will know to put the baby to that breast first the next time. The pin of course would be moved after each feeding.

Supplemental Feedings The use of supplemental feedings is generally to be discouraged during the 3 to 4 weeks the milk supply is being established because they interfere with stimulation of milk production and because their frequent use may result in the token breast-feeding discussed earlier in this chapter. If supplemental formula is given during this time, it might be given with a dropper so that the infant does not learn to prefer the rubber nipple to the breast. When this preference is established, it is very difficult to maintain the breast milk supply long enough to reaccustom the infant to the breast. If a dropper is used, a plastic one, as is available in drugstores, should be used rather than a glass one with a rubber tip attached to it. The rubber tip may rather easily be sucked off the dropper and could cause an intestinal obstruction.

It is usually desirable for the infant to receive an occasional bottle-feeding once the breast milk supply is well established, so that the mother can be away from the infant if she desires to be or in case of an emergency.

Manual Expression of Milk Manual expression of milk can be accomplished by supporting the breast with one hand and grasping the areola with the thumb and fingers of the other hand. Squeezing the thumb and fingers together should result in expression of milk. The mother should rotate the thumb and fingers so that all ampulae under the areola are compressed. When the milk ceases to flow readily, it may help to massage the breast, beginning near the axilla and working across the breast and progressively closer to the nipple. This helps move milk which is high in the breast, especially when engorgement is present. Manual expression may be used to be sure that the breast is completely emptied after each nursing period, and it can be used to express milk when nursing must be interrupted for any reason.

Nursery Care of the Breast-Fed Baby

Care of the breast-fed babies in the nursery should be essentially the same as for other babies except the infants should not be given formula in the nursery if they can be taken to their mothers frequently for feeding. Obviously, if policy prohibits taking the baby to the mother on demand, it may be necessary to offer some formula at times. An attempt should be made first, however, to satisfy the infant with sterile water, which is less likely than formula to interfere with hunger at feeding times.

Countryman recommends that the newborn be allowed to nurse the breast within an hour after delivery.[22] This, she states, helps in early establishment of milk production. There is evidence, also, that the colostrum functions as a laxative, speeding the elimination of meconium from the intestinal tract, a phenomenon which seems to decrease jaundice in the newborn (see Chapter 9, Moderate Hyperbilrubinemia, Resorption from the Gastrointestinal Tract).

BOTTLE-FEEDING

Bottle-feeding a baby has a few problems different from those of breast-feeding. The preparation of formula takes time for the new mother to do, and she may worry about having enough prepared when the baby needs it, especially since new mothers usually have difficulty organizing themselves at first. There are many prepared formulas on the market, but generally they are relatively expensive. Care must be used by the nurse to be sure that mothers who intend to bottle-feed have adequate instruction about sterilizing bottles and preparing a formula that they are likely to be able to afford. Referrals to community health nurses for continued help in the home should be made as needed. Bottle-feeding equipment need not be exorbitantly expensive. Glass bottles and nipples are available for a nominal cost. Simple sterilizers which are heated on the cooking stove are also inexpensive, or they can be improvised satisfactorily. A container taller than the bottles and a lid to cover it are the essential materials for improvising a sterilizer.

Terminal Sterilization

The easiest method of sterilization is terminal sterilization. The bottles and nipples are washed in clean water (it is best to wash them separately from the family dishes so that they do not get a film of grease on them). The formula is prepared according to directions. The bottles are filled with the formula in quantities which the mother thinks the baby will drink at one feeding. Then the nipples are attached with their covers and the bottles are placed in the sterilizer with about 3 inches of water in the pan. The bottle caps should be put on loosely. The cover to the sterilizer is added, and the bottles are boiled for 25 minutes. The time should be counted from the time the water actually starts boiling. After the boiling time is finished, the bottles are allowed to cool just until they can be handled easily, the caps are tightened, and then they are refrigerated. (Bottles should not be allowed to stay at room temperature for long periods of time.) If the mother does not have refrigeration available, or if she cannot manage the sterilization consistently, then it might be better for her to use one of the prepared formulas in powdered form. Powdered formulas are less expensive than the liquid prepared formulas, and the unused portion will not spoil before it is mixed with water. Some of the mothers could use clean rather than sterile technique, if they would be sure to wash everything well before preparing the formula and if they have an approved water supply. Well water should not be used without sterilization, however. All mothers need to be taught the reasons behind procedures, not simply the procedures.

Aseptic Method of Sterilization

The aseptic method of sterilization may be used. In this method the bottles and nipples are washed and then sterilized by boiling for 5 minutes. They are left in the boiled water while the formula is being prepared. A pan of water to be used in mixing the formula is also boiled for 5 minutes, and then this water is mixed with the concentrated milk or formula as prescribed by the doctor. If canned milk or canned formulas are used, the opened can must be stored in the refrigerator and the unused portion discarded or used in general family cooking after 24 hours. Being careful not to contaminate the bottle or the formula, the formula is added to the bottles and then refrigerated.

Problems in Bottle-Feeding

One thing that is difficult for all mothers to do is to discard the formula left in the baby's bottle after a feeding. This formula need not be thrown away. It can be used in cooking for the family, but it should not be given to the baby at a later time because of the possibility of organisms growing in it.

Another problem in bottle-feeding is the mother's tendency to be overly concerned about the volume of formula taken at any one feeding. The mother should know that the baby's hunger will vary from one time to the next and that the infant will take different amounts of formula at different times.

A problem faced by all mothers but perhaps more often worrisome to mothers who bottle-feed is the matter of schedules. There is still enough literature available to convince many mothers that babies are supposed to be fed every 4 hours. This myth is promulgated through hospital practice which brought infants to the mother on 4-hour intervals and kept them separated in the interim. She may not have any idea how much the baby is awake or crying between feedings in the hospital. Mothers need some instruction in the reasons babies cry and how to tell if they are hungry. Babies do cry because they are uncomfortable, lonely, or tense, and because they are hungry. If they root or chew on a fist, they are probably hungry and need to be fed, regardless of how long it has been since the last feeding. However, the mothers need to know, also, that there is a tendency to overfeed babies and that babies are not able to distinguish between hunger and intestinal discomfort as a result of overfeeding. When they need to burp, they may behave as though they were hungry. If only an hour or two has elapsed since the last bottle, the mother should try burping the baby and testing to see whether there might be reasons other than hunger for the crying.

Techniques of Bottle-Feeding

The techniques of bottle-feeding require a few instructions to a first-time mother. The mother needs to know that the baby should be held for feedings. A baby who is unable to hold his or her own bottle should never be left with a propped bottle, both because of the danger of aspiration and because of the need for the warmth of human contact to begin to build relationships. The bottle should be held in such a way that there is always milk and no air in the nipple (see Figure 5-4). In addition, the baby needs to be burped frequently during the feeding. Initially, the baby should be burped at least after every ounce of formula. As the baby gets older, burping will be necessary less often. If bottles with disposable liners are used, less air is swallowed and less frequent burping is required. The baby may be placed on the mother's shoulder for burping. If the nurse burps a baby, it is better for her to hold him upright in her lap rather than putting the baby on her shoulder (see Figure 5-5). In this position, the nurse can observe spitting up and avoid a wet back. The baby is less exposed to the nurse's nasal organisms, also. A mother may prefer the sitting position, too. As with breast feeding, the mother should adopt a relaxed, unhurried manner and take time to enjoy her baby.

TEACHING THE NEW PARENTS

The teaching needs of new parents are extensive. The specific information needed, the manner of its presentation, and the effects of such teaching, however, vary with the individual and from one social group to another. While the traditional approach to postpartum teaching is a more or less formalized one, indications are that such is not the most effective for several groups.[23,24,25] Groups that do not seem to profit from traditional methods include adolescent, low-income, and black mothers. (Studies as to the effectiveness of the traditional approach for middle-income mothers are not

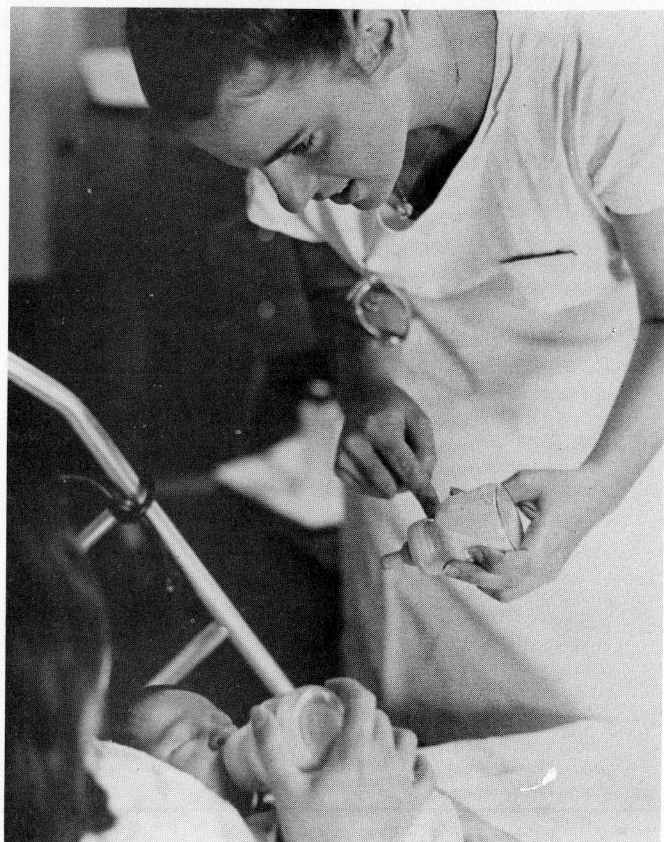

Figure 5-4 Always hold a baby bottle so that milk fills the nipple. *(Photo: Penelope Ann Peirce.)*

available to this author at this time; thus, no conclusions on that regard can be drawn.)

The Process of Teaching

Before examining specific content which should be included in teaching, it is important to consider the teaching-learning process. Basically, this process includes (1) the identification of a teaching need, (2) motivation of the learner, (3) the preparation of objectives, (4) the adoption of a teaching method, (5) the teaching-learning sequence, and (6) evaluation of the learning.

Identification of a Teaching Need The learner, the teacher, or a third party may identify a teaching need. When the learner identifies the need, he

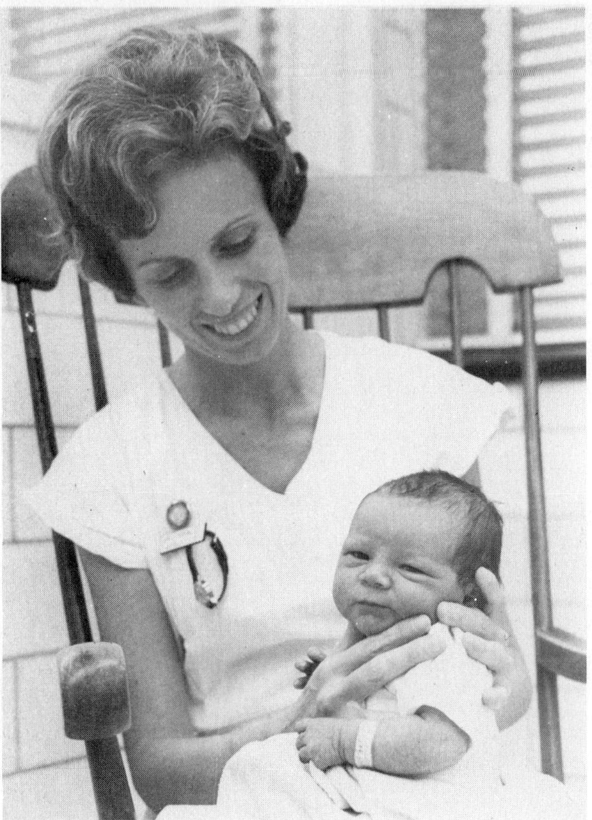

Figure 5-5 It is better for nurses to burp babies in a sitting position on their laps. Notice how the baby's head is supported. *(Photo: Penelope Ann Peirce.)*

or she may bring this need to the attention of a potential teacher or may seek the information through independent efforts. Such behaviors as asking questions, voicing doubts, or expressing fears and anxieties may indicate the individual's desire for information. When the teacher identifies a teaching need, he or she must bring this need to the attention of the learner. (Nurses may identify teaching needs by observing the physical condition of their patients and by observing patient behavior.) This may be done with a well-timed question, by diplomatically pointing out an error the learner is making, or by stating the need as the teacher sees it. It should be emphasized, however, that the teacher should take care not to make students defensive, nor undermine their self-confidence, nor raise their anxiety in indicating to them their teaching needs, as doing so interferes with subsequent learning. When a third party identifies a teaching need, he or she usually either calls the need to the attention of the learner or requests the teacher to intervene. Again, tact and diplomacy are of utmost importance.

Motivation of the Learner One of the most important jobs of the teacher is to assess and enhance the motivation of the learner. Indeed, if the learner is not motivated to learn, the best teaching in the world goes for naught. Self-motivation is by far the most effective. People can learn almost anything if they want to, but they may be led through class after class without learning if they do not wish to. Learners who identify their own need for learning are the most likely to learn; thus, it is best if at all possible to give students an opportunity to participate in determining content areas to be learned. The teacher will frequently suggest content that is needed, but perhaps students can help in setting priorities. Students can be motivated to learn because of their respect for the authority who says they need to learn a certain subject, because they want to please the teacher, or because the material to be learned is required for accomplishing a future goal. While fear and anxiety may at times motivate learning, they are never conducive to a positive student-teacher relationship and have little justifiable place in the teaching of patients. Generally, learning is most effective and most long-lasting if it is accomplished in a comfortable relationship with a warm, supportive teacher who is sensitive to the needs and interests of the student.

The Preparation of Objectives One of the most often omitted steps in the teaching-learning process is the preparation of specific objectives. Teachers tend to begin giving information without any real planning, especially in clinical teaching. (This is not to say that the spontaneous answering of questions is not appropriate.) The result is that some material which the student may need is omitted, and the teacher comes away from the experience not really knowing whether the student has learned or not. Common errors which occur as a result of this practice are the presentation of too much material at one time and the presentation of material in a disordered fashion. While it is not necessary to write down objectives for every teaching experience, it is advisable to do so for every organized class, whether the class is designed for a group or an individual.

It might be a good idea to have general teaching objectives in mind for all postpartum patients and to have these available on a card file or chart so that as spontaneous teaching occurs, the objectives which have been accomplished may be noted. Such an organized approach to patient teaching would be helpful for improving discharge planning and referrals to community-based nurses. (It is important in making notations of learning to be sure that learning has actually occurred and not merely that a teaching effort was made. It is the learning, not the teaching that is important!)

The preparation of objectives is time-consuming but not difficult. The objectives should be written as student objectives, that is, in terms of what the *student* is to do. This is different from the teacher objective, which is written in terms of what the teacher is to do. Secondly, the objective should be written in behavioral terms. The behaviors should be concrete, specific, and easily measured or observed. For instance, "To prepare formula correctly according to the standardized terminal sterilization procedure" is a behavioral student objective. In this instance it would be necessary to indicate what standardized procedure is to be used, but most often a description of one is given to the mother during her hospital stay. In most instances, it would also be necessary to clarify what is meant by "correctly," especially if there are critical points which must be adhered to, such as boiling the bottles for 25 minutes. A more detailed objective for a formula preparation might be as follows. The student should state the steps for terminal sterilization of formula in a logical order including the following critical points:

1 Wash hands before starting.
2 Wash all articles to be used in hot, soapy water.
3 Rinse all articles in clear water.
4 Mix formula correctly (give specifics according to formula being used).
5 Fill bottles to appropriate levels (determined by intake of infant).
6 Screw on bottle caps loosely.
7 Cover the sterilizer.
8 Boil for 25 minutes.
9 Refrigerate formula as soon as bottles can be handled comfortably.

It is frequently desirable to state the conditions under which the student will perform the behaviors listed in the objective and to what extent errors are allowed for successful completion of the objective. For instance, in the above objective, there is quite a bit difference in the learning required if the mother is to list the steps of formula preparation from memory or if she is allowed to refer to written material as she explains the process. (For most patient teaching, allowing patients to refer to written material which they will be taking home is desirable.) There should be some indications also of variations which would be allowed in the procedure. For instance, should the formula be mixed up before or after the bottles are washed, or is either permissible? Would the same flexibility be allowed for the time for boiling the formula? Such decisions made before the teaching begins will help clarify the critical points and ensure that patients learn those things which they really need to know. The nurse should be careful not to insist dogmatically on any particular points for which there is no real reason. A knowledge of personal biases is essential here.

It should become obvious that adequate preparation of objectives requires a thorough knowledge of the subject; however, once they are written, good objectives simplify the remainder of the teaching-learning process.

For the novice teacher, perhaps it is easiest to establish one or two very general objectives and then to study the subject before attempting to write detailed ones. In the above instance, the preliminary objective might have been "To learn formula preparation."

Adoption of a Learning Method In deciding on a teaching method, it is important to determine what kind of learning is required. Learning has been divided into three categories or domains[26]: cognitive—the acquisition of intellectual information and conceptual skills; affective—the adoption of certain attitudes and feelings; and psychomotor—the learning of motor skills. Nursing instruction may include all three. Generally, intellectual learning is done by the methods the student is familiar with—lecture, reading, group or individual discussion, films, audiovisual aids, programmed instruction, and the like. For patient teaching, lecture is probably the least desirable and should be used infrequently.

The affective domain is a very important one for nurses to recognize. Much of health care is greatly influenced by the patient's attitudes and feelings. A mother may be able to repeat the reasons for having her infant immunized, but if she is basically afraid of "shots," she may never get around to doing it. Changes in attitude and feeling are rather difficult to accomplish. The best approach seems to be one of perceptive listening and supportive counseling until the patient is able to work through the attitude or feeling which is interfering with appropriate behaviors. Arguing or pressuring are rarely effective.

Finally, the learning of motor skills is best accomplished by demonstration, practice, and return demonstration. A mother needs to show that she has learned the skill, not merely be able to talk about it.

The Teaching-Learning Sequence When the teacher has completed the above steps, it is time to engage the learner in the teaching-learning sequence. This is best done when both are well rested and free of the need to be doing something else. (Do not begin teaching 10 minutes before shift change unless you are able and willing to miss "report" and stay late to finish the job.) A quiet area, away from distractions, is most satisfactory, though an effective environment can be made simply by pulling a curtain around the mother's bed. Be sure all materials are on hand before beginning, and then proceed with the plan, but do not become so involved with the imparting of information that you become unaware of a change in the learner's need for teaching. It may be more appropriate to discard a plan and deal with feelings that have surfaced than to continue with content, no matter how well organized. Keep the teaching session short. Stop when the mother seems tired even if the whole lesson has not been covered. Encourage questions throughout the lesson, and do not be afraid to digress when a need for a digression is indicated. Clinical teaching is at best very free and flexible.

Evaluation The final step in any teaching program is to evaluate the learning that has taken place. If the original objectives are well written, evaluation is merely a matter of comparing the end behaviors with the original objectives. If objectives are not well stated, then it is a mattter of judging the student's progress against a vague idea in the instructor's mind. Such judgments may be very astute, or they may be mostly a matter of guesswork.

Content to be Taught

Traditionally, classes for new parents have covered the baby bath, feeding, layette, family planning, and home care of the mother. While these are the general topics of information mothers need to know, it has been shown that there is a wide variation from one subculture to another and from one individual to another as to what the *mother* has felt she needs to know.[27] It has been further shown that mothers tend to remember and use only that information which they feel is important.[28] For instance, among some groups it is customary to bathe the infant with oil rather than water. Mothers in this group who received the traditional instruction on baby baths still bathed their infants in oil. They felt that the rashes that frequently developed as a sequel to this practice were "normal" since all babies in their acquaintance developed the same kind of rash. Hence, it can be seen that these mothers did not change their behaviors on the basis of teaching. Listening to the mother's plans for bathing her baby and helping her recognize the consequences of her method (the rash) are far more likely to make a change in the behavior than the traditional bath demonstration. Mothers who have grown up with younger siblings and nieces and nephews in the home do not generally feel the need for instruction on the techniques of baby baths. On the other hand, mothers who have had little contact with infants do want to learn techniques. The point here is simply that one cannot presuppose what the mother needs to know.

The nurse should make an assessment of the mother's knowledge and identify areas where more information is needed. Such need areas might be identified from misinformation which the mother has or from a lack of knowledge in a particular area, or the nurse may provide *anticipatory guidance;* that is, the nurse may anticipate a problem which commonly occurs and provide the mother with some information on handling it before the problem is apparent to the mother. Anticipatory guidance is most effective with middle-income mothers who are accustomed to thinking in terms of future events. Mothers from poverty situations are more "now" oriented and tend to let tomorrow take care of itself. Even for middle-income mothers it is important, however, to elicit their interest before giving them a lot of information in anticipating problems. They will profit little from the instruction if they are merely being polite in listening. The nurse should also be aware of the possibility of creating a problem where one does not exist. If the mother is by culture and expectations accustomed to paternal nonparticipation in child care, the nurse should not create a problem by insisting that all fathers must participate in the care of their children. It is also important for nurses to give information that is not in conflict with instructions the mother will be receiving from her doctor. Perhaps a notebook containing specific instructions of the doctors using a particular hospital service could be kept. Topics which should be considered in assessing teaching needs are listed in Table 5-1.

Timing and Pacing

It is equally important to be aware of the proper time to do patient teaching. A mother who is feeling badly or who is in the taking-in phase in assuming her maternal role (see Chapter 6, Assumption of the Maternal Role) is not ready to learn to care for her infant. The mother must first recover from the labor and delivery (this includes talking about her memories of the experience repeatedly) and identify her infant as an individual

Table 5-1 Content Suggested for Assessing Teaching Needs of New Parents

Physical and Emotional Needs of the Mother
- Fatigue levels and how to combat them
- Care of the episiotomy
- Bowel hygiene
- Exercises
- Breast care
- Personal hygiene (when to take tub bath, wash hair, care of vaginal discharge, etc.)
- Organization of household tasks to save time and energy
- Setting priorities at home
- Understanding the "blues"
- Family planning
- 6-week postpartum check up

Physical Characteristics of the Newborn
- Behavior (especially reflexes, hiccuping, crying, etc.)
- Physical appearance (especially crossed eyes, cord, shape of head)
- Sleeping and eating patterns

Emotional Needs of the Newborn
- Need for holding and cuddling
- Dangers of bottle propping
- What is a "spoiled" baby?

Skills of Mothering
- Holding, dressing and undressing, bathing
- Formula preparation and feeding techniques (including breast-feeding, if appropriate)
- Cord care
- Selection and care of baby clothes

Needs of Other Family Members
- Need of the father for attention
- Participation in child care by the father
- Dealing with siblings (see Chapter 6, Needs of Siblings)

(by inspecting, fingering, and comparing the infant to members of the family), before she is ready to learn to care for her baby.

Special Target Groups

In many families, it is not the mother who provides most of the care of the infant. Many times it is the grandmother or an aunt or perhaps a housekeeper who will be primarily responsible for the care of the infant. In these instances, especially when the grandmother is the primary caretaker, it does little good to teach only the mother. This is particularly true when the mother is very young. For the most part, what the grandmother says is law, regardless of the mother's views, and the views of a stranger (the nurse) may be totally ignored. If the nurse can make arrangements to speak with the grandmother, it might be possible to effect change, though often these women have reared several children and are not so open to suggestion as the young mothers. The nurse might be best advised, if the grandmother resists suggestions, to try to establish a positive relationship with the grandmother in the hope that she can begin to see health professionals as helpers rather than critics. Then, a community-based nurse may be able to do effective teaching.

The father should be encouraged to participate in the teaching-learning with his wife if he desires. This will recognize his role in the family and facilitate his acceptance of the father role.

Postpartum teaching has in many instances become an automatic response with little regard to the individual needs of the learners. When done this way, it may be viewed as a rather mundane chore. This is unfortunate, because it can be one of the most challenging and satisfying responsibilities of the nurse.

REFERENCES

1 Madeline H. Schmitt, "Superiority of Breast-Feeding—Fact or Fancy," in Mary H. Browning and Edith P. Lewis (comps.), *Maternal and Newborn Care: Nursing Interventions,* American Journal of Nursing, New York, 1973, pp. 186–196.

2 Niles Newton, "Psychologic Differences between Breast and Bottle Feeding," *The American Journal of Clinical Nutrition,* August 1971, pp. 993–1004.

3 Schmitt, op. cit., p. 193.

4 Sharon Serena Joseph and Rana Limbo Peck, "Postpartum Needs of the Family," in Joy Princeton Clausen, Margaret Hemp Flock, Bonnie Ford, Marilyn A. Green, and Elsa S. Popiel (eds.), *Maternity Nursing Today,* McGraw-Hill, New York, 1973, p. 570.

5 Mary Lou Moore, *The Newborn and the Nurse,* Saunders, Philadelphia, 1972, p. 195.

6 Janet Hardy, "Medical Care of the Newborn," in Robert E. Cooke (ed.), *The Biologic Basis of Pediatric Practice,* McGraw-Hill, New York, 1968, p. 1486.

7 Barbara Barlow, Thomas V. Santulli, William C. Heird, Jane Pitt, William A. Blanc, and John N. Schullinger, "An Experimental Study of Acute Neonatal Entercolitis—The Importance of Breast Milk," *Journal of Pediatric Surgery,* October 1974, pp. 587–595.

8 Hardy, op. cit., pp. 1486–1487.

9 Schmitt, op. cit., p. 188.

10 Ibid.

11 Ashley Montagu, *Touching: The Human Significance of the Skin,* Harper & Row, New York, 1971.

12 Newton, op. cit.

13 Ibid., p. 1001.

14 L. L. Langley, Ira R. Telford, and John B. Christensen, *Dynamic Anatomy and Physiology,* McGraw-Hill, New York, 1969, p. 788.

15 Joseph and Peck, op. cit., p. 590.

16 American Academy of Pediatrics, Committee on the Fetus and the Newborn, *Standards and Recommendations for Hospital Care of Newborn Infants,* American Academy of Pediatrics, Evanston, Ill., 1971, p. 31.

17 George R. Barnes, Anton N. Lethin, Jr., Edith B. Jackson, and Nilda Shea, "Management of Breast Feeding," *Journal of the American Medical Association,* Jan. 17, 1953, p. 194.

18 Newton, op. cit., p. 995.

19 La Leche League, *The Womanly Art of Breast Feeding,* La Leche League International, Franklin Park, Ill., 1963, p. 63.

20 Joseph and Peck, op. cit., p. 584.

21 Ibid.

22 Betty A. Countryman, "Hospital Care of the Breast-fed Newborn," *American Journal of Nursing,* December 1971, pp. 2365–2371.

23 Margaret Spaulding, "Adapting Postpartum Teaching to Mothers' Low-Income Life-Styles," *Current Concepts in Clinical Nursing,* vol. 2, Mosby, St. Louis, 1969, pp. 280–291.

24 Janice E. Banard, "Peer Group Instruction for Primigravid Adolescents," *Nursing Outlook,* August 1970, pp. 42–43.

25 Helen Dixie Koldjeski, "Concerns of Antepartal Mothers Expressed in Group Teaching Experiences and Implications for Nursing Practice," *ANA Clinical Sessions,* 1966, Appleton-Century-Crofts, New York, 1967, pp. 117–124.

26 Benjamin S. Bloom (ed.), *Taxonomy of Educational Objectives: The Classification of Educational Goals. Handbook I: Cognitive Domain,* McKay, New York, 1956.

27 Spaulding, op. cit.

28 Ibid.

BIBLIOGRAPHY

Adams, Martha: "Early Concerns of Primigravida Mothers Regarding Infant Care Activities," *Nursing Research,* Spring 1963, pp. 72–77.

American Academy of Pediatrics, Committee on the Fetus and the Newborn, *Standards and Recommendations for Hospital Care of the Newborn Infant,* American Academy of Pediatrics, Evanston, Ill., 1971.

Banard, Janice E.: "Peer Group Instruction for Primigravid Adolescents," *Nursing Outlook,* August 1970, pp. 42–43.

Barlow, Barbara, Thomas V. Santulli, William C. Heird, Jane Pitt, William A. Blanc, and John N. Schullinger: "An Experimental Study of Acute Neonatal Entercolitis—The Importance of Breast Milk," *Journal of Pediatric Surgery,* October 1974, pp. 587–595.

Barnes, George R., Anton N. Lethin, Jr., Edith B. Jackson, and Nilda Shea: "Management of Breast Feeding," *Journal of the American Medical Association,* Jan. 17, 1953, pp. 192–199.

Bloom, Benjamin S. (ed.): *Taxonomy of Educational Objectives: The Classification of Educational Goals, Handbook I: Cognitive Domain,* McKay, New York, 1956.

Countryman, Betty Ann: "Breast Care in the Early Puerperium," *Journal of Obstetric, Gynecologic and Neonatal Nursing,* September/October 1973, pp. 36–40.

———: "Hospital Care of the Breast-fed Newborn," *American Journal of Nursing,* December 1971, pp. 2365–2371.

Crow, Roberta Monroe: "Why My Babies Are Bottle Fed," in Mary H. Browning and Edith P. Lewis, (comps.), *Maternal and Newborn Care: Nursing Interventions,* American Journal of Nursing, New York, 1973, pp. 211–213.

Eiger, Marvin S., and Sally W. Olds: *The Complete Book of Breastfeeding,* Bantam Books, New York, 1973.

Gardner, William U.: "Mammary Gland," in Roy O. Greep (ed.), *Histology,* McGraw-Hill, New York, 1966, pp. 667–676.

Hardy, Janet,: "Medical Care of the Newborn," in Robert E. Cooke (ed.), *The Biologic Basis of Pediatric Practice,* McGraw-Hill, New York, 1968, pp. 1467–1490.

Joseph, Sharon Serena, and Rana Limbo Peck: "Postpartum Needs of the Family," in Joy Princeton Clausen, Margaret Hemp Flock, Bonnie Ford, Marilyn A. Green, and Elsa S. Popiel (eds.), *Maternity Nursing Today,* McGraw-Hill, New York, 1973, pp. 553–614.

Koldjeski, Helen Dixie: "Concerns of Antepartal Mothers Expressed in Group Teaching Experiences and Implications for Nursing Practice," *ANA Clinical Sessions,* 1966, Appleton-Century-Crofts, New York, 1967, pp. 117–124.

La Leche League: *The Womanly Art of Breastfeeding,* La Leche League International, Franklin Park, Ill., 1963.

Langley, L. L., Ira R. Telford, and John B. Christensen: *Dynamic Anatomy and Physiology,* McGraw-Hill, New York, 1969.

Montagu, Ashley: *Touching: The Human Significance of the Skin,* Harper & Row, New York, 1971.

Moore, Mary Lou,: *The Newborn and the Nurse,* Saunders, Philadelphia, 1972.

Murdagh, Sister Angela, and L. Ellen Miller: "Helping the Breast-feeding Mother," in Mary H. Browning and Edith P. Lewis (comps.), *Maternal and Newborn Care: Nursing Interventions,* American Journal of Nursing, New York, 1973, pp. 202–210.

Newton, Niles: "Psychologic Differences between Breast and Bottle Feeding," *The American Journal of Clinical Nutrition,* August 1971, pp. 993–1004.

Nunnally, Dianne Moore: "A New Approach to Helping Mothers Breastfeed,"

Journal of Obstetric, Gynecologic and Neonatal Nursing, July/August 1974, pp. 34–35.

Redman, Barbara K.: *The Process of Patient Teaching in Nursing,* Mosby, St. Louis, 1972.

Scahill, Mary C.: "Helping the Mother Solve Problems with Feeding Her Infant," *Journal of Obstetric, Gynecologic and Neonatal Nursing,* March/April 1975, pp. 51–54.

Schmitt, Madeline H.: "Superiority of Breast-Feeding—Fact or Fancy," in Mary H. Browning and Edith P. Lewis (comps.), *Maternal and Newborn Care: Nursing Interventions,* American Journal of Nursing, New York, 1973, pp. 186–196.

Spaulding, Margaret: "Adapting Postpartum Teaching to Mothers' Low-Income Life-Styles," *Current Concepts in Clinical Nursing,* vol. 2, Mosby, St. Louis, 1969, pp. 280–291.

Tompson, Marian: "The Convenience of Breast Feeding," *American Journal of Clinical Nutrition,* August 1971, pp. 991–992.

"What Parents Worry about in Their Newborn Infants," *Medical Times,* January 1972, pp. 51, 57–59.

Chapter 6

The Infant's Family

In considering the family, it is important to note that most of the research available on the development of parental roles, and certainly the experience of this author, are centered on a relatively homogenous subcultural group—the socioeconomically middle-class, traditional American family. While many of the findings from study of this group undoubtedly hold true for other groups, their universality should not be presumed. The nursing practitioner must be always alert to the uniqueness of the individual family and to the normal variations which contribute to that individuality. It is with regret that neither the scope of this book nor the expertise of this author permits a thorough exploration of all family forms. Students are directed to the special reference list at the end of the chapter for suggested readings through which to increase their understanding of family form and function.

THE PARENT-CHILD RELATIONSHIP

The parent-child relationship does not begin with the birth of the infant. Many aspects of the actual relationship have been molded by the life experiences of the parents long before they thought seriously about becoming parents. Mother-child and father-child relationships develop somewhat differently because of the biological reality of pregnancy. For this reason the two are discussed separately here; however, it should be noted that the father probably will have some of the same developmental experiences as the mother, especially after delivery of the child.

BEGINNINGS OF THE MOTHER-INFANT RELATIONSHIP

The earliest influences on the mother-infant relationship are the experiences the mother has had as an infant and small child, herself. Her intuitive responses to her infant will be determined primarily by the kind of mothering she received as an infant and by the concept of mother which she developed as she grew from a young child, through adolescence, into womanhood. Her overall self-concept as a person and as a female person will affect her ability to relate to her child, also. Successes or failures in her total life experience will have conditioned her to expect success or failure in her mothering role. Her relationship with her husband and the happiness of their marriage may profoundly affect her responsiveness to her infant. Whether or not the child was desired and the extent to which its arrival is seen as a joyous occasion or an inconvenience will also influence the development of the relationship between mother and child.

Major Psychological Tasks of Pregnancy

There are four major psychological tasks of pregnancy which begin shaping the relationship between a mother and a specific infant.[1]

Fusion The first of these is called *fusion,* which is the bonding of mother and child into one being. In order to accomplish this task, the mother must accept the fact of her pregnancy and begin to relate to the embryo as a part of herself. For most women, the wish to become pregnant is a "someday" wish. The diagnosis of pregnancy (even on a presumptive basis) changes that vague, future someday to now.[2] The resulting emotional response is usually a mixed one—some joy, some regret. The vagueness of the early physical signs of pregnancy add to the difficulty in accepting its reality. A physical counterpart to fusion occurs when the embryo is implanted in the lining of the wall of the uterus about a week after conception. Failure of this physical act to occur would result in miscarriage of the embryo; failure of the psychological task to be completed may lead to a sense of detachment and a lack of emotional response to the infant after delivery. Fusion forms *bonds of attachment* between the mother and her infant which are never completely lost from the relationship, although they change in intensity and character with the growth and development of the child. It is these bonds of attachment which stimulate maternal love for the child.

Separation The second task of pregnancy is that of beginning the process of psychological *separation* from the child which will continue for a number of years after birth. The mother must both retain her identification with the child and simultaneously begin to perceive and relate to the child as a separate individual. Ironically, quickening assists the mother in accomplishing both the task of separation and the task of fusion. The movement of the fetus proves his or her existence and thus facilitates fusion. At the same time it is a sign of the presence of an individual whose body can move independently of the mother. Most expectant mothers enjoy the movement of their babies and readily establish with them a bond which is characterized by a sense of privacy and intimacy. This relationship may in fact be so satisfying to the mother that she is quite reluctant to give it up. Her reluctance is probably one indication of successful accomplishment of the earlier task of fusion. As the pregnancy progresses, however, the discomforts increase, and even the woman who thoroughly enjoys the state of pregnancy will eventually come to desire its end. In addition to the discomforts of the last weeks of pregnancy, the focus of expectations upon a "due date" helps to prepare the mother for the event of physical separation. Eagerness to know the sex of the child and the anticipation of the birth shared with family and friends also encourage the desire for separation. Both fusion and separation play an important role in the early mother-child relationship, and both are functional parts of that relationship for the life span of the mother and child. A tension in the mother-child relationship is thus established: a tension between the need to hold on (fusion) and the need to release (separation). This tension exists throughout the lifetime of mother and child, and successful mothering is greatly dependent upon the mother's ability to find and maintain the appropriate balance between these forces in concert with the child's needs to grow and develop.

Identity as Mother The third task of the pregnant woman is to begin to *view herself as a mother.* This task is accomplished by fantasizing and by seeking information. Rubin denotes three stages in prenatal reaction to the mother role:[3] (1) role rejection, as evidenced by the woman's inability to imagine herself as a mother, (2) role contemplation, as evidenced by the woman's fantasizing herself in that role, and (3) role seeking, as evidenced by a search for information and behavioral models to copy. These stages provide helpful data for nurses who are responsible for prenatal care.

The task of formulating a self-concept as mother is not completed in the first pregnancy, however, as it requires time in living and growing with a child before a woman really begins to adopt the mother role as a part of herself. For many women, the automatic, unconscious acceptance of self as mother is greatly enhanced when the second pregnancy is experienced. Some women, particularly young or immature ones, seem never to see themselves as mothers, rather playing more the role of babysitter or older sister to their children.

An important component of the mother's self-concept is her expectations of herself as a mother. To a great extent, her expectations were formed when she was small by the way she saw her own mother. She may have related to her mother as a role model to be copied, or she may have rejected her mother as a role model and formed either opposing expectations or a composite of expectations from other sources. Female nurses may function as role models of the mothering one when a woman's self-concept as a mother is not well established. This is one way nurses may exert positive influences upon the development of healthy mother-child relationships.

How well the mother can meet her expectations of herself as a mother will determine to a great extent whether she will view herself as a competent, "good" mother or as an incompetent, "bad" mother. The extent to which she sees herself as a good or bad mother will, in turn, influence her ability to separate from her child successfully. If she has misgivings about her own competence, she may try to control the child inappropriately in order to prove by the child's model behavior that she is a good mother; or she may fail to exert any controls on the child at all, becoming a willing, though resentful, slave and tolerating behavior which can only make her angry. Her anger increases her feelings of incompetence, to which she responds by increasing her attempts to pacify the child, which in turn perpetuates the cycle. The child becomes very confused by the overt solicitous behavior and the covert anger and hostility which he or she senses within the relationship. The child's reaction to this confusion tends to be one of anxiety and insecurity, which often lead to increasing demands for proof of love from the mother. These increasing demands further increase the mother's frustration and thereby increase the unhealthiness of the cycle.

Childbirth Fantasies The fourth major task of pregnancy is to *deal with the fantasies and fears of childbirth.* Prenatal parent education is a great help in the accomplishment of this task. Willingness to attend to it increases as the desire for separation increases toward the end of pregnancy. However, both the woman who is afraid of labor and the woman who does not want the child she is carrying may "put off" preparing themselves psychologically for labor and delivery until labor actually begins. These are the women who are most likely to consider the experience as a psychologically traumatic one. This perception of trauma may in turn impede the establishment of the early mother-child relationship after birth.

THE FATHER AND CHILD

While the mother is experiencing her pregnancy and preparing herself for her new role as mother, the expectant father has work to do, also. He, too, is formulating a new identity, although for most fathers this new identity does not seem tangible until they actually see the baby. As with the mother, the father's intuitive responses and expectations of himself as father are primarily determined by his early childhood experiences.

While his wife is preparing herself during pregnancy to be the primary caretaker for the infant, the father is assuming responsibility as chief breadwinner. According to psychoanalytic theory, the development of the boy toward maturity requires not only heterosexual maturation and biological fatherhood but also acceptance of the protector-provider role and demonstration of empathy and tenderness in his relationship with his offspring.[4] Ironically, the drive to be a good provider may interfere with the ability to be empathetic and tender with his children. In our modern society, the means of livelihood, unlike earlier agrarian pursuits, requires the father to be away from home and family, thus decreasing the contact between father and child which is necessary for building relationships. Some young couples are attempting to overcome this problem by more nearly sharing the child-care and breadwinner functions. This solution to the problem would seem to present the possibility of conflict as regard to the father's role as provider; certainly adjustment in role expectations is necessary for both parents. Such role diffusion has been experienced by many young couples prior to parenthood with the increase in early marriages and the extended periods of time spent in the pursuit of education. (The socioeconomic and subcultural heritage of the family greatly influences such role expectations, however, and the student should be familiar with the cultural experience of the parents involved.)

The father's role during pregnancy and in the early part of the child's life is somewhat contradictory: the mother increasingly needs his emotional support and physical assistance with tasks around the house, and yet to a great extent, he is excluded from meaningful participation in major events of the pregnancy and early infancy of the child. He feels the baby move in utero only when his wife calls the movement to his attention. He is most often excluded from the labor and delivery unit of the hospital, and thus does not participate in his child's birth. In many hospitals his only contact with his infant is to look at him or her through a glass window. When the baby goes home, he finds that his wife is totally absorbed in the care of the infant and that she is irritable and fatigued. His mother-in-law may become a household resident for a while, perhaps further separating him from his wife and child.

Unless special effort is made to include the father in the infant's care, some fathers retreat to a "safe distance" from the relative chaos which reigns during those early weeks at home and become psychologically if not actually "absentee fathers." These men may assume the provider role almost exclusively to the detriment of their relationships with their wives as well as their children. Nursing actions which encourage fathers to become emotionally involved with their children and supportive of their wives in their mothering role, thus, can make a positive contribution to the present and future mental health of the family in cultural groups where the husband's participation is deemed desirable. (In some families such fatherly participation would result in a loss of esteem for both parents because it would violate role expectations.)

THE IMMEDIATE NEWBORN PERIOD

When the baby is born, the relationship between the parents and child continues to develop. Now the parents have an objective reality with which to relate as well as the baby of their fantasies. It must be remembered that the relationship between parents and children is only partially based in reality. In part, every child is fulfillment of fantasy: the child represents fulfillment of the parents' dreams and ambitions, is seen as an extension of self which will endure beyond the parents' lifetimes, and may even represent an especially loved or feared person in the parents' lives.

Elaboration of Prenatal Themes

The themes which were begun in pregnancy are now elaborated. Fusion is manifested by the mother's continuing view of the baby as an extension of herself, as demonstrated by her great concern for perfection in the infant and by her extreme reactions to even minor imperfections. Fusion is further demonstrated by the mother's normal tendency to feel somewhat lost or empty after delivery, as though she had given up a physical part of herself, which to some extent is fact.

The theme of separation is greatly enhanced by the delivery of the infant. Now, the mother can begin to identify the baby's uniqueness as a separate individual. The first thing she usually wants to know is the sex of the child. Even in the immediate newborn period, parents relate to infants differently according to their sex. After the mother establishes the sex of the child, she will usually attempt to identify features of the baby which remind her of various relatives. In this way, she forms a composite picture in her mind of the baby's identity. As she looks at the baby, she also traces the outline of his or her features, particular the facial features, with her finger, as though to establish them firmly in her mind.

The third theme which was begun in pregnancy, that of establishing the mother's self-concept as a mother, is also greatly affected by the delivery of the baby. If the mother has successfully delivered a healthy, normal baby, her feelings of self-esteem are enhanced, and she can proceed with relating to her infant with expectations of success in her mother role. If, however, the baby was preterm, sick, or had a congenital anomaly, the mother's feelings of self-esteem are damaged, and a reaction of grief and guilt intrudes upon and may very well interrupt the normal establishment of the maternal-child relationship.

Establishment of Affectional Bonds

Two new tasks must be initiated in the immediate newborn period. One of these is the establishment of *affectional bonds.* Rather strong affectional bonds, which are precursors to feelings of love for the infant, appear immediately after the delivery of the child as an extension of fusion, but they are greatly enhanced by actual physical contact with the child. In fact, there is evidence to suggest that these bonds are seriously weakened and may be lost entirely by prolonged physical separation of mother and infant.[5] Of particular help in establishing affectional bonds is the mother's opportunity to have eye contact with her baby[6] (see Figure 6-1). Infants participate in the establishment of affectional bonds by the searching movements of their eyes as they try to focus on the environment around them. Whether or not the infant actually can see the mother is doubtful, but this gives her the impression that the child is looking for her and looking toward her, which increases her emotional response to the child. It is interesting to note here that the first part of the face to which the infant responds, though this comes some weeks later, is also the eyes.[7] Young infants seem to respond just as positively to a mask which contains only eyes as they do to the complete human face.

Holding and caressing the infant also increases the establishment of affectional bonds. Tactile contact with the newborn in the early days of life may actually be a necessary experience for mothers to develop keen awareness and sensitivity to their babies' needs (see Figure 6-2).In a study done at Case Western Reserve University, it was found that mothers who were allowed to hold their infants for increased amounts of time in the first few days after birth demonstrated more sensitivity to the needs of the infant later when the children came to clinics for health supervision.[8] The same kind of response was first noted in animal studies, and it is thought that perhaps this is an important aspect of the early mother-child relationship in humans as well.

Establishment of Mutuality

The second major task which must be begun in the newborn period is the establishment of *mutuality* between the mother and infant. Mutuality is really the beginning of interpersonal interaction between the two and forms the foundation for the development of trust. It involves both the mother's ability to sense and meet the needs of the infant and the infant's ability to communicate needs and to reward the mother with satisfaction responses, such as relaxing and falling asleep, when those needs have been met. One aspect of mutuality is the establishment of a rhythm of activity which is

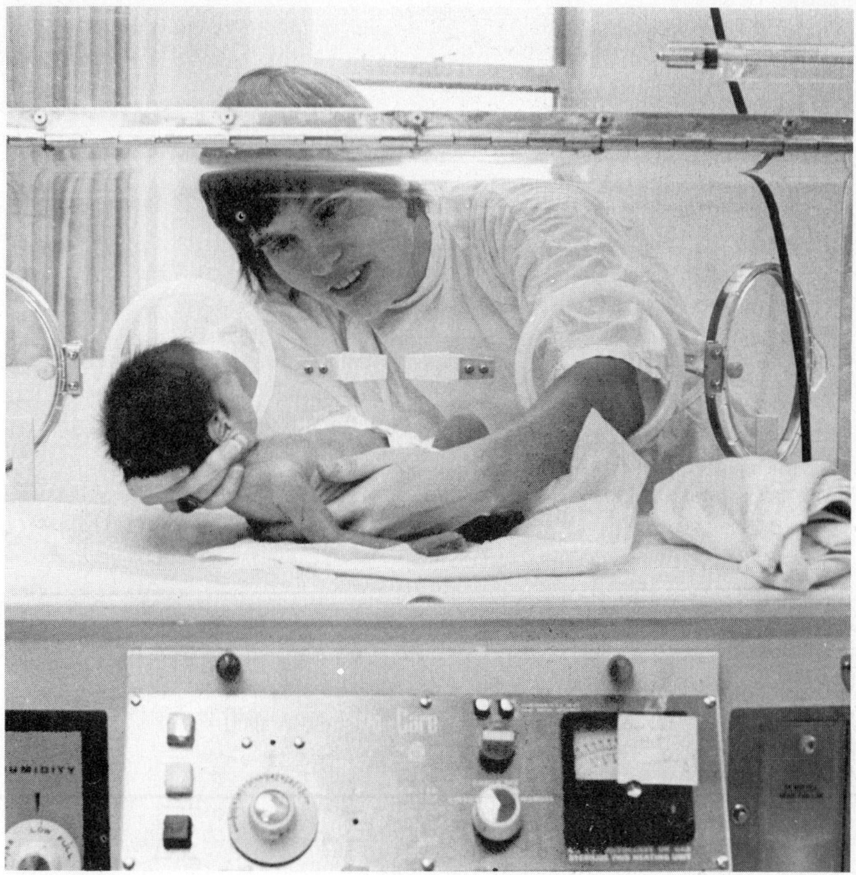

Figure 6-1 Mothers need eye contact with their infants to establish affectional bonds. (*From G. Scipien et al., Comprehensive Pediatric Nursing, McGraw-Hill, New York, 1975, p. 351, by permission.*)

comfortable for both. Some babies are naturally at birth more active than others.

Dr. T. Brazleton, in his book *Infants and Mothers* (see reference list), has described in great detail the development of mother-child relationships in three very different mother-infant couples. The striking differences which he related are all within the range of the normal and are all primarily differences in the inherent activity patterns of the infants. Dr. Brazelton gives many excellent examples of just how the infant's behavior affects his mother's reaction to him and the consequences of the mother's behavior in the overall development of the child. This book is highly recommended to students and others who wish to develop understanding in depth of the interactional patterns of infants and their parents.

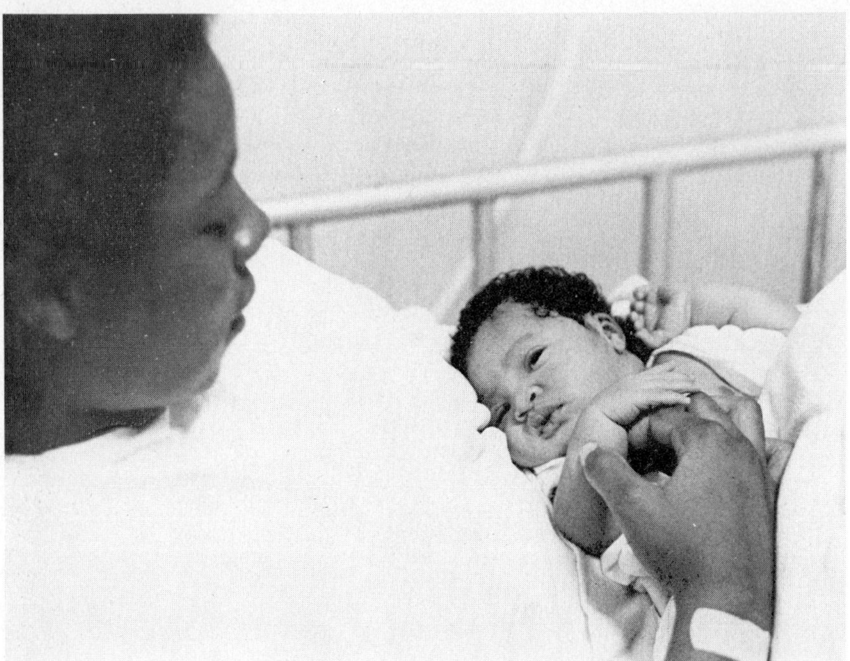

Figure 6-2 A mother holds her baby a few minutes after delivery. The baby in this picture is still in the first period of reactivity. Note that the mother is using her fingertips to explore her baby (fingering). (*Photo: Penelope Ann Peirce.*)

It is crucial in the development of mutuality that the new mother learn to identify behavioral differences in her infant and to react to them in a positive, constructive way. Here the nurse can make a significant contribution. By learning to identify specific differences in babies, the nurse can develop a wide range of experience from which to assist the parents in identifying specific characteristics of their infants. Carrol Farrar recommends observing for such characteristics as how the infant indicates an internal need such as hunger, satisfaction responses, specific methods of quieting the infant, and responses to specific stimuli.[9]

The nurse should be careful in discussing observations with the mother. The mother should not be overwhelmed with too much data, and the mother should have an opportunity to share her own observations. The nurse's approach should be gentle and tactful. A new mother's shaky self-esteem can be easily disturbed by an unsympathetic show of professional competence.

Empathic Perception

One tool which the mother and infant use to help establish the relationship of mutuality is called *empathic perception,* which is an unconscious awareness of each other that facilitates the development of communication between the two. Neither the mother nor the infant is consciously aware of the signals which they are transmitting and receiving, but both participate in the communication. For instance, the baby's cry soon develops different qualities which cue the mother as to the problem which the baby is experiencing. Although the mother probably could not explain to an outsider exactly what is different about the cries, she can identify and respond to their differences sufficiently to take specific action appropriate to meeting the infant's needs. Similarly, the infant senses the mother's comfort or discomfort in this role and responds in turn with comfort or discomfort.

Touch is very important in communicating the mother's comfort or discomfort with her baby. There are several components of touch which seem to be important.[10,11] One of these is temperature. If the mother feels comfortable with the baby, she will enfold him, holding him close to her body and transmitting to him her body heat, which is reminiscent of the intrauterine environment. This association helps the baby relax and become quiet, a satisfaction response, which helps her in turn to relax and be more comfortable with the baby. Conversely, the baby can sense muscle tension in the mother, which causes discomfort. The baby responds to this discomfort with fussiness, crying, and tension of his own. The mother then feels more tense, the baby's tension increases, and in this way a disruptive cycle may be initiated.

Montagu has suggested rather strongly that rocking chairs are a great adjunct to the care of infants, especially in establishing and maintaining mutuality, and subsequently, trust.[12] He feels that rocking chairs recreate the motion which the infant was used to in utero and that rocking gives the infant a sense of relatedness and companionship with the mother because of the pressure of her body as they sway back and forth. Mothers are also usually more relaxed in a rocking chair, and rocking is a soothing motion for the mother as well as for the baby, thus enhancing their mutual relaxation and comfort. Also, rocking has an hypnotic effect which is soothing to the immature central nervous system, further increasing the infant's relaxation. Montagu believes that rocking also improves the infant's circulation, respiration, and digestion, all of which contribute to an increased sense of well-being and help facilitate satisfaction responses.

The Feeding Cycle

Probably the most important single event in the infant's life, as far as establishment of trust is concerned, is the feeding cycle. It is important that the nurse understand the behavioral components of this cycle. Initially, the infant arouses from a state of sleep because of awareness of discomfort. The baby, of course, cannot identify the cause for the discomfort, but will respond to it with increased physical activity, agitation, and crying. When the infant becomes agitated, he may be able to get his hand to his mouth and begin sucking, which is one way of alerting his mother to the nature of his discomfort. The mother responds to the crying by going to the infant and picking him up. If she recognizes that the infant is hungry, she will prepare him for feeding and then provide him with either the breast or bottle. The baby responds to objects touching his cheek by *rooting,* that is, by turning his head toward the object and attempting to grasp it in his mouth. The mother can assist the baby in locating and grasping the nipple, and then the infant takes the active role in sucking and swallowing as he participates in meeting his own need for food. Finally, as the infant takes in the milk and satisfies his hunger, his activity decreases, and he drifts into a deep, relaxed sleep. The mother sees this satisfaction response and feels increased self-esteem and pleasure in her mothering role.

It is important to note here that sucking is in itself a pleasurable activity, functioning both to release tension and to provide sensory pleasure for the infant. Infants have both a need for food and a need to suck. Normally, they satisfy their need to suck while feeding, although they will usually suck more than is actually needed just to take in enough milk to meet their need for food.

Very young infants have no capacity whatsoever to relieve their own tensions without outside assistance. Only as they communicate their needs and receive maternal responses will they begin to trust that their needs will be met, and only as this cycle is repeated numerous times will this trust become a part of their life expectations. Some mothers, particularly first-time mothers, in their desire to meet their infants' needs are very apt to overfeed the babies, thinking that any time they cry they need to be fed. These mothers need assistance in identifying other kinds of needs their infants have, such as relief from pressure caused by lying in one position too long, relief from being too warm or too cold, the need for socializing, or the need for relief from some other kind of physical discomfort besides hunger.

ROLE TRANSITION

Alice Rossi characterizes the transition from nonparent to parent as the most difficult role transition a person, particularly a woman, faces in an entire lifetime.[13] She compares this transition to role transitions in marriage and occupational settings. According to her viewpoint, there are four stages in the role cycle: the anticipatory stage, the honeymoon stage, the plateau stage, and the disengagement-termination stage.

The Anticipatory Stage

The *anticipatory stage* in the marriage role is the engagement period when the couple are learning to know each other and perhaps setting up an apartment for occupancy following marriage. In the occupational role, the anticipatory stage encompasses the training or educational period which actually precedes the acceptance of the role. In the parenthood role, the anticipatory stage is the period of pregnancy. Rossi points out that the pregnancy offers the couple no clear way either to get to know the infant or really to practice parenting skills.

The Honeymoon Stage

The *honeymoon stage* in marriage is an indefinite period beginning with the wedding ceremony and ending at a nonspecific time, depending on the couple. It is characterized by intimacy and close contact through which bonds of affection become firmly established. A similar period can be identified in the work world when the new employee is enthusiastic about the job and is to some extent immersed in it. In the parental role, the honeymoon period is also that time when bonds of attachment are established.

The Plateau Stage

The *plateau stage* is that period in which the work of the role is carried out. In marriage and parenting it usually encompasses that time when the home is established, children are reared, and at least the father's career is established, and often the mother's as well. In the occupational setting, it is the full assumption of the work role.

The Disengagement-Termination Stage

Finally, the *disengagement-termination stage* occurs when for one reason or another a role is relinquished. This could happen at retirement, or simply when a change of jobs occurs, at the death of a spouse, or at the time of divorce. The parent role is never relinquished entirely, short of death, but, many parents feel a lifting of the responsibility when a child marries or leaves home to become self-supporting.

Difficulties in Assuming the Parental Role

There are a number of difficulties inherent in the assumption of the parental role. The first difficulty is that in spite of modern contraceptives, the assumption of the parental role may not have been planned, and it may not be desired. In spite of abortion laws which make it legally acceptable to terminate a pregnancy, there are many people who could not for religious or emotional reasons bring themselves to terminate their pregnancies. Thus, many children are born whose arrival is not heralded by tidings of great joy. Another problem is that, although other roles may be assumed and rejected at will, parenthood may not for the most part be rejected once it is established. As Rossi so eloquently states, "We can have ex-spouses and ex-jobs but not ex-children."[14] She goes on to point out that as a rule, later-born children are anticipated with less enthusiasm than the first and that actual satisfaction in the parenting role seems to decrease with time. She makes the same statement about the housekeeping role of the wife—that with the passage of time, it is less and less enjoyed. This is not to say that some parents do not enjoy their children more as they get older or that for some parents, large families are not a source of joy and satisfaction, but that at least for the average middle-class American family, the eager anticipation of and pleasure in parenting seems to decrease as the number of children increases. If one looks at the demands made on the parent, especially the mother, by increasing numbers of children, it is easy to see how this could be true.

Finally, the transition to parenthood is made more difficult because there is so little actual training available during the anticipatory stage and because the assumption of the role is abrupt. The new mother has very little time to learn her role before she has complete and total responsibility for the infant's care.

Such guides to infant care as are available tend to be contradictory, and by warning of the harm that can result from parental errors, they tend to undermine the self-confidence of the mother in following her maternal instincts in providing for her child. Thus, relaxed intuitive responses have to a great extent been replaced by tense, anxious hovering.

At the time the new mother assumes total responsibility for the care of her infant, she is physically and emotionally still recovering from the trauma of the labor and delivery experience. Because of the mobility of our society and the relative isolation of the nuclear family, the new mother is likely to be separated from female relatives who traditionally have assisted during this transition period. It seems quite possible that the person least able emotionally and physically to assume the total responsibility for a new infant (and the attendant chores of running the house and dealing with older siblings) is the new mother; and yet this is the person to whom the responsibility falls. There is a real need for investigation of ways to provide assistance to new mothers so that they can have a recovery period before taking on the full responsibilities of infant care and household management. Perhaps the practice in our grandmother's day of experiencing a period of confinement, when the new mother was not expected to do anything except rest and nurse the baby, has some merit which should be reconsidered.

Assumption of the Maternal Role

Reva Rubin, an outstanding nurse educator in maternity nursing, has investigated very thoroughly the process through which a new mother assumes the maternal role. Rubin has defined three phases in the assumption of this role and has described clearly three stages in maternal touch which indicate to the observer where the mother is in the assumption of that role.[15] The three phases in the assumption of the role are the *taking-in phase,* the *taking-hold phase,* and the *letting-go phase.* Although these phases are most often described in terms of the days in which they may be expected to be present, there is no set time schedule which a particular mother will follow. All mothers follow the same general sequence of events, but multiparas move from one phase to the next much more rapidly than do primiparas. There may be movement back and forth from one phase to another during the first few days after delivery. The mother is likely to move back to an earlier phase when she is experiencing physical discomforts or if she becomes overly fatigued.

The Taking-in Phase The *taking-in phase* is a period when the mother is oriented primarily to her own needs. She is quite passive and has very great dependency needs, which must be met if she is to be able to give to her child later. She may be quite talkative about her memories of labor and delivery as though trying to incorporate them into her life experience. During this phase, if the baby is brought to her, she will make little effort to reach for him. Rather, she waits passively for the child to be placed in her arms. Her passivity is not due to a lack of interest in the baby, but rather an indication of her strong dependency needs. It is much more important at this time that these dependency needs be met than for her to be given much responsibility for her baby's care. During this time, however, she is taking in information to help identify her baby—using primarily fingertip contact. *Fingering* is the first stage of maternal touch. The mother will often lay the baby on the bed and have no physical contact with him other than with her fingertips. This behavior is a part of the identification process, and it is both an indication of her feeling of strangeness with the baby and evidence of her awakening interest.

Although the taking-in phase is predominant only in the first 2 or 3 days after delivery, it is likely to recur when the mother is fatigued or emotionally distressed, as often happens after discharge from the hospital. There are times throughout the life cycle of the mother when she needs to be relieved of responsibility for child care, if only for a few hours.

The Taking-hold Phase The *taking-hold phase* becomes predominant for most primiparas about the third day after delivery, though it may be observed *briefly* much earlier than that. It tends to predominate earlier for multiparas, as a rule. During this phase, the mother is acutely interested in her baby and his care. At this time, the mother can profit from encouragement and assistance in the identification process. The nurse can assist the new mother in identifying her infant by helping her see the uniqueness of her child. Observations of the baby's behavior in the nursery can be shared with the mother at this time. It is especially important to share observations that will help her in identifying and meeting her child's needs. (How does he indicate hunger? Does he have special behaviors for fatigue?)

As the new mother, particularly the primipara, begins to hold her infant, she seems very awkward and holds the infant stiffly in her arms away from direct contact with her body, and frequently in positions that are uncomfortable both for her and for the baby. It is not unusual to see a new mother supporting her baby's head stiffly on the tips of her fingers rather than in the palm of her hand or in the crook of her arm. As the mother becomes more comfortable with her baby, she begins to use the palms of her hands for contact with him. This stage of *total hand contact* with the baby is the second stage of maternal touch. Only when the mother becomes really at ease, will she begin to relax her arms and enfold the baby close to her body. This *enfolding* is the third stage of maternal touch. As a rule, the more satisfying the mother-child relationship at any particular time, the closer the mother will hold the child. Distance, awkwardness, and tension in holding the baby, then are clues that supportive nursing intervention is needed. (It is interesting to note that the stages of maternal touch are repeated over and over again as the mother and child share their lives. When the mother is angry with the child, for instance, there is increased distance in their physical relationship. When she is frightened for her child or feeling very affectionate, she tends to hold him or her very close to her body. After a prolonged or anxiety-provoking separation, the first contacts may be rather tentative, especially when the mother is unsure of herself, as after her child has had surgery.)

Teaching is best done when the mother is thoroughly at ease with her baby. The teaching can be paced by observing how the mother handles the infant. As she is learning a new procedure, she repeats the stages of touch, beginning with fingertip contact and awkwardness. When she becomes comfortable with the procedure, she uses her palms and the enfolding contact. She should be allowed to become thoroughly at ease with one procedure before a new one is introduced. (From a teaching point of view, it is unfortunate that new mothers are discharged from the hospital so soon after their babies' births. A greater availability or a broader use of community-based nurses would help with this problem.)

It is important to note when teaching new mothers that during the taking-hold phase of the maternal role, they tend to expect perfection from themselves. Any difficulty with a task is often seen as total failure. An unthinking nurse can add to the mother's feeling of inadequacy by being "too efficient." For instance, if a mother is having difficulty feeding her baby and the nurse confidently takes the child from her and quickly quiets and feeds him, the mother may feel that she will never be so competent as the nurse. It is more helpful for the nurse to assist and encourage the mother to do the task at hand than to do it for her.

The Letting-go Phase As the mother begins to assume the mothering functions, the third phase, the *letting-go phase* becomes evident. During this phase the mother must finally accept her physical separation from her infant. In addition, she experiences a different kind of separation. She must separate herself from her former role as a childless person. Never again, barring the death of her child, will she be childless. For several years, she must accommodate her life to the relative helplessness of the infant and small child. This may mean giving up, at least temporarily, much of the freedom and autonomy to which she may have become accustomed. This aspect of motherhood may be especially difficult if the new mother has only recently separated herself from the controls of her parents, or if she has participated in a satisfying career to which she does not plan to return right away. Even if she does plan to continue working soon after her baby is born, she must cope with the complex problems such as providing adequate mother substitutes during the child's early years. The new mother must also take on a considerably heavier work load than she has been accustomed to, even if she has older children. Each new baby brings additional middle-of-the night feedings and mountains of clothes to launder, even if one is already managing a sizable household. Rubin has characterized this phase as being one of grieving. The grief is focused primarily on the lost role or status, as the new mother moves through the transition to motherhood.[16] It seems quite likely that the "baby blues," the depressive intervals experienced by most new mothers, are at least in part attributable to the grief which accompanies role change. This third phase may last for several weeks, and it is possible for the mother to experience brief periods of depression related to her mothering role at times of stress whenever the needs of the children exceed her ability to meet them.

The Father

Relatively little has been written about role transition for the father, specifically. An interesting study by A. Doreen Jorday indicates that participation in prenatal classes, assisting his wife during labor and delivery, and holding his infant soon after delivery all enhance the establishment of the father-child relationship and the development of the father's sense of fatherhood.[17] Beyond these few observations, it might be hypothesized that the father's role transition proceeds along lines similar to that of the mother, but further study must be done.

THE FIRST WEEKS AT HOME

Much has been written, and sung, and said about the joys of parenthood and its deep satisfactions, which are very real; however, little is mentioned in popular literature about the stresses of parenthood, which are also very real. The following material is presented not to paint a gloomy picture but to balance the rosy and frequently unrealistic picture of parenthood which most people develop as they grow up. The introduction of a new baby into a family is a stressful period, and currently one for which very little professional help is available. Perhaps the future will be a time when the skills

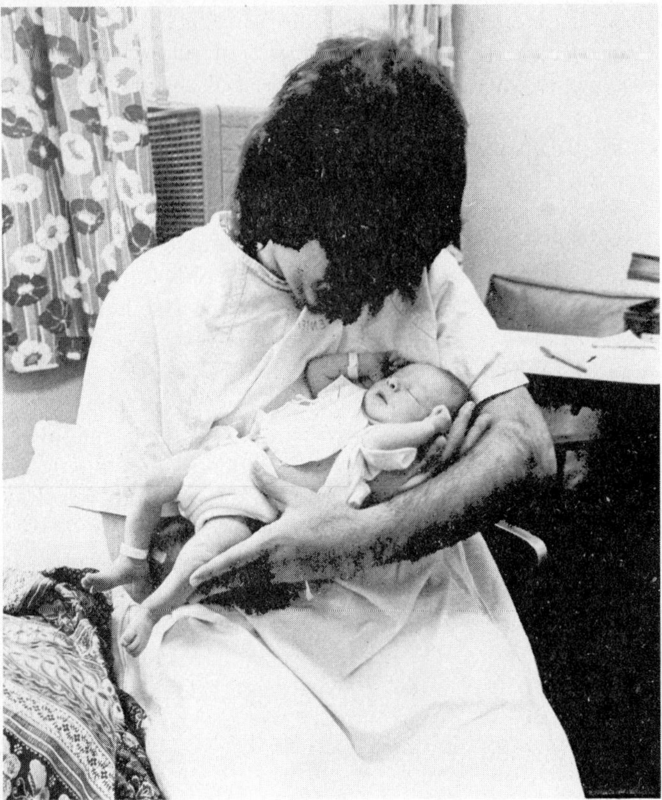

Figure 6-3 Fathers, too, need physical contact with their infants in order to form affectional bonds. This father is holding his infant for the first time. (*Photo: Penelope Ann Peirce.*)

which the nurse holds, uniquely, can be used to decrease the stress of this period.

One of the most disillusioning periods in a woman's life is the first few weeks of her first child's life. All her fantasies of being an ideal mother soon give way to extreme fatigue and utter frustration. The calm, orderly household she has envisioned becomes a nightmare of dirty diapers, unwashed dishes, and general clutter. Instead of smiling sweetly as she bathes and feeds her baby, she finds herself, much to her own horror, screaming at the infant for crying and feeling as though she surely has been possessed by some demon. Let us examine some of the causes for this distress.

Complete Dependence of the Baby

The first fact that must be considered is the complete and total dependence of the infant upon others for his care. This is a well-known fact. What is not so often stated or understood by new mothers is that the needs of the infant far exceed the mother's abilities to meet them. Alice Rossi is perhaps the most outspoken on this point.[18] Drawing from such noted authors as Therese Benedek, she concludes that there is a great discrepency between the infant's need for mothering and the mother's need to mother. An associated problem for the young mother of today is the mobile society which often places her hundreds of miles from relatives who otherwise could help. Critics of Rossi have stated that her observations seem to be true primarily for middle-class mothers but that most of them do not hold true for other subcultures. Be this as it may, the conclusions drawn by Rossi do seem to be true for a large group of mothers.

Boredom

There are valid reasons why a young woman might not find the mothering role satisfying. Many young women are highly educated and have enjoyed periods of productive and stimulating work prior to marriage and motherhood. Caring for an infant may seem extremely routine and unstimulating to these women. In contrast, a very young woman who has not yet completed her adolescence may find the job of caring for an infant totally overwhelming.

Unrealistic Expectations

Commercial advertising and the mass media have built images of motherhood that are highly unrealistic and unattainable in real life, while at the same time holding up fantasies of a happier, richer life if only one could have more money, get out from under the children, or own certain products. For many young women, these fantasies may appear to be more real than their own lives, and they may come to view the normal frustrations of parenthood, which they were not prepared to expect, as evidence of their own failure as parents or as some sort of "rotten deal" from life. Lacking supportive figures who can reassure them of the worth of what they are doing, many of these young women try to escape from their roles as mothers, or else they find that their self-esteem begins decreasing and continues in this trend for several years as they are more and more unable to live up to their idealized standards.

More realistic preparation for parenthood and a supportive relationship with a community-based nurse could perhaps prevent such negative attitudes about mothering. Perhaps the place to start is to recognize that no mother, no matter how mature, can possibly meet all the needs of her children all the time. The needs of the mother as a person, and the needs of the parents as a couple must at times take precedence over the needs of the child or children.

The Mother's Need for Sleep

One need that many mothers often try to ignore is their own need for rest and sleep. Even when they are aware of their need, it may not be possible for them to meet it without outside assistance. Hence sleep deprivation is a part of all mothers' lives to some extent. For mothers of newborns, it can become a rather severe problem. The newborn arouses from sleep primarily because of hunger. For a breast-fed baby, the intervals of sleep between feedings may be as little as 2 hours for the first month. Even the bottle-fed baby does not adhere to a neat 4-hour schedule. An adult, on the other hand, is accustomed to periods of several hours of sleep without interruption.

Williams notes that sleep needs increase during pregnancy but that the mother's ability to rest comfortably and get her sleep decreases toward term.[19] In addition, Williams indicates that the physical exertion of labor and delivery causes an energy deficit which takes about 6 weeks to be overcome. To compound the problem, the postpartum stay in the hospital provides the new mother with less sleep than she ordinarily got at home before she became pregnant. All this leaves the mother with a tremendous energy and sleep deficit which will increase sharply during the first few weeks she is at home with the infant.

Effects of Sleep Deprivation

Sleep deprivation has been studied to some extent, primarily with healthy volunteers. Changes in mood and even in mental functioning have been noted. A pattern of responses has been identified by Murry in progressive sleep deprivation.[20] Fairly early in the deprivation, the person exhibits increased anxiety which is thought to be due possibly to the person's fear of detrimental effects from the loss of sleep. The prevailing mood is one of apathy and depression. There is a progressive decrease in talkativeness and sociability of the individual as withdrawal and narrowing of interests occurs. Irritability is characteristic of the sleep-deprived person, whose frustrations may be expressed by overt aggression. In extreme sleep deprivation, there may be mental confusion, paranoid delusions, and illogical thought patterns. Anyone who works with new mothers will soon realize that many of the described characteristics are prominent in their behavior during the first few weeks after the birth of a baby. Unfortunately, very few mothers have any professional contacts during the first month after the baby is born.

To further complicate the matter, the new mother finds that when the baby does go to sleep she is left lying in her bed wide-awake and unable to fall asleep.

The dynamics of this situation involve need arousal and inability to meet the need. Frustration occurs when the satisfaction of a need is blocked by a seemingly insurmountable object. The result of the frustrations is anger and resentment, which cause increased body tension. In this instance, the mother's need for sleep is blocked by the baby's need for food. The mother struggles to meet her baby's needs and in the process increases her own body tension. Insomnia is the result of the tension in her body. Kahn found in experiments with college students that exercises which resulted in progressive relaxation of body muscles were helpful in decreasing the time required by insomniac students to fall asleep.[21] Hence, the recommendation earlier in this book to teach new mothers techniques for progressive relaxation as a means of helping to alleviate some of the sleep deprivation which inevitably accompanies the care of a newborn. (See Chapter 5, Breast-Feeding, Fatigue.)

Sleep deprivation can become a severe problem when there is more than one child in the family. One mother kept a record of her sleep patterns, and on one particular night she recorded the following:

9:30 P.M.: I went to sleep.
11:00 P.M.: Susie (newborn) awoke.
12:15 A.M.: Susie went back to sleep.
2:00 A.M.: Susie awoke.
2:20 A.M.: Susie went back to sleep.
2:50 A.M.: Jimmy (older child) awoke with a nightmare.
4:00 A.M.: Jimmy went back to sleep.
5:00 A.M.: Susie awoke.
5:20 A.M.: Susie went back to sleep.
7:00 A.M.: Susie awake.
7:30 A.M.: Jimmy got up for the day.

The longest period of time this mother had between periods of being up with her children was 1 hour and 45 minutes. During this same night, the mother also recorded feelings of intense anger at the baby and an episode of yelling at the baby. She said she actually felt like throwing the baby across the room. This feeling is not particularly unusual in the first weeks after bringing a new baby home. In this particular household, the mother was fortunate to have a husband present who was willing to take over for a few hours and allow her to sleep. If he could not have done this, the mother might well have acted in ways that would have been at least emotionally traumatic for her children. New mothers often cite periods when they experience paranoid-type feelings and when they begin to think they will never have a life of their own again. One mother said that just seeing her husband sleeping or hearing him snore while she was up with the baby could evoke feelings of rage toward him.

Husbands, on the other hand, are usually not aware of the sleep problems their wives are experiencing, and they may be extremely bewildered by the personality changes which occur. If they withdraw from their wives at this time or fight with them (a natural response to irritability and aggression), the whole problem is compounded.

Needs of Siblings

Besides contending with their own needs and the needs of the infant, most mothers at one time or another have older children who also have needs to be considered in making the transition home with a new baby. Concern for the needs of the siblings should begin before the birth of the baby, and their preparation for the event should be carefully planned.

Preparation for the Baby Preparation of a child for the birth of a sibling should be geared to the age of the child and his or her experience. Advance preparation should not be made too early, as time passes very slowly for a child. During the last month or two of the pregnancy, the mother might let her older child feel the baby move and talk about the fact of its existence in her uterus. This is a fine time, incidentally, to do a little sex education, depending upon the age of the child. As physical preparations for the baby are made, such as fixing up a room, the older child should be allowed to help in ways appropriate for his or her age.

If the older child is to be moved from a crib, or to a new room, however, these changes should be made 5 or 6 months in advance of the baby's birth with the emphasis being placed on the child's growing up and needing a new room or bed, so that the feeling of being displaced by the baby does not occur. If the toddler is just beginning to be old enough for toilet training about the time the baby is expected, it is better to put off the training until

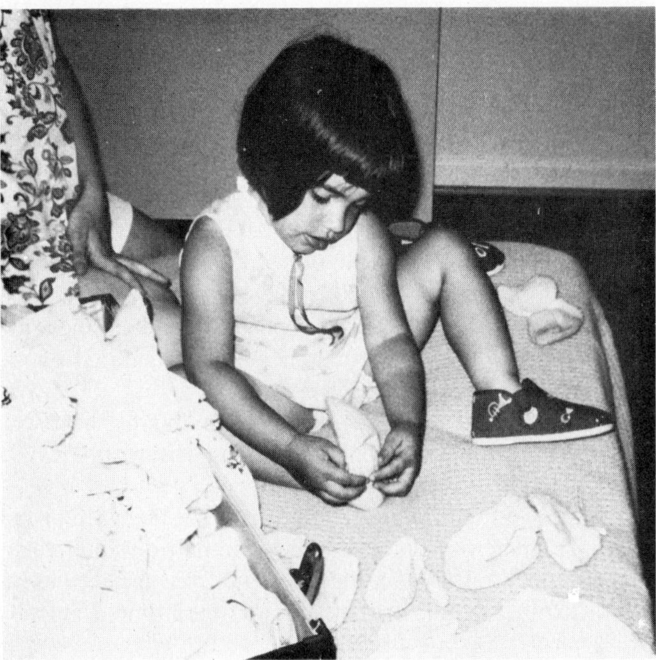

Figure 6-4 A toddler needs to help prepare for a new baby. The child here has taken time out from unpacking baby clothes to see if she can wear them herself.

adjustment to the infant has been made, as regression is expected and the child may feel he is being toilet-trained because of the baby. This will definitely slow down the training process and may also create problems in the mother-child relationship. If the child is well past the training period when the baby comes, there may be temporary regression to wetting, but it is not likely to be prolonged if the mother can accept it calmly and matter-of-factly as "something that just happens when a new baby comes to live in a house."

It is helpful to give older children an opportunity to be around a young baby for short periods of time so that they have some idea of what a baby is really like. All too often, children expect their baby brothers or sisters to be able to run and play with them. They may indeed feel cheated when the baby arrives and can only cry and take up mother's time and attention.

Of utmost importance in preparing a child for the birth of a baby is to anticipate and discuss negative feelings which are very likely to occur. *All* children have some feelings of anger and jealousy toward a rival, especially one that takes so much of their parent's time and attention away from them (see Figure 6-5). When there are several children in the family, the younger ones may also resent the attention the older children pay to the baby. The important point here, is to keep communications open so that the child can express anger openly rather than having to hide it and possibly hurting the baby when the mother is not looking. It is important to tell the child directly that all children have these feelings and that the mother understands. The mother should also invite the child to share his or her feelings with her when they are bothersome, and she must be ready to listen and accept the feelings when they occur whether or not that time is convenient for her. It should be pointed out here that accepting angry feelings toward the baby is not the same thing as accepting hurtful behavior. Children must know that they will not be allowed to hurt the baby in any way. They will in most instances be relieved to know that the mother is strong enough to prevent their hurting the infant. Often they are themselves fearful of their anger and aggressive tendencies.

After the Baby Comes Home Some mothers have found it helpful to give the older child a baby doll to care for alongside the mother as she cares for the baby (see Figure 6-6). This seems to be especially well accepted if the older child is a girl. It should be considered for older boy children, as well, however, unless the parents (most often the father) have such negative reactions to seeing a boy play with dolls that it could not be treated casually. Here again, depending on the age of the children in question, anything which encourages the older child to identify with the mother will help decrease the inevitable regression and anger. Especially helpful are opportunities for the older child to "help" the mother in the baby's care. With an

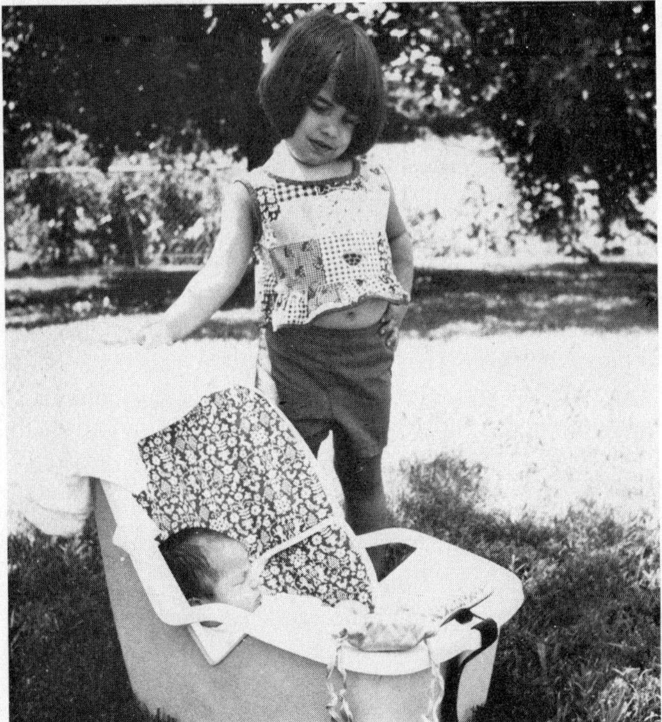

Figure 6-5 Toddlers have mixed emotions about new babies.

adult sitting next to him, even an older toddler can hold an infant and give her a bottle. (See Figure 6-7.) Such experiences help to instill a sense of accomplishment in the older child and provide a model of acceptable behavior toward the baby.

Allowing the child new privileges, such as engaging in water play or visiting a playmate alone, may also help. One family made a point of allowing the older child to "help" with the grocery shopping while the baby, who was "too little" to go, was left at home with a babysitter. Another family planned special activity for just the older child and the father. (See Figure 6-8.) The mother, too, should spend some time alone with the older child so that the family does not become divided into two "camps."

Keeping the child happily occupied with interesting and satisfying activities will help decrease the hostility and hurt that is felt at being "displaced" by the new baby, but it does not make it all go away. One child was found by her mother sitting on the back steps crying softly to herself during the second week after the baby came home. When asked what was wrong, the child said very sadly, "I wish somebody would talk to me." Other chil-

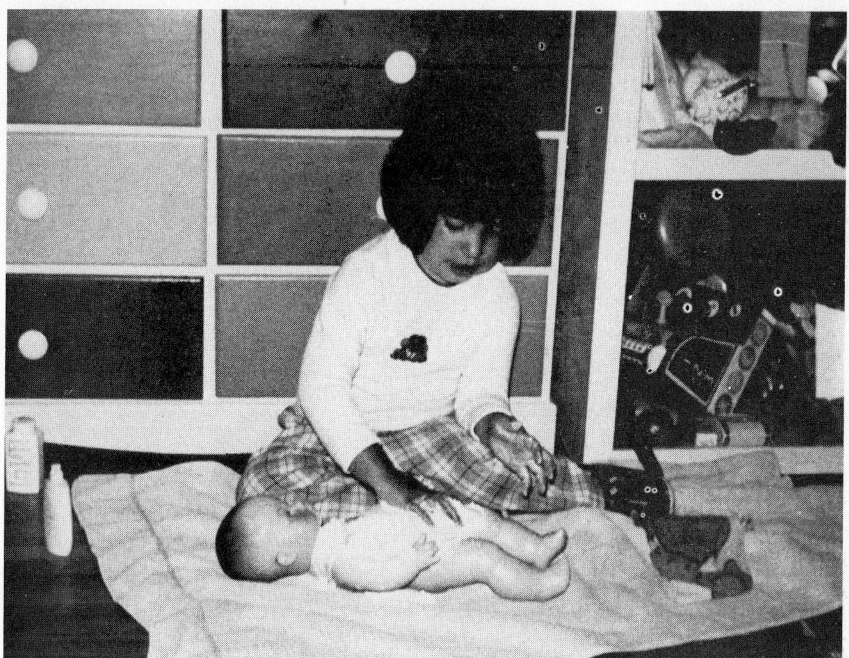

Figure 6-6 It is helpful for toddlers to have a doll to care for, as their mother cares for the new baby. Here the girl powders her doll liberally.

dren are very direct in acting out their feelings about the baby. One little girl, who was about 5 years old, actually carried her baby brother over to the house of a neighbor and "gave him away." It is not uncommon for children to tell their mother to put the baby to bed or to stop feeding him because he is full. The mother needs to recognize and acknowledge the feelings that underlie such statements. Sometimes it is helpful for the mother to say something like this: "It's awfully hard for kids when their mothers have to spend all their time taking care of the baby, isn't it? Big kids often wish the baby would go away. Sometimes they think they would like to give the baby to someone else or even to hurt it. I understand how you feel, and it's okay to feel that way, but I will never let you hurt Susie (or Jimmy, or Billy), just as I won't let anyone hurt you." Obviously, all this might not be said at one time; the mother doesn't want to lecture the child, but comments of this type can be very helpful. Sometimes children cannot acknowledge their feelings openly. One child told her mother that her *doll* was very angry with *her* mother. Even though this child never acknowledged her own anger, the mother was able to deal with it by talking about it in terms of the way "most kids" feel.

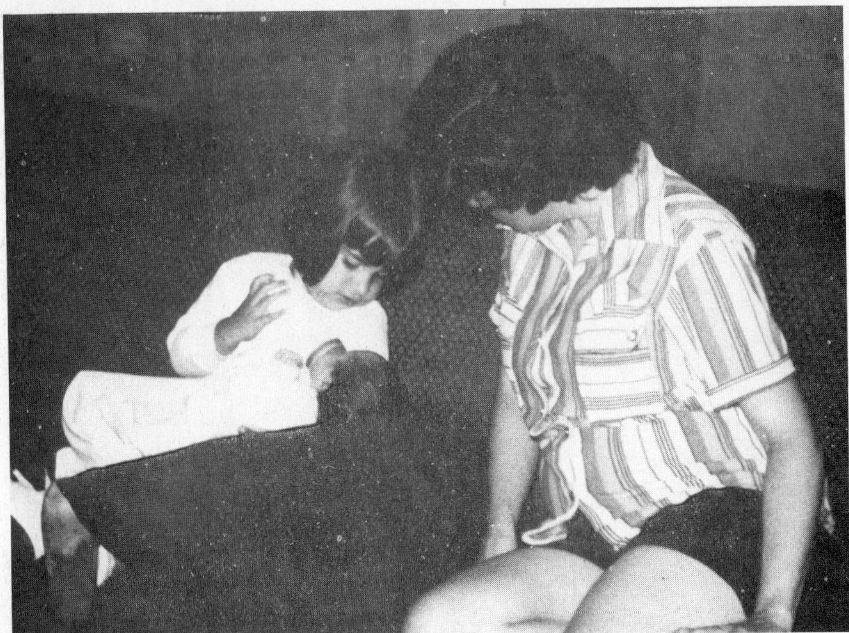

Figure 6-7 With the baby's head supported on a pillow and the mother sitting within reach, a toddler gives "her" baby a bottle.

Protecting the Baby Regardless of how hard parents try to help the older child cope with the situation, the reality of it is that there is another child in the family and the older child needs time to make appropriate adjustments. It is important for the parents to be aware of the potential for physical harm from the older child. The harm may or may not be intentional. For instance, a toddler could hurt a baby by dropping a hard toy into the baby's crib while actually trying to be nice and share his toys. In any event, it is probably wise to provide some kind of physical barrier between a toddler and an infant. Folding gates across the door to the baby's room will prevent a toddler or preschooler from entering the room without the mother's knowledge. The baby should also spend time with the total family, however. Placing the infant in the middle of a large playpen provides protection from accidental bumps and bruises. A young child probably should not be left in the same room with a baby without supervision. An infant should never be left on a chair or counter in an infant seat, as these are easily tipped over by curious toddlers.

Not all confrontations can be prevented by physical barriers, however. In the end, mothers will probably have to set definite limits on the older children's behavior. Rules need to remain consistent, just as they did before the baby's birth. Open defiance of household rules cannot be tolerated for

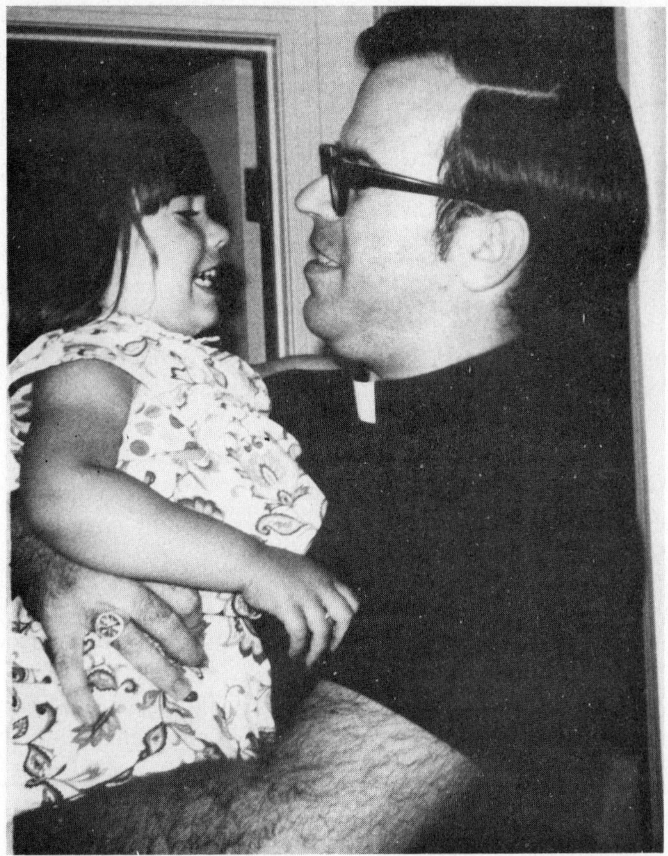

Figure 6-8 Special fun with Daddy helps to ease the adjustment of an older child to the addition of an infant to the family. Note that this child is wearing the maternity top her mother was wearing in Figure 6-4. This helps her to identify with her mother.

long if the family is to survive. While some leniency may be needed at first, it should be remembered that an older child receives security from the limits parents set and enforce consistently. Lots of praise for appropriate behavior will help take the sting out of the necessary reprimands.

Children's Concerns

Most children are concerned about physical differences between themselves and the baby. This is especially true if the two are of opposite sexes. Girls really do wonder why they do not have a penis, and boys, as well, may be concerned about a baby sister who does not have one. One little boy was very distressed when his mother changed his sister's diaper. Finally he blurted out, "Mommy, she don't have no teeth and no penis." Many children are worried about an umbilical cord which is still attached when the baby comes home. They need to know what it is and what its function was and that it is no longer needed, so that when it falls off they do not become alarmed.

It is interesting to note that children seem to go through an identification process in learning to relate to their brothers and sisters, just as their parents do. They like to touch the baby and to spend long periods looking at him. Sometimes they simply comment on the characteristics of the infant such as, "He has fingers and toes!" This may be especially true if they have not had much experience with young babies. If the baby smiles while the older child is watching (even though the smile is a nonspecific satisfaction response), it helps to tell the child that the baby likes him or her. This helps the older child form positive feelings for the infant, just as it helps mothers establish mutuality.

Visitors When friends come to see the new baby, there may be other problems to consider. Often they bring gifts to the infant, and the older child may feel even more neglected. Some mothers keep on hand some dime-store toys already wrapped up and ready to give to the older child. It is best that this is not done every time a gift is given to the baby, however, or the child will learn to expect it every time. The toys might also be used at other times to ward off restlessness or to reward especially good behavior.

Sometimes friends do rather thoughtless things. Children can be very deeply hurt when a special friend of theirs merely speaks to them and then spends all the time playing with the baby. Parents need to be especially alert to this possibility, as the child may either withdraw or suddenly become very "naughty." A technique frequently used by adults in relating to the older child when a baby is new is to ask if they can take the baby home with them. This can be very upsetting to older children because they secretly wish someone would do just that. Yet, if someone takes the baby away, what assurance would they have that it might not happen to them, too? Parents need to be very firm and direct in stating (for the child's benefit, as the adults obviously don't mean what they are saying) that no one will ever be allowed to take any of their children away from them.

Helping an older child accept a new brother or sister can be very trying for parents, but it also can be very interesting and satisfying, especially if the older child is old enough to share his or her thoughts and feelings.

REFERENCES

1 Grite Bibring, Thomas F. Dwyer, Dorothy S. Huntington, and Arthur F. Valenstein, "A Study of the Psychological Processes in Pregnancy and of the Earliest Mother-Child Relationship," *The Psychoanalytic Study of the Child,* vol. 16, 1959, pp. 9–72.

2 Reva Rubin, "Cognitive Style," *American Journal of Nursing,* March 1970, p. 505.

3 Ibid., p. 506.

4 Therese Benedek, "Fatherhood and Providing," in E. James Anthony and Therese Benedek (eds.), *Parenthood, Its Psychology and Psychopathology,* Little, Brown, Boston, 1970, p. 175.

5 Marshall H. Klaus and John H. Kennel, "Mothers Separated from Their Newborn Infants," *Pediatric Clinics of North America,* November 1970, pp. 1015–1037.

6 K. Robson, "The Role of Eye to Eye Contact in Maternal-Infant Attachment," *Journal of Child Psychology and Psychiatry,* May 1967, p. 13.

7 Theodore Litz, "Infancy," *The Person: His Development throughout the Life Cycle,* Basic Books, New York, 1968, 117–158.

8 Klaus and Kennel, op. cit.

9 Carol Ann Farrar, "A Data Collection Procedure to Assess Behavioral Individuality in the Neonate," *Journal of Obstetric, Gynecologic and Neonatal Nursing,* May/June 1974, pp. 15–20.

10 Lienne D. Tempesta, "The Importance of Touch in the Care of Newborns," *Journal of Obstetric, Gynecologic and Neonatal Nursing,* September–October 1972, pp. 27–28.

11 Ashley Montagu, "Tender, Loving Care," *Touching: The Human Significance of the Skin,* Harper & Row, New York, 1971, pp. 92–165.

12 Montagu, op. cit.

13 Alice Rossi, "Transition to Parenthood," *Journal of Marriage and the Family,* vol. 30, 1968, pp. 26–39.

14 Ibid., p. 32.

15 Sharon Serena Joseph and Rana Limbo Peck, "Postpartum Needs of the Family," in Joy Princeton Clausen, Margaret Hemp Flock, Bonnie Ford, Marilyn A. Green, and Elsa S. Popiel (eds.), *Maternity Nursing Today,* McGraw-Hill, New York, 1973, pp. 554–557.

16 Joy Clausen, "The Fourth Stage of Labor," in Joy Princeton Clausen, Margaret Hemp Flock, Bonnie Ford, Marilyn A. Green, and Elsa S. Popiel (eds.), *Maternity Nursing Today,* McGraw-Hill, New York, 1973, p. 531.

17 A. Doreen Jordan, "Evaluation of a Family-centered Maternity Care Hospital Program," *Journal of Obstetric, Gynecologic and Neonatal Nursing,* part I, January–February 1973, pp. 13–35; part II, March–April 1973, pp. 15–27.

18 Gerald Handel, "Sociological Aspects of Parenthood," in Debra P. Hymovich and Martha Underwood Barnard (eds.), *Family Health Care,* McGraw-Hill, New York, 1973, p. 90.

19 Barbara J. Williams, "Sleep Needs during the Maternity Cycle," in Mary H. Browning and Edith P. Lewis (comps.), *Maternal and Newborn Care: Nursing Interventions,* American Journal of Nursing, New York, 1973, pp. 34–39.

20 Edward J. Murray, "Personality Adjustment during Sleep Deprivation," *Sleep, Dreams, and Arousal,* Appleton-Century-Crofts, New York, 1965, pp. 211–246.

21 Michael Kahn, Bruce L. Baker, and J. M. Weiss, "Treatment of Insomnia by Relaxation Training," in Jerome Kagan, Marshall M. Haeth, and Catherine Caldwell (eds.), *Psychology: Adapted Readings,* Harcourt Brace Jovanovich, New York, 1971, p. 301.

BIBLIOGRAPHY

Benedek, Therese: "Fatherhood and Providing," in E. James Anthony and Therese Benedek (eds.), *Parenthood, Its Psychology and Psychopathology,* Little, Brown, Boston, 1970, pp. 167–183.

———: "Motherhood and Nurturing," in E. James Anthony and Therese Benedek (eds.), *Parenthood, Its Psychology and Psychopathology,* Little, Brown, Boston, 1970, pp. 153–165.

Bibring, Grite, Thomas F. Dwyer, Dorothy S. Huntington, and Arthur F. Valenstein: "A Study of the Psychological Processes in Pregnancy and the Earliest Mother-Child Relationship," *The Psychoanalytic Study of the Child,* vol. 16, 1959, pp. 9–72.

Bowman, Henry A.: *Marriage for Moderns,* McGraw-Hill, New York, 1970.

Brazelton, T. Berry: *Infants and Mothers,* Dell, New York, 1969.

Clausen, Joy: "The Fourth Stage of Labor," in Joy Princeton Clausen, Margaret Hemp Flock, Bonnie Ford, Marilyn A. Green, and Elsa S. Popiel (eds.), *Maternity Nursing Today,* McGraw-Hill, New York, 1973, pp. 527–552.

Committee on Public Education: *The Joys and Sorrows of Parenthood,* Group for the Advancement of Psychiatry, New York, 1973.

Farrar, Carol Ann: "A Data Collection Procedure to Assess Behavioral Individuality in the Neonate," *Journal of Obstetric, Gynecologic and Neonatal Nursing,* May/June 1974, pp. 15–20.

Handel, Gerald: "Sociological Aspects of Parenthood," in Debra P. Hymovich and Martha Underwood Barnard (eds.), *Family Health Care,* McGraw-Hill, New York, 1973, pp. 77–92.

Jessner, Lucie, Edith Weigert, James L. Foy: "The Development of Parental Attitudes during Pregnancy," in E. James Anthony and Therese Benedek (eds.), *Parenthood, Its Psychology and Psychopathology,* Little, Brown, Boston, 1970, pp. 209–244.

Jordan, A. Doreen: "Evaluation of a Family-centered Maternity Care Hospital Program," *Journal of Obstetric, Gynecologic and Neonatal Nursing,* part I, January–February 1973, pp. 13–35; part II, March–April 1973, pp. 15–27.

Joseph, Sharon Serena and Rana Limbo Peck: "Postpartum Needs of the Family," in Joy Princeton Clausen, Margaret Hemp Flock, Bonnie Ford, Marilyn A. Green, and Elsa S. Popiel (eds.), *Maternity Nursing Today,* McGraw-Hill, New York, 1973, pp. 553–614.

Kahn, Michael, Bruce L. Baker, and J. M. Weiss: "Treatment of Insomnia by Relaxation Training," in Jerome Kagan, M. Haeth Marshall, and Catherine Caldwell (eds.), *Psychology: Adapted Readings,* Harcourt Brace Jovanovich, New York, 1971, pp. 301–305.

Klaus, Marshall H., and John H. Kennel: "Mothers Separated from Their Newborn Infants," *Pediatric Clinics of North America,* November 1970, pp. 1015–1037.

Litz, Theodore: "Infancy," *The Person: His Development throughout the Life Cycle,* Basic Books, New York, 1968, pp. 93–116.

Maebius, Nancy K.: "The Nurse and the Expanding Family: A Mother's Viewpoint," in Debra P. Hymovich and Martha Underwood Barnard (eds.), *Family Health Care,* McGraw-Hill, New York, 1973, pp. 198–210.

Montagu, Ashley: *Touching: The Human Significance of the Skin,* Harper & Row, New York, 1971.

Murray, Edward J.: "Personality Adjustment during Sleep Deprivation," *Sleep, Dreams, and Arousal,* Appleton-Century-Crofts, New York, 1965, pp. 211–246.

O'Grady, Roberta S.: "Feeding Behavior in Infants," *American Journal of Nursing,* April 1971, pp. 736–739.

Robson, K.: "The Role of Eye to Eye Contact in Maternal-Infant Attachment," *Journal of Child Psychology and Psychiatry,* May 1967, pp. 13–25.

Rossi, Alice: "Transition to Parenthood," *Journal of Marriage and Family,* vol. 30, 1968, pp. 26–39.

Rubin, Reva: "Basic Maternal Behavior," *Nursing Outlook,* November 1961, pp. 683–686.

———: "Cognitive Style," *American Journal of Nursing,* March 1970, pp. 502–508.

———: "Puerperal Change," *Nursing Outlook,* December 1961, pp. 753–755.

Tempesta, Lienne D.: "The Importance of Touch in the Care of Newborns," *Journal of Obstetric, Gynecologic and Neonatal Nursing,* September–October 1972, pp. 27–28.

Williams, Barbara J.: "Sleep Needs during the Maternity Cycle," in Mary H. Browning and Edith P. Lewis (comps.), *Maternal and Newborn Care: Nursing Interventions,* American Journal of Nursing, New York, 1973, pp. 34–39.

Winnicott, Donald W.: "The Mother-Infant Experience of Mutuality," in E. James Anthony and Therese Benedek (eds.), *Parenthood, Its Psychology and Psychopathology,* Little, Brown, Boston, 1970, pp. 245–256.

Suggested Supplemental References on the Family

Bee, Helen L.: *Social Issues in Developmental Psychology,* Harper & Row, New York, 1974, part II, "Separation of Mother and Child, and Alternative Care," pp. 93–216; part III, "The Effects of Poverty," pp. 217–300.

Bernard, Jessie: *Marriage and Family among Negroes,* Prentice-Hall, Englewood Cliffs, N.J., 1966.

Browning, Mary H., and Edith P. Lewis (comps.): *Maternal and Newborn Care: Nursing Interventions,* American Journal of Nursing, New York, 1973, sec. V, "Adolescent and/or Unwed Parenthood," pp. 223–258.

Glasser, Paul H., and Lois N. Glasser: *Family in Crisis,* Harper & Row, New York, 1970. (Covers poverty, disorganization of the family, illness, and disability.)

Hymovich, Debra, and Martha Underwood Barnard (eds.): *Family Health Care,* McGraw-Hill, New York, 1973, sec. I, "The Family: General Considerations," pp. 1–166. (Covers family systems, law, sociology, economics, nursing, Mexican-American families, low-income families.)

Montagu, Ashley: *Touching: The Human Significance of the Skin,* Harper & Row, New York. 1972, sec. 7, "Culture and Contact," pp. 253–335.

Rainwater, Lee: *And the Poor Get Children,* Quadrangle, Chicago, 1960.

Reinhardt, Adina M., and Mildred D. Quinn (eds.): *Family-centered Community Nursing: A Sociocultural Framework,* Mosby, St. Louis, 1973. (Covers expanded role of the nurse, major behavioral science concepts, community dynamics, collaboration in providing services, Navajo Indians, Mexican-Americans, and Blacks.)

Satir, Virginia: *Peoplemaking,* Science and Behavior Books, Palo Alto, Calif. 1972. (Covers communication techniques helpful in dealing with families.)

Skolnick, Arlene: *The Intimate Environment: Exploring Marriage and the Family, and Instruction Manual,* Little, Brown, Boston, 1973. (Explores family as a problematic unit of society; looks at definitions, different life styles, and the impact of history and values on the family.)

——— and Jerome H. Skolnick: *Intimacy, Family, and Society,* Little, Brown, Boston, 1974, "The Parental Mystique," pp. 360–434. (Covers maternal role, parental guilt, battered children, day care.)

Sussman, Marvin B.: *Sourcebook in Marriage and the Family,* Houghton Mifflin, Boston, 1974, sec. 1, "Definitions, Meanings, and Networks of Families," pp. 1–42; sec. 2, "Nontraditional Family Forms in the 1970's," pp. 43–101 (covers open marriage, group marriage, communal family, one-parent family, complications of changing forms); sec. 5, "Family–Non-Family Linkages," pp. 233–301 (covers kinship bureacracy, low-income, health care, mental health).

Toffler, Alvin: *Future Shock,* Bantam, New York, 1971, chap. 11, "The Fractured Family," pp. 238–262.

Willie, Charles V. (ed.): *The Family Life of Black People,* Merrill, New York, 1970.

Chapter 7

The High-Risk Infant

The concept of the high-risk individual is a very useful one, but difficult to define. Basically, an individual is considered to be high-risk if he or she has a greater chance than average of developing a disease or other pathological condition (such as a congenital anomaly) or if his or her chances of survival are low. When one speaks of a high-risk pregnancy, one usually implies that the chances of delivering a normal term baby are somewhat less than average. A high-risk infant may be the product of such a high-risk pregnancy or may be the product of a "normal" pregnancy in which unexpected complications developed. Sometimes, also, an apparently normal term infant is designated a high-risk infant after birth because of some condition which develops then.

USEFULNESS OF DETERMINING RISK STATUS

The usefulness of designating high-risk individuals lies in the extra precautions that can be taken (1) to prevent pathology from occurring and/or (2) to provide the best possible medical management of conditions which cannot be prevented.

It is possible, for instance, to predict the probability of the occurrence of certain hereditary conditions (such as hemophilia). The prospective parents then can decide whether or not they want to take the risk of having a child. It is also possible through amniocentesis (withdrawal of some amnionic fluid to study the fetal cells floating in it) to determine whether or not a particular fetus is, indeed, affected by a major chromosomal abnormality, such as some forms of Down's syndrome. In such a case, the decision whether or not to terminate a pregnancy may be made with a reasonably accurate prediction of what the baby will be like if carried to term. In instances where blood incompatibility is the risk factor (such as when the mother is Rh negative and the father is Rh positive), it is possible through studies of maternal blood serum and the amnionic fluid to determine whether or not the fetus is affected by the problem, and to what extent. An affected fetus may be treated in utero to reverse some of the pathology, or the pregnancy may be terminated a few weeks before term in order to prevent permanent damage to the fetus. Mention has already been made of fetal monitoring as a means of identifying fetuses who are experiencing stress during labor and delivery so that medical intervention may prevent total decompensation. Preventive measures may be taken from another point of view, also. There are certain substances, such as some drugs and some viruses, which are known to be damaging to the fetus during the early weeks of development. Preventing contact of the mother with these substances is a way of preventing pathology from occurring in the fetus.

Sometimes it is not possible to prevent insult to the fetus. At such times, the aim of identifying the high-risk infant is to prevent the condition from worsening and to prevent the development of complications.

RISK FACTORS

The number of factors which may be cited in identifying a high-risk newborn is very great. Rather than attempt to list them all here, attention shall be turned to a brief explanation of how certain kinds of factors may cause damage, and to a summary of major classes of factors. A few illustrative examples of conditions will be given, but no attempt will be made to consider all possible conditions or even all the major ones. Those readers who wish to examine lists of causative agents should see Korones[1] or Klaus and Fanaroff[2] or other appropriate references.

GENETIC DAMAGE

Genetic damage can occur when the structure of either the genes or the chromosomes is altered. This alteration results in a change in the cellular proteins manufactured, since their manufacture is directed by the genes.

Cellular Proteins

Proteins in the form of enzymes govern all cellular activity. Organic proteins are long chains of amino acids called *polypeptide chains,* which have a peculiar "backbone" of polyglycine, glycine being one of the simplist amino acids. Other amino acids are attached to the backbone and laterally to each other to form filaments of matter which are looped and twisted to form complex organic proteins, often containing hundreds of amino acids.

The ability of the protein to function depends upon its molecules having the correct amino acids arranged in a specific order. An individual must have hundreds of thousands of correct proteins in order to live. How is the manufacture of these proteins determined?

Genes

The manufacture of proteins within the cell is controlled by the genes. Current theory holds that there are two kinds of genes: structural genes, which control protein manufacture, and regulator genes, which control the activity of the structural genes. (Not all genes are functional at the same time.) The structural genes are what are popularly called simply "genes," which control hair color, eye color, etc. We know now that they exert this control through determining the proteins that are made. According to the one gene–one protein theory, there is one gene for every protein manufactured by the body.

DNA

Structural genes may also be defined as *a linear segment of chromosomal DNA which controls the manufacture of one cellular protein.* DNA is the substance of the chromosomes. It forms a double strand of material bound laterally and longitudinally and spiraled around itself to form a helix which looks much like a twisted ladder (see Figure 7-1).

The DNA is formed of nucleotides. Nucleotides are submolecular units composed of a *phosphate group* [phosphoric acid (H_3PO_4) minus one, two, or three of its hydrogen atoms], a *simple sugar, and a group of atoms arranged into rings,* either a purine (one ring) or a pyrimidine (two rings). Each strand of DNA has a backbone made up of the sugar and phosphate groups. These backbones form the supports for the helix. Joining them together are the "ring" groups, the purines and pyrimidines, which are attached to each other so that each "rung" of the helix ladder is exactly three rings wide.

In DNA there are two *purines, adenine* (A) and *guanine* (G), and two *pyrimidines, cystosine* (C) and *thymine* (T). Since adenine, a purine, is always bonded to thymine, a pyrimidine, and guanine, a purine, is always bonded to cytosine, a pyrimidine, the three-ring width of the helix is maintained. During cellular reproduction (either mieosis or mitosis), the DNA helix

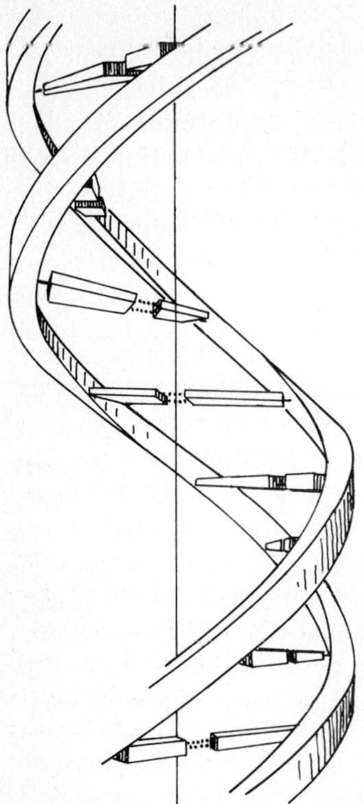

Figure 7-1 The DNA helix is like a spiral "ladder." (*From J. B. Stanbury et al., The Metabolic Basis of Inherited Disease, McGraw-Hill, New York, 1972, p. 31, by permission.*)

straightens out and the individual strands of DNA separate, and *replication* occurs. During replication, a complementary strand of DNA is produced for each of the two original strands. Each new chromosome that is formed by this process, then, should be an exact duplicate of the original one. Since a structural gene may be defined as a linear segment of chromosomal DNA which controls the manufacture of one cellular protein, and since the alignment of amino acids in the protein produced depends directly upon the alignment of the nucleotides in the gene, it becomes apparent that "correct" replication of chromosomal DNA is essential to the life of the individual.

Factors That May Affect Chromosomal Replication

There are many factors which may affect chromosomal (DNA) replication.[3] For instance, in cells experimentally starved of thymine, another compound, 5-bromouracil, may be substituted for thymine in the new DNA strands formed during replication. The nucleotide thus formed then combines with guanine rather than adenine, as thymine normally does. This process changes the resulting complementary DNA strand and thus would alter the protein whose manufacture is controlled by that gene.

Physical agents may also affect DNA. X-rays, for instance, may break DNA chains or alter one or more of the nucleotides. Thus drastic changes may occur in future generations of cells formed by the damaged DNA. If the damaged cells are the reproductive cells, the damage is passed on to future generations if indeed, survival is possible.

Factors That May Affect DNA Functional Influence

The functional influence of the DNA may also be altered, especially by viruses.[4] It is interesting to note here how viruses function in bacterial cells. (Presumably similar events occur when a virus invades a human cell.) The virus particle is essentially DNA contained within a protein coat. The virus attaches itself to the surface of the bacterium. (Specific viruses affect specific bacteria.) The protein coat of the virus remains outside the bacterial cell, but the DNA is injected into the cytoplasm. Because of factors that are not clearly understood, the cell then ceases to form proteins based on the bacterial DNA in the nucleus. Instead, it begins forming viral proteins and new viral DNA as directed by the viral DNA. Soon the new viral DNA and viral protein combine and new viruses are produced. The cell eventually bursts and the new viruses infect other cells. Possibly, a similar viral substitution of DNA is the mechanism through which virus infections of the embryo can cause the devastating congenital anomalies that some viruses cause. It is important to note here, however, that in order for the above sequence to occur, the cell must be *competent;* that is, it must be able to accept the viral DNA and function under its direction. Not all cells are competent. Those that are competent may be so only at certain stages in their life cycles. Thus, harmful viral infections of the fetus during the first trimester of pregnancy cause much more damage, as a rule, than the same viral infections in the third trimester.

Chromosomal Aberrations

Besides the changes that can occur due to damage or alteration in the DNA helixes, aberrations involving whole chromosomes may occur. Basically, there are two types of errors: either an excess of chromosomal material or an absence of some that should be present. According to Summitt and Atnip, at least 1 baby in every 200 that are born live has some significant chromosomal abnormality.[5] Either the excess of genetic material or its lack results in drastic consequences for the infant. Most are mentally retarded and many have physical deformities as well, if indeed, they survive at all. In addition, it is thought that in at least 25 percent of all spontaneous abortions, the fetus has a significant chromosomal abnormality.

Karyotypes Chromosomal abnormalities can be identified by microscopic studies of cells taken from the patient. The cells are cultured, and during the metaphase stage of mitosis (somatic cell division) the cells are "fixed," and microphotographs are taken. The chromosomes are visible microscopically, and individual chromosomes can be identified by their size and shape. The chromosomes in the microphotograph are cut out and placed in order according to a standard which has been developed. This arrangement is called a *karyotype* (see Figure 7-2). In the karyotype the chromosomes are arranged in pairs from the largest to the smallest. It is the assumption that in each pair there is one chromosome from each of the individual's parents. You will note that some of the chromosomes in Figure 7-2 are grouped rather than paired. Although the chromosomes which belong to these groups can be readily differentiated from others in other pairs or groups, individual pairs within the group cannot be differentiated with certainty. In the karyotype, there are 22 pairs of chromosomes which are numbered or grouped, plus an X and Y chromosome if the patient is male and two X chromosomes if the person studied is female. The 22 numbered pairs are called *autosomes,* and they are the same in both sexes. The unnumbered pair is the pair of sex chromosomes. Genetic disorders, those carried by genes alone, may not be identified by the study of a karyotype because

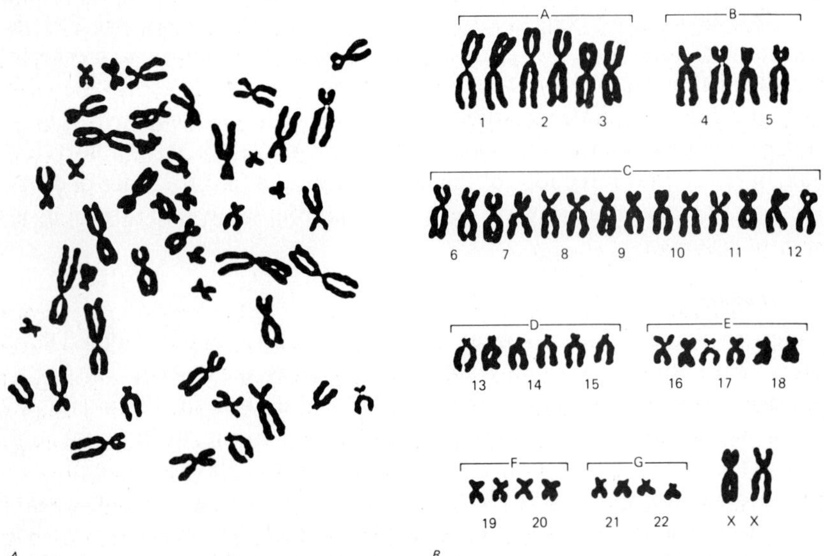

Figure 7-2 Human chromosomes are arranged to form a karyotype for chromosomal analysis. (*From G. Scipien et al., Comprehensive Pediatric Nursing, McGraw-Hill, New York, 1975, p. 89, by permission.*)

the genes themselves are not visible. Chromosomal disorders, however, can be diagnosed by this method.

Trisomy The most common form of chromosomal abnormality is the condition known as *trisomy*. In this condition, there are three chromosomes in one of the "pairs." The pathologic mechanism responsible for this condition is *nondisjunction*. During *meiosis* (gamete formation), when the chromosomes normally separate and migrate to opposite poles, one pair fails to do so, and both chromosomes of that pair migrate to the same pole. The resulting gametes would have either a total of 22 or 24 chromosomes, depending upon the daughter cell from which they develop. The first syndrome to be identified as being caused by autosomal trisomy (trisomy of chromosomes other than the sex chromosomes) is Down's syndrome. This trisomy involves the twenty-first pair of chromosomes and so is called trisomy 21. Children with Down's syndrome are mentally retarded, and they have a characteristic facial appearance and a number of other physical characteristics, including short hands and fingers and a wide space between the first toes of each foot. They are subject to a number of illnesses and usually require lifelong care.

Trisomy can also involve the sex chromosomes. In Turner's syndrome, for instance, a girl is born with only one X chromosome rather than the normal pair. These girls are sterile, and they generally have characteristic abnormalities, such as a broad chest with widely spaced nipples, short stature, webbed neck, low hair line in the back, and congential heart disease. Some of the girls are retarded as well. The ovaries are not present, and sexual development is minimal or does not occur at all. In Klinefelter's syndrome, male children are born with two or more X chromosomes in addition to the normal Y chromosome. These boys fail to develop normally at puberty, and they also are sterile. About one-fourth of them are mentally retarded. Other trisomies have been identified, but the mechanism behind them is essentially the same.

Translocation In some instances of Down's syndrome, trisomy is not present. Instead, the long arm of the "extra" chromosome of the twenty-first pair is attached to a nonhomologous chromosome in place of its short arm. This may occur spontaneously for no apparent reason, or the child may have a parent who is designated a *translocation heterozygote* but has no symptoms. The translocation heterozygote is a person who has only 45 chromosomes. One of the twenty-first pair is missing, but the long arm of the missing twenty-first chromosome is attached to another chromosome in place of its short arm. The translocation heterozygote has essentially the normal total genetic mass, since it is thought that the missing short arm of the recipient chromosome is insignificant in its genetic content. The children of a translocation heterozygote stand a 50-50 chance of being affected by the condition, depending upon which chromosomes they inherit.

Mosaicism Mosaicism is a condition in which the autosomal cells of an individual show more than one chromosomal pattern. The mechanism behind it is a *mitotic* nondisjunction that occurs after fertilization, resulting in abnormal numbers of chromosomes in different daughter cells. If the nondisjunction occurs in the first mitotic division of the fertilized egg, there will be two lines of cells in the individual, half with 47 chromosomes and half with 45. If the nondisjunction occurs later, there will be some cells with the normal component of chromosomes, and others with 47 chromosomes, and still others with 45 chromosomes. The resulting abnormalities will vary depending on the cells affected.

Deletion The loss of a whole chromosome does not seem to be compatible with life. In some instances, however, the loss of a part of a chromosome has been found in individuals showing mosaicism. The best-known syndrome of this type is the cri-du-chat syndrome, which derives its name from the peculiar cry of the infant, which sounds very much like that of a kitten. A portion of a chromosome in pair 5 is missing. The infant is mentally retarded and has both prenatal and postnatal growth retardation. A characteristic facial appearance is present along with shortening of the metacarpals and metatarsals.

Polyploidy Polyploidy is the condition of having a multiple of 23 chromosomes other than the normal 46. Triploidy (69 chromosomes) has been found in some severely retarded individuals. This condition is usually found in conjunction with mosaicism for the normal number of chromosomes. One child has been reported who had 92 chromosomes.[6]

The causes of chromosomal abnormalities have not been determined precisely, but maternal age seems to be a factor, as does irradiation of the gonads and possibly the ingestion of LSD or other drugs. A genetic predisposition to nondisjunction may occur, also, and viruses have been implicated in chromosomal damage in lower forms of life.

GENETIC COUNSELING

Genetic counseling is a form of counseling in which prospective parents are advised of their probability, based on family history and chromosomal studies, of producing a child with a chromosomal abnormality and/or a genetically inherited disease. Couples who seek this kind of counseling usually either have had a child with congenital anomalies or have a family history of a serious disease or abnormality.

If the condition under consideration is known to be a genetic one, such as cystic fibrosis, in which no chromosomal abnormalities are involved, then chromosomal studies are not done. Instead, a careful family history is taken and the couple is advised of the risk based on the laws of inheritance.

The Laws of Inheritance

For each gene in the autosomal chromosomes inherited from the mother there is a corresponding gene on the homologous chromosome inherited from the father. For a particular trait, if the gene inherited from one parent is dominant, the child will have the trait regardless of whether a corresponding like gene is inherited from the other parent. If the gene is recessive, however, the child must inherit like genes from both parents to inherit the trait. A slightly different condition is present in the sex chromosomes, however, in that the Y chromosome does not have as much genetic material the X chromosome because it is smaller. (The X chromosome is thought to carry the disease trait.) Recessive genes carried on the X chromosome will give the trait to all boys in which it is present, but not to girls who have inherited a corresponding "normal" gene on the X chromosome donated to them by their fathers. Girls could inherit a recessive trait carried on the X chromosome only if both the X chromosomes they receive carry the same recessive gene. Sex-linked dominant traits may be inherited when the dominant gene is inherited on only one X chromosome.

Some diseases are well known by their mode of inheritence. Osteogenesis imperfecta, a condition characterized by fragility of the skeletal system, is an autosomal dominant trait. Cystic fibrosis, a metabolic disease, is an autosomal recessive trait. Hemophilia is a sex-linked recessive trait, while a condition known as hypophosphatemic vitamin D–resistant rickets is a sex-linked dominant trait.

The risks for a particular couple depend upon both the mode of transmission and, in the case of sex-linked dominant conditions, whether it is the mother or father who is affected. In autosomal dominant traits, it is also important whether the affected parent is carrying dominant genes on both chromosomes or only one. At this time it is not possible to make this determination, since individual genes cannot be studied per se, but it is thought that in most cases, the affected parent has only one dominant gene for a disease condition. When this is true, there is a 50-50 chance that a particular child will have the trait. When the trait is autosomal recessive, the risks for any particular pregnancy is 25 percent, since the child must inherit the condition from both parents.

In sex-linked dominant traits, if the affected parent is the mother, there is a 50 percent risk with each pregnancy, since the trait is carried on the X chromosome, and she will give one X chromosome to each child. If the affected parent is the father, then none of his sons will carry the trait, but all his daughters will. An affected father cannot pass a sex-linked recessive trait on to his sons, but half his daughters will carry the gene in an asymptomatic form. A carrier daughter will pass the trait to half of her sons, on the average. Half of her daughters, on the average, will be normal and half will be carriers, as she is.

Genetic Counseling in Chromosomal Abnormalities

There is no way at this time to know whether or not a specific fetus is affected by a specific genetic trait, since specific gene analysis is not possible. It is possible, however, to identify with surety most of the chromosomal abnormalities from studies of fetal cells prior to the birth of the infant. In a procedure called *amniocentesis,* a needle is inserted, through the mother's abdominal wall, into the amnionic cavity and amnionic fluid is withdrawn. There are always some fetal cells floating in the amnionic fluid. These cells can be cultured and a karyotype of the fetus made. In this way it is possible to determine whether or not a given fetus is carrying a trisomy or a translocation. Such a study could make possible a decision for or against a therapeutic abortion, for instance.

In terms of future conceptions of children in families who have had one child with a chromosomal abnormality, chromosomal studies of the parents are important. For instance, if a child is born with Down's syndrome, it is very important for future planning to determine both the chromosomal makeup of the child and that of the parents. If Down's syndrome is caused by translocation in a particular child, it is important to discover whether one of the parents is a translocation heterozygote. If so, the risks of having a second child with the syndrome are 10 to 20 percent. (These rates do not follow the risk ratios of genetic inheritance.) On the other hand, if translocation is the cause and neither parent is a translocation heterozygote, then the chances of a recurrence are only 0.5 to 1.0 percent.[7]

If the cause of Down's syndrome is trisomy 21, the risk of recurrence is closely related to maternal age. The risk of a woman 15 to 24 years of age having a child with Down's syndrome is only 1 in 1,500. The risks for a woman over 44 years of age is 1 in 50. In such situations it is advisable to do chromosomal studies of all fetuses of subsequent pregnancies. In fact, Summitt and Atnip mention that it is recommended by many authorities that *any* woman who becomes pregnant after the age of 40 have chromosomal studies of the fetus done.[8]

PRENATAL AND POSTNATAL RISK FACTORS

Assuming that a normal ovum and a normal sperm are united to form a normal zygote, it is still possible for "things to go wrong." Tissues may fail to grow when they should; they may grow too much and thus distort the normal pattern; tissues that should be resorbed by the embryo may not be; those which should not be resorbed may be.

The causes for all the possible errors in development are not clear; however, a few large categories of risk factors have been identified. One type of risk factor has to do with the environment in which the embryo is developing. If the mother suffers from certain diseases, especially endocrine or metabolic disease, cardiovascular disease, renal disease, neoplastic disease, or anemia, the embryo is endangered. If the mother is unusually small in stature (less than 60 inches tall), if she is more than 20 percent over or under weight, or if she is over 35 or under 16 years of age at the time of conception, the infant is at risk. If the mother is exposed to toxins such as lead fumes or if she takes certain drugs or smokes heavily, the embryo is a high-risk embryo. If the mother is poorly nourished or if she comes from a poverty condition, the embryo is at risk. Some complications of pregnancy cause the infant to be considered high-risk. Such conditions as toxemia of pregnancy, polyhydramnios or oligohydramnios, or previous obstetric complications are examples of these factors. Risk factors during labor and delivery have been discussed in some detail in Chapter 4, Identification of Risk Factors, but to summarize them, any factor which decreases oxygenation of the fetus (such as maternal hypotension or uterine tetany), any factor which makes passage of the fetus through the pelvis more hazardous (such as contracted pelvis or abnormal lie of the fetus), preterm delivery, or delay of delivery past 42 weeks may put the infant at risk. Birth trauma, the development of sepsis, respiratory depression, or low Apgar scores are all examples of postdelivery risk factors.

Besides noting that a risk factor is present, it is also important to be aware of when the risk factor was introduced. Figure 7-3 shows critical periods of time that specific systems of the embryo are likely to be damaged.

The major categories of risk factors have been summarized in Table 7-1. The factors listed in the table, though not exhaustive, should serve as a guide for the nurse who is alert to the possibility of delivery of a high-risk infant. Nurses can play a major role in identification of high-risk infants both before and after their births.

IMPACT OF THE HIGH-RISK INFANT ON THE FAMILY

The birth of an infant is usually a joyful event. The delivery of a high-risk infant, in contrast, is usually an event associated with great fear and anxiety. Such fear and anxiety may influence the parent-child relationship for years to come.

In considering the reactions of parents to their high-risk infants, it seems helpful to consider three classes of high-risk infants: (1) those who seem essentially normal, but whose intact survival due to preterm or post-

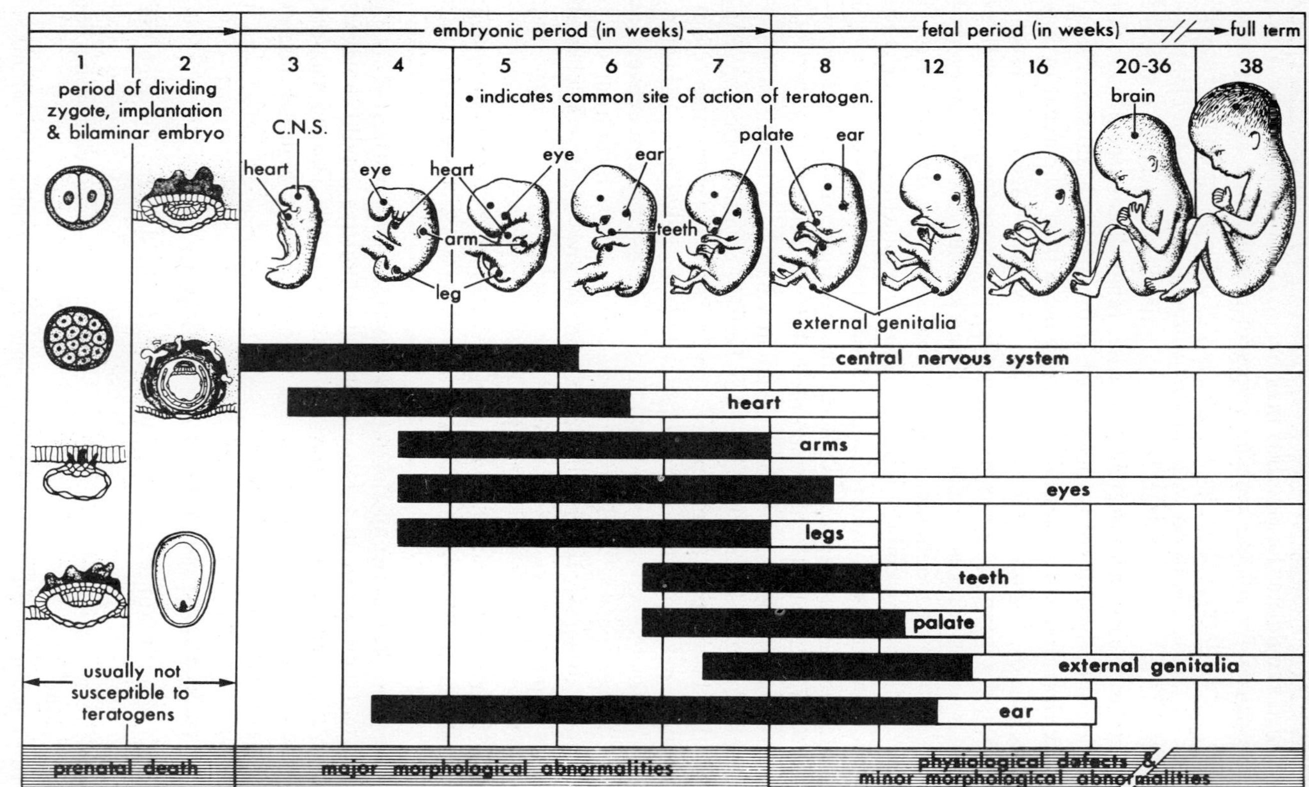

Figure 7-3 Body systems are most likely to be damaged seriously at specific critical times in fetal development. (*From K. L. Moore, Before We Are Born, Basic Embryology and Birth Defects, Saunders, Philadelphia, 1974, by permission.*)

Table 7-1 Risk Factors Summarized

Chronic maternal disease
Infection of the mother during the first trimester or at labor and delivery
Maternal ingestion of drugs other than those prescribed by the obstetrician
Exposure to industrial or other toxins
Less than optimal socioeconomic conditions
Extremes in maternal age (under 16 or over 35 years)
Previous or present obstetric complications
Complications of labor and delivery
Aberrations in growth-gestational age relationships or preterm or postterm delivery
Presence of multiple fetuses (twins, etc.)
Presence of anomalies or signs of illness in the infant after birth
Low Apgar score at 5 minutes
Abnormalities of the placenta or umbilical cord

term delivery or other high-risk factors is in question, (2) those who have obvious deformities or who have diagnosed genetic or chromosomal disorders, and (3) stillborns or those who die within the first minutes after birth.

Infants Whose Survival Is in Question

Infants in this group are those whose survival is in question for a number of hours or days, but for whom full, healthy lives can be expected if they do survive.

If the infant is preterm, the experience of the mother differs from that of the "normal" mother from the onset of labor. It has been noted that mothers in early labor seem unable to recognize the symptoms of labor.[9] They may have to rush to the hospital at the last minute. They frequently receive little or no medication during labor, and they are usually cared for with a sense of urgency and of concern for the outcome. The mother sees the worried looks on the faces of personnel, whether or not she overhears their hushed conversations. When the baby does arrive, he or she may or may not cry right away. Usually the infant is rushed to a special-care nursery before the mother has a chance to see him or her, and often she is separated from the baby for several days, if not weeks, after birth. The mother may or may not be given information about the infant's condition and prognosis. She spends many lonely hours as other mothers receive their babies for feedings several times a day. In the meantime, she is struggling to cope with the sense of loss she is experiencing. She was not ready to separate from her infant. She had not had time to deal with the developmental task of separation. She will probaby be in a state of shock and grief for some time. In addition, her husband is experiencing a grief reaction.

These parents, like those of any infant whose survival is in question, seem to be held in suspended animation. They cannot move forward to establish affectional bonds with the child because they fear the possible loss. They cannot begin grieving because survival is still a possibility. They may vacillate emotionally from strong hope of survival and certainty of a bright future to deep depression and fear of loss. These parents especially need frequent, truthful information on how the infant is progressing. Keeping them "in the dark" does not protect them; rather, it gives them no reality with which to relate, leaving them at the mercies of their fantasies. Giving them false reports of progress or false reassurrance is cruel and unkind and is usually done to spare personnel the problem of dealing with their own feelings. If death occurs, it is much easier to accept if its possibility has been realistically anticipated than if the possibility of death has been denied. Many parents wish to see and touch their infants, even when they are not expected to live. This is generally thought to be advisable if the parents wish it, since it helps them cope with a real baby or a real loss rather than a fantasy. Seitz and Warrick state very emphatically that this indeed is a parent's right and privilege, not to be denied.[10] Sandra Eckes emphasizes the need for infant-parent contact in preparing parents to care for the infant after discharge.[11]

Psychological Tasks of the Parents There are basically four psychological tasks of the parents of infants whose survival is in question. First, they must tolerate and cope with what David Kaplan terms a "withdrawal-hope conflict."[12] Second, they must come to terms with their failure to produce a healthy, term baby. This is particularly true in the case of the birth of a preterm infant, whose physical appearance may be very disappointing. Third, they must begin to establish affectional bonds when the infant's survival is assured, or they must begin the grief process in the case of his death. And finally, they must deal with the temporary precautions needed for the care of the infant because of his high-risk condition and begin relating to him as a totally normal child when this is appropriate, or they must work through the grief process and move on to accept the loss in the event of the infant's death. It is important that these tasks are accomplished in the order they are presented here. Fathers generally go through the same stages as mothers, though their pace may differ from the mother's depending upon the amount of contact they have with their infants and with the health care team.

Gerald Caplan has identified parental behaviors and categorized them as either healthy or unhealthy in terms of expected future outcomes.[13] Healthy responses include the seeking of specific information about the infant's condition and prognosis and the recognition and acceptance of negative feelings about the infant and his birth. Unhealthy responses include both denial of the seriousness of the infant's condition and movement into a state of anticipatory grief with the conviction that the infant will die imminently or in early childhood. If the mother progresses to the state of anticipatory grief, she tends to withdraw from the infant and may lose the bonds of attachment established by fusion during pregnancy. She tends to avoid any contact with the infant and does not attempt to find out about his or her progress. Personnel may interpret such behavior as evidence that she does not care about her child, when in reality, she cares so much that she cannot bear to face the possibility of loss. This mother needs a lot of help in reestablishing a relationship with her infant.

Other parental behaviors have been identified as signifying probable future problems[14]: the inability to respond with hope once the baby begins to improve, the inability to share with each other their fears and negative feelings about the baby, and the inability to utilize the support which is available. The lack of available support systems within the family or the community also puts the family at risk.

The Parent-Child Relationship There is evidence that the relationships of preterm infants and their parents are different from the relationships of term infants and their parents. Although extensive studies have not been done, it is frequently observed that parents of infants or children who have been seriously ill early in their lives have great difficulty relating to their infants as they get older. These parents find it especially hard to set limits on the children's behavior and may tolerate extremely disruptive and aggressive behavior. Ironically, the same parents may find it hard to give their children the normal freedoms in playing with other children and in developing skills of independence. Many times these parents become unduly concerned with bodily functions and may worry about a minor illness long after the child has recovered from it.

In addition to the above general observations about parent-child relationships, several specific syndromes have been observed to be highly associated with preterm delivery. One such syndrome is the failure-to-thrive syndrome, a puzzling failure of the infant to grow normally when no organic reason can be found. In its extreme, the infant may die. Infants who are institutionalized soon after birth frequently suffer from severe forms of this syndrome and very often do not survive. Infants cared for by their mothers usually do not exhibit such severe growth retardation, but they may require hospitalization and special care. Since these babies usually do well in the hospital setting, the syndrome is thought to be due to disturbances in the mother-child relationship.

In addition, many battered children were preterm infants. Klaus and Fanaroff feel that the reason for this disturbance of the mother-child relationship, as well as many others, is the separation from their infants usually experienced by these mothers.[15] It is hypothesized that affectional bonds fail to become established adequately.

Physical Separation from the Infant Much concern has been expressed in recent literature about the effects of the separation of parents from their high-risk infants on the formation of affectional bonds, especially between mother and child. Experimentation with animals has shown that there is, for many species, a period of time soon after birth when the mother and her offspring must be together physically if she is to accept and care for it later. Although the work with human mothers is not conclusive, there is considerable evidence that physical separation for a prolonged period after birth may indeed affect the responses of the mothers as they begin to care for their infants.[16] Of particular importance is the ability to have eye contact with the infant. Especially important is assumption of the "enface" position, with the mother's and infant's eyes meeting in the same vertical plane. (See Figure 6-1.) This eye-to-eye contact is possible as early as the first period of reactivity, immediately after birth. Such contact is thought to stimulate the formation of affectional bonds with the infant and to encourage caretaking responses. Klaus and Faronoff have found that mothers who were allowed to enter the high-risk nursery and touch their infants soon after delivery and throughout their stay there showed more warmth and responsiveness to their infants as late as 6 months after delivery than mothers who were denied entrance to the nursery.[17] The question is far from settled, but there seems to be a definite trend toward encouraging increased contact between mothers and their newborn infants.

Assisting the Family in Coping with a Preterm Delivery

Louise Warrick has written an article that is of agreat value in planning care for the family of the high-risk infant.[18] In it she describes care as it is given at New York Hospital–Cornell University Medical Center. The student or nurse responsible for helping parents should read the original article; but briefly, the nursing care as she describes it is as follows.

To begin with, parents are encouraged to spend as much time as possible with their infants. (They are barred from the nursery only when they are ill or if there is infectious disease in their home.) While the mother is still in the hospital, the nursery nurse visits her and assesses her emotional state and the attitude she has about her experience and her infant. This assessment includes a review of the mother's perceptions and feelings about the labor and delivery experience. (The mother cannot focus on the baby until she has incorporated the labor and delivery experience into her life.) If the mother did not hear her baby cry, or if she saw him only as a limp blue baby, the infant's ability to function normally is explained (realistically). A booklet explaining the nursery procedures and equipment is given to the mother, and the nurse goes over it with the mother if she is ready to discuss it. A very important principle of care is to pace the teaching to the mother's readiness to learn.

On the first visit to see the baby in the nursery, the nurse assigned to the family accompanies the mother and, if possible, the father, as well. Mothers' responses to the nursery vary widely. Some mothers will want to be physically close to their babies immediately. Others are afraid to cross the threshhold of the doorway. The nurse explains to the mother the normal lag in maternal feelings, especially if the infant's condition is guarded or if the mother has experienced a long period of separation.

It is particularly important to note the mother's verbal comments about the infant's appearance. If the mother describes the infant in terms of animal characteristics, such as "a skinned chicken," or in terms of a corpse, it is felt that she is not ready to be encouraged to care for the child. Rather, the nurse should focus her attentions on the mother's feelings about herself as a wife and mother, being especially attentive to expressions of guilt or depression. Only after the mother works through such feelings can she turn her attention to the care of her infant.

On the initial visit to the nursery, if the mother does not wish to touch the infant, the nurse undresses the baby. Together, the nurse and the mother examine the infant, carefully noting his or her completeness and normal function. When the mother begins to touch her infant, she starts with poking motions (fingering) and then gradually progress to palmar and full-hand contact. Some mothers progress through these stages in a few minutes; others may take several days or possibly several weeks to make the same progression. It is important to allow the mother to proceed at her own rate and not to rush her.

After the mother is comfortable with physical contact with her infant, the nurse may help the mother particpate in mothering procedures, such as feeding the infant. At this time, too, it will be observed that the mother begins the work of identifying her infant. The "corner has been turned" when the baby is perceived to have his father's nose or her grandmother's eyes, rather than looking liked a "drowned rat." Then, the nurse knows that the mother has begun building a healthy mother-child relationship and can take on more responsibility for the infant's care.

At this time the mother will usually share spontaneous comments such as, "It is so good to know he is going to make it," and she begins to make concrete plans for the infant's homecoming. The nurse can help by pointing out to the mother the little steps of progress that the infant makes, such as a decrease in the amount of oxygen needed or the discontinuation of an intravenous feeding. Soon the mother will begin interacting with the infant and talking in the intimate relaxed way mothers usually talk to their newborns.

While the attention has been focused on the mother and infant, the father is included in care when possible. Brothers and sisters of the infant are not forgotten, either. Pictures may be taken by the parents to take home to the older children to help them cope with their disappointment in not having a baby at home. If pictures of their infant would be too disturbing, a standardized picture of a preterm infant is given to the parents. The children need to be told that negative feelings they might have had about the coming baby could not have influenced the early arrival. Children can carry a tremendous burden of guilt because of their inability to understand cause-and-effect relationships in instances like this. They need to know, also, that what happened to the baby cannot happen to them, as they may not understand this point. After the frightening equipment is removed from the infant, the siblings are encouraged to visit the hospital and view the infant through the nursery window. The children should be encouraged, also, to help in the preparations for the infant to come home.

Early contact between parent and infant is to be encouraged. However, there may be problems as a result of the infant's immaturity. Johnson and Grubbs point out that while early contact between mother and infant is desirable, some of the characteristics of the preterm infant may be very frightening to the mother if she has not been prepared for them.[19] An exaggerated Moro reflex, for instance, may convince the mother that her touch causes the infant pain. A mother who believes this understandably decreases the amount of physical contact she has with the infant, to the detriment of both the mother-infant relationship and the infant's later development. The generally poor respiratory efforts of the infant along with the use of monitors may convice the mother that the infant will never be dependable in maintaining respiratory function. Some mothers are afraid to take their infants home for this reason. Others have been known to sleep with their infants for months at home so that they will have them close by in case they stop breathing.

The infant may be especially unable to reward the mother for her eager ministrations. If, for instance, the infant cannot suck well, she may be unsuccessful in feeding him, or may have to wait several days or even weeks before she is allowed to try. Fear that the infant may choke may continue long after choking ceases to be a realistic problem. Some mothers are especially disappointed when their infants, due to immaturity of the grasp reflex, fail to hold their fingers when they place them in the baby's hand.

Nurses must be constantly aware of mothers' expectations and strive to help them base their expectations on realistic data and knowledge of their infant's true condition. It is especially helpful for the mother to learn to evaluate her mothering skills in terms of her baby's specific abilities to respond, rather than the abilities of the average term newborn.

Emotional Needs of the Infant While attention is often directed to the infant's physical survival and to the needs of the parents, it is vital that the infant's emotional needs not be overlooked. The basic task of the infant is to establish a sense of trust in his or her environment and to begin to perceive human interaction as a pleasurable experience. It is difficult for the infant to do this when so much of this experience is negative—being poked and prodded, injected, and infused. The infant may even become conditioned to anticipate pain rather than pleasure when a person approaches the incubator, because so often such an approach heralds some form of discomfort. Some infants who have been treated for high-risk conditions do indeed demonstrate behaviors that would indicate such conditioning.[20] They prefer to look at ceiling lights rather than at the person caring for them, and they may decrease their crying behavior as though in a state of depression.

Besides the uncomfortable experiences, the infant may also be denied the normal pleasures, such as sucking, cuddling, and visually exploring the environment. (His vision may be greatly distorted by the sides of the incubator.) The infant may be bombarded with auditory stimuli and at the same time unable to hear clearly her mother's voice, due to the noise of the incubator motor and other nursery noises.

Attempts have been made to remedy some of these problems by the use of water beds and by the introduction of recordings of maternal heart beats and voices into the incubator. Much more work needs to be done. Nurses are in a position to contribute significantly to research in this area.

Infants with Obvious Defects

The parents of infants with obvious defects may have profound problems with which to deal. Some defects are totally correctable, others partially, and many not at all. The basic process through which the parents must pass is similar to that of parents of "normal" preterm infants, however, and the degree of the reaction of the parents may not be related directly to the severity of the defect. Some parents may react very intensely to the presence of a correctable foot deformity, whereas other parents may be able to accept the presence of a facial deformity with surprising equanimity. The prior relationship between the parents, their maturity, the meaning which this particular child holds for them, and the significance to them of the affected part all affect their reaction. Generally, visible deformities are harder to accept than internal ones, and facial deformities are harder to accept than those involving other parts of the body. All parents whose babies have an anomaly, however, must work through a grief process. They must mourn the loss of the expected perfect child and learn to accept the reality of the child they have delivered. If the infant's survival is in question they must deal, in addition, with the tension of the hope for its survival and the wish for its death. Many parents are alarmed to discover that at some time they do indeed wish for the death of their severely handicapped infant. They must be told that this is a normal and expected reaction, if they are to deal with their guilt satisfactorily.

The Grief Process: The Shock Phase The grief process has been described in a number of different but similar phases. The initial reaction is one of shock and denial. The resulting feeling of numbness may last from several hours to several days and may recur at intervals for a period of weeks. For some parents of a child with serious congenital anomalies, a degree of denial may become a part of the relationship between the parent and child. The relationship between a mother and her 8-year-old child with hyperteliorism (widely spaced eyes) and related mild retardation is a good example of this denial. This mother told the worker at the mental health center where she had taken the child for testing that surgery was scheduled which would make this child look just like her 10-year-old sister (who was a very pretty, normal child). This same mother, also, became very angry when testing indicated that the child was indeed mildly mentally retarded. Rather than place her in the recommended special education program in the public school, the mother tried to get her enrolled in a private school for average to very bright children. She insisted that the child would do well in school if only she got the right teacher. Mercer indicates in her work that the use of fantasies to accomplish denial is a fairly common method of coping with anomalies.[21] These fantasies usually take the form of an expectation of perfect surgical correction or superior compensatory intellectual development.

Unrealistic fantasies of this type should never be reinforced with false reassurance. Nor should they be "jerked away" from the parents by harsh argument or brutal presentation of "the facts." Rather, the parent should be led gently and kindly toward acceptance of the realities that exist. Such comments as, "After surgery there will be a scar, but it will fade in time," or "Jimmy may never have full use of his left hand, but he will learn to compensate with his right one," are examples of the kinds of statements that may be helpful in bringing parents back to reality. It is, perhaps, more helpful in the *immediate* neonatal period to accept unrealistic expectations of the child's later years just as one accepts the presentation of a baseball glove to a 2-day-old infant boy. Many parents need to deny the reality of their child's defects early in their relationship, because they are just beginning to react to what has happened to them. All parents of children with serious defects need continued contact with knowledgeable professionals throughout their child's life, or at least until a repairable defect has been corrected. Then, ironically, the parent's biggest problem may be in accepting the normality of their child.

Awareness of Reality When the parents finally begin to relate to the reality of their defective child, they will go through three phases described by Kubler-Ross as the "why me?" phase, the "If I" phase, and the "How can I?" phase.[22]

The "Why me?" phase is primarily one of intense anger which may be directed toward God or Fate, toward medical personnel, toward the spouse, or toward the infant. If the infant survives, this anger may become a frequently expressed component of the parent-child relationship as the parent deals not only with the normal frustrations of parenthood, but also with the added financial and physical strain of caring for a child with a defect. Parents need to know that anger is normal in this situation, and they need to learn to deal with it in ways that are not harmful either to themselves or to their child. So many people have been conditioned to believe that "good parents" never become angry with their children that they fail to deal realistically with the normal anger component of parenting. Parents of children with birth defects may feel so much guilt that they are unable to accept even the possibility that they might feel angry. These parents frequently fail to set limits for their children, and, indeed, they may allow the child to tyrannize them.

The "If I" phase is basically one of fantasy. The parents may try to figure out what they did wrong that caused the problem, and they may also attempt to work out a bargain through which some sort of penance on their part will restore wholeness to the child. Tactfully pointing out that the mother's failure to eat liver could not have caused a cleft lip, or that accepting no social invitations for the next year will have no affect on the child's condition, may be helpful.

The "How can I?" phase is primarily a period of depression during which the parents feel they are totally unable to cope with the reality of their child. Staying with the parents and encouraging them to express their feelings are helpful during this time. Crying should not only be permitted, but indeed encouraged. Most parents feel a blow to their self-esteem as parents and individually as men and women when they produce a less than perfect child.

During this time the parents may not have any energy for even looking at their child, let alone trying to care for him. Responsibilities should not be pushed on them when they are depressed, but some activity, even if only walking in their room or going to the lounge for a cup of coffee, may be helpful in mobilizing their energies to move out of the depression. Helping them see their strengths and planning care so that they can have small successes, perhaps in just caring for their own needs at first, will help them through this period. One of the tasks of parents during this stage of grief is to emancipate themselves from the fantasized perfect child which they had expected. In order to do this, they need to relive these fantasies over and over and to tell and retell stories about the pregnancy and labor and delivery. Personnel should encourage these kinds of expressions as evidence that grief work is being done.

Acceptance of Reality Finally, ideally, the parents will begin to accept reality. This is a process that has to be continued throughout the child's lifetime. For some parents, as the child reaches each of the major milestones of development, the grief process must begin over and over, as they realize the child's limitations. One father of a retarded child described his life as one of "chronic sorrow." Acceptance of reality, then, is not a sudden flash of insight and understanding, but rather a long and usually a painful process. The degree of acceptance likely to be observed during a short hospital maternity stay is small indeed. Planning for the immediate care of the child is about the best that can be hoped for in such a short time. It seems unfortunate that so often discharge from the hospital means the end of frequent contact with nurses who could be so helpful to these parents.

The Infant Who Is Stillborn or Dies Soon after Birth

Discovery that she is carrying a dead child is a very painful and traumatic experience for any woman.[22] Most mothers hope that there has been something wrong with the diagnosis and that in the end everything will be all right. Some accept the doctor's diagnosis and simply wish for the ordeal to be over. Some strongly deny the doctor's diagnosis and continue to plan for the baby as though everything were fine. For all these mothers, the experience of labor and delivery will be a traumatic event. They may be very afraid of what they will deliver, and they will feel the futility of having to experience the stresses of labor when they know there is no hope for the infant. Staff personnel, too, may find that working with these mothers is very hard on them emotionally. Unfortunately, many times they avoid the mother in order to avoid their own pain. These mothers will go through the same grief process described above, but for them there is no baby to take home. It has been found that they need to know something about their babies, however, such as the color of hair, sex, and weight.[23] They may wish to see their baby. Seitz and Warrick feel they should be allowed to do so if they wish, with some preparation as to what they are likely to see.[24] Then they can relate to the dead infant as a person, rather than as a monster of some sort. Usually fantasies are much worse than reality in this regard. Parents whose infants die shortly after birth experience the grief process, just as do parents of stillborns.

The Needs of Siblings The needs of siblings of the stillborn must be considered also. They, too, have been looking forward to the expected baby. It is especially important that they not be left out of the grief process. The common reaction of the grieving parents is to "spare" the children. In reality, by not sharing their grief, they only isolate the children and teach them that there are some things that cannot be discussed between them. Children need to know that they are in no way responsible for the death of the baby and that they are in no danger of dying. It is especially important that they not be sent away for the duration of the crisis. They need to know that they will always be an important part of the family and that their parents still love and care about them. It is best, also, that they not be told a "story" rather than the truth about the baby's death, as they are likely to be confused by anything but the simplest facts. Children can often handle such a crisis more philosophically than can their parents. Sometimes their attitude can actually be a comfort to their parents.

REFERENCES

1 Sheldon B. Korones, *High Risk Newborn Infants: The Basis for Intensive Nursing Care,* Mosby, St. Louis, 1972, pp. 38–42.

2 Marshall H. Klaus and Avroy A. Fanaroff (eds.), *Care of the High-Risk Neonate,* Saunders, Philadelphia, 1973, pp. 314–416.

3 Mahlon B. Hoagland, "Coding, Information Transfer, and Protein Synthesis," in John B. Stanbury, James B. Wyngaarden, and Donald S. Frederickson (eds.), *The Metabolic Basis of Inherited Disease,* McGraw-Hill, New York, 1972, p. 35.

4 Ibid.

5 Robert L. Summitt and Robert L. Atnip, "Autosomal Abnormalities," in James G. Hughes (ed.), *Synopsis of Pediatrics,* Mosby, St. Louis, 1971, p. 71.

6 Ibid., p. 92.

7 Ibid., pp. 79–80.

8 Ibid., p. 74.

9 Don R. Dubois, "Indications of an Unhealthy Relationship between Parents and Premature Infants," *Journal of Obstetric, Gynecologic and Neonatal Nursing,* May/June 1975, p. 22.

10 Pauline M. Seitz and Louise H. Warrick, "Perinatal Death: The Grieving Mother," *American Journal of Nursing,* November 1974, pp. 2028–2033.

11 Sandra Eckes, "The Significance of Increased Early Contact between Mother and Newborn Infant," *Journal of Obstetric, Gynecologic and Neonatal Nursing,* July/August 1974, pp. 42–44.

12 Dubois, loc. cit.

13 Gerald Caplan, Edward Mason, and David Kaplan, "Four Studies of Crisis in Parents of Prematures," *Community Mental Health Journal,* Summer 1965, p. 153.

14 Dubois, op. cit., p. 23.

15 Marshall Klaus and John Kennell, "Care of the Mother," in Klaus and Fanaroff (eds.), op. cit., p. 106.

16 Ibid., pp. 98–118.

17 Ibid., p. 102.

18 Louise H. Warrick, "Family-centered Care in the Premature Nursery," *American Journal of Nursing,* November 1971, pp. 2134–2138.

19 Suzanne Hall Johnson and Judith Pierson Grubbs, "The Premature Infant's Reflex Behaviors: Effect on Maternal-Child Relationships," *Journal of Obstetric, Gynecologic and Neonatal Nursing,* May/June 1975, pp. 15–20.

20 Jane M. Brightman and Stephanie Clatworthy, "Care of the High-Risk Infant and His Family," in Joy Princeton Clausen, Margaret Hemp Flock, Bonnie Ford, Marilyn M. Green, and Elsa S. Popiel (eds.), *Maternity Nursing Today*, McGraw-Hill, New York, 1973, p. 861.

21 Ramona T. Mercer, "Mother's Responses to Their Infants with Defects," *Nursing Research,* March/April 1974, pp. 133–137.

22 Seitz and Warrick, op. cit., p. 2028.

23 Sylvia Bruce, "Reactions of Nurses and Mothers to Stillbirths," *Nursing Outlook,* February 1962, pp. 88–91.

24 Seitz and Warrick, op. cit., pp. 2031–2032.

BIBLIOGRAPHY

Bruce, Sylvia: "Reactions of Nurses and Mothers to Stillbirths," *Nursing Outlook,* February 1962, pp. 88–91.

Caplan, Gerald, Edward Mason, and David Kaplan: "Four Studies of Crisis in Parents of Prematures," *Community Mental Health Journal,* Summer 1965, pp. 149–160.

Dubois, Don R.: "Indications of an Unhealthy Relationship between Parents and Premature Infants," *Journal of Obstetric, Gynecologic and Neonatal Nursing,* May/June 1975, pp. 21–24.

Eckes, Sandra: "The Significance of Increased Early Contact between Mother and Newborn Infant," *Journal of Obstetric, Gynecologic and Neonatal Nursing,* July/August 1974, pp. 42–44.

Goodman, Melainie Balestra: "Two Mother's Reactions to the Deaths of Their Premature Infants," *Journal of Obstetric, Gynecologic and Neonatal Nursing,* May/June 1975, pp. 25–27.

Hardgrove, Carol, and Louise H. Warrick: "How Shall We Tell the Children?" *American Journal of Nursing,* March 1974, pp. 448–450.

Hoagland, Mahlon B.: "Coding, Information Transfer and Protein Synthesis," in John B. Stanbury, James B. Wyngaarden, and Donald S. Fredrickson (eds.), *The Metabolic Basis of Inherited Disease,* McGraw-Hill, New York, 1972, pp. 29–51.

Johnson, Suzanne Hall, and Judith Pierson Grubbs: "The Premature Infant's Reflex Behaviors: Effect on Maternal-Child Relationship," *Journal of Obstetric, Gynecologic and Neonatal Nursing,* May/June 1975, pp. 15–20.

Klaus, Marshall H., and Avroy A. Fanaroff (eds.): *Care of the High-Risk Neonate,* Saunders, Philadelphia, 1973.

——— and John Kennell: "Care of the Mother," in Marshall H. Klaus and Avroy A. Fanaroff (eds.), *Care of the High-Risk Neonate,* Saunders, Philadelphia, 1973, pp. 98–118.

Korones, Sheldon B.: *High-Risk Newborn Infants: The Basis for Intensive Nursing Care,* Mosby, St. Louis, 1972.

Mercer, Ramona T.: "Mother's Responses to Their Infants with Defects," *Nursing Research,* March-April 1974, pp. 133–137.

———: "Two Fathers' Early Responses to the Birth of a Daughter with a Defect," *Maternal-Child Nursing Journal,* Summer 1974, pp. 77–86.

Seitz, Pauline M., and Louise H. Warrick: "Perinatal Death: The Grieving Mother," *American Journal of Nursing,* November 1974, pp. 2028–2033.

Summitt, Robert L., and Robert L. Atnip: "Autosomal Abnormalities," in James G. Hughes (ed.), *Synopsis of Pediatrics,* Mosby, St. Louis, 1971, pp. 70–95.

Warrick, Louise H.: "Family-centered Care in the Premature Nursery," *American Journal of Nursing,* November 1971, pp. 2134–2138.

Chapter 8

Care of the Normal Preterm Infant

CLASSIFICATION OF NEWBORN INFANTS

The identification of the "premature infant" has until recently been a relatively simple matter. Any infant who weighed less than 2,500 g (5½ lb) was considered to be premature. As neonatology has developed, however, it has become evident that such a simple means of classifying infants is highly inadequate. In its place, there is developing now an elaborate system for classifying newborn infants. Three basic parameters are usually considered: gestational age, weight, and intrauterine growth pattern.

Gestational Age

Gestational age is most often calculated from the mother's memory of the first day of the last normal menstrual period preceding the pregnancy. It should be noted, however, that the difference between the menstrual age and the fertilization age of the fetus may vary as much as a week even when the mother's memory is accurate. In addition, there is often some inaccuracy in the mother's memory, unless she happens to write down the date, or unless she is especially aware of it for some other reason. When the mother's accuracy is questionable, the gestational age may be estimated by the obstetrician by such criteria as the size of the uterus (early in the pregnancy) or the date of the first audible heart sounds (20 weeks with an ordinary stethoscope)[1] or by an elaborate scoring system applied to the infant after birth. The gestational age may also be estimated by studies of certain components of the amnionic fluid, by fetal x-rays, and by ultrasound studies of fetal size. *Calculated* gestational age refers to the age as determined by the mother's memory of dates, and *estimated* gestational age refers to the estimates made by the obstetrician or based upon assessment of the infant after birth. The World Health Organization recommends that the age given refer to completed weeks of gestation.[2] Hence, gestational age of 34 weeks means that the infant has completed 34 weeks of development but has not yet reached 35 weeks of age. The nomenclature denoting gestational age has eliminated the term *premature* because it is generally used inaccurately. Gestational age is now expressed as *preterm, term,* and *postterm.* Preterm is generally accepted as less than 38 (completed) weeks of gestation; term refers to 38 to 42 weeks of gestation; and postterm refers to more than 42 weeks of gestation.[3]

Birth Weight

In considering the birth weight of the infant, many factors must be taken into consideration. It has long been recognized that the size of an infant may be directly related to the size of the parents and to their ethnic background and socioeconomic status. Until recently, however, there was no accurate way to compensate for these factors. Even now, in practice, such factors may not be considered specifically. Tanner feels that it is important to adjust the actual birth weight of the infant on the basis of the height and midpregnancy weight of the mother and according to sex and birth order of the infant, and he has devised an interesting system for doing this.[4] The sex of the infant is often, though not universally, considered in determination of the normality of birth weight, but the other factors Tanner suggests seem generally not to be considered.

Nationally and internationally, the term *low birth weight* is currently used for all infants weighing less than 2,500 g at birth. In 1968 the AAP Committee on the Fetus and the Newborn, recommended the use of numerical weight groups, such as under 2,500 g, over 2,500 g, without descriptive terms.[5]

Intrauterine Growth

Measurement of the infant's weight and gestational age are not sufficient to predict his risk potential. It is important also to compare the two and make a determination of the appropriateness of weight for gestational age. Infants, thus, may be classified "small for gestation age" (small for dates), "appropriate for gestational age" (appropriate for dates), or "large for gestational age" (large for dates). It makes a considerable difference in survival rates whether the infant is preterm and appropriate for gestational age, or preterm and small for gestational age. This determination is usually made with the Colorado Growth Chart or an adaptation of it. Figure 8-1 shows an adaptation of the chart which indicates mortality rates as well as norms for weights. The importance of determining normality of gestational growth lies in the fact that small-for-dates babies have a tendency to develop specific complications not ordinarily seen in babies who are the appropriate size for their gestational age. These complications will be discussed in detail in Chapter 9.

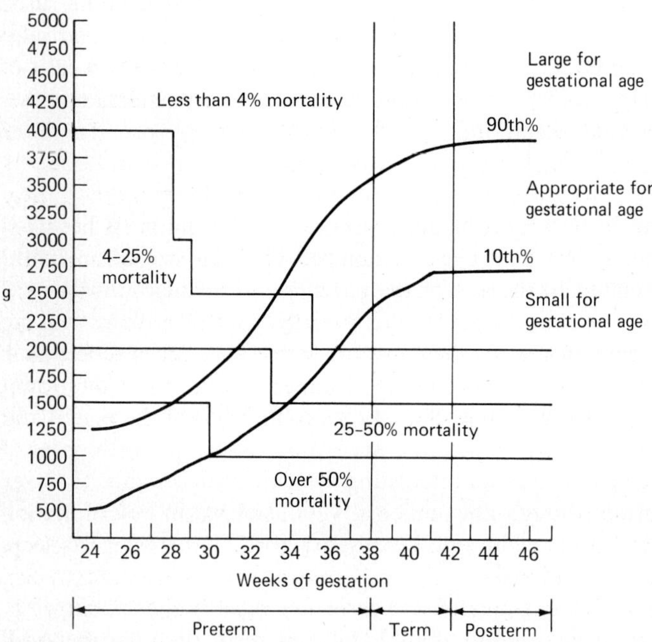

Figure 8-1 An infant's mortality risk can be determined by considering the birth weight and gestational age. (*From F. C. Battaglia and L. O. Lubchenco, "A Practical Classification of Newborn Infants by Weight and Gestational Age," Journal of Pediatrics, vol. 71, pp. 159–163, 1967, by permission.*)

Gestational Age Determination from Observations of the Infant Because of the possibility of inaccuracy in the mother's memory of menstrual dates, several systems of scoring have been developed for determining the age of the infant from direct observation. The information obtained from these observations also provides a great deal of information about the physical characteristics of the infant at various ages. Doing the evaluations, therefore, is of great value to the student in learning about infants, as well as to the infant in making possible more appropriate care.

In comparing several means of estimating gestational age, Finnstrom has concluded that of several methods studied, the most accurate results could be obtained from a combination of two of the following methods: measuring head circumference, observing external signs, and performing neurological tests.[6] The results obtained are accurate to within 2½ weeks. He cautions that the external signs tend to lose their accuracy after the first week of extrauterine life. When only one method of scoring is to be used, the external signs seem to be most useful for the first week of life, with the neurological exam giving more accurate results after the first week of life. Finnstrom and others point out that both the external signs and the neurologic tests give results that are to some degree in error for small-for-dates infants.[7] Lubchenco notes that in these babies, breast tissue development is usually smaller than would otherwise be expected for the gestational age, but sole creases and desquamation of the skin may be more like that of infants who are older than the calculated age of the small-for-dates infant.[8] Conditions which affect the intrauterine environment may affect other external characteristics, also. Daughters of diabetic mothers, for instance, may have more mature genitalia than would otherwise be expected for their true gestational age. Nurses who perform examinations for determining gestational age should keep the possibility of such differences in mind in evaluating their results.

Chemical Determination of Gestational Age The possibility of chemical determination of gestational age is being explored. Tests on cord blood and on amnionic fluid offer possibilities. Of particular promise are studies involving fetal hemoglobin and fetal serum concentrations of certain immunoglobulins. In assays of amnionic fluid, the ratio of lecithin to sphinogomyelin (both phospholipids) seems to be most promising in determining fetal maturity.[9] (If the ratio is 2.0, or more, the infant's gestational age is probably 35 weeks or more.[10])

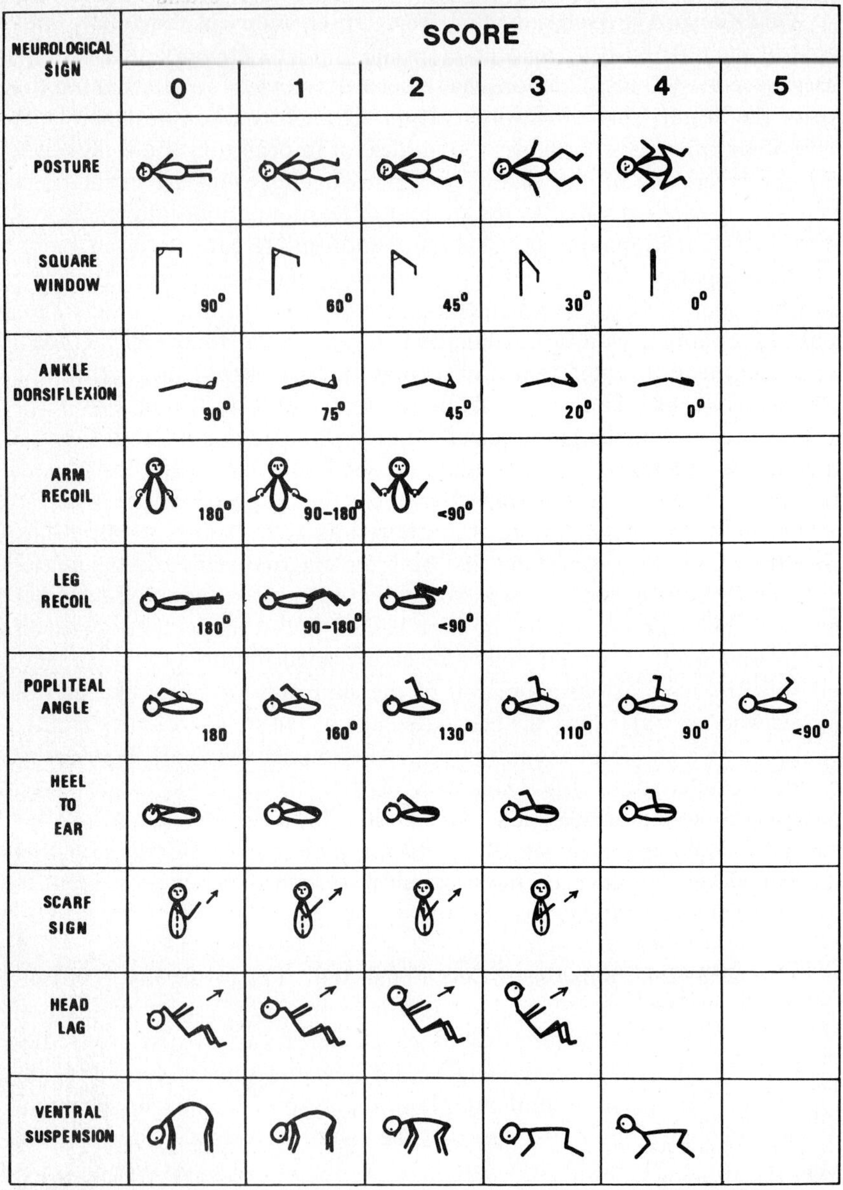

NEUROLOGICAL SIGN	SCORE 0	1	2	3	4	5
POSTURE						
SQUARE WINDOW	90°	60°	45°	30°	0°	
ANKLE DORSIFLEXION	90°	75°	45°	20°	0°	
ARM RECOIL	180°	90–180°	<90°			
LEG RECOIL	180°	90–180°	<90°			
POPLITEAL ANGLE	180	160°	130°	110°	90°	<90°
HEEL TO EAR						
SCARF SIGN						
HEAD LAG						
VENTRAL SUSPENSION						

Figure 8-2 Scoring system for neurologic criteria. (*From L. M. S. Dubowitz, V. Dubowitz, and C. Goldberg, Clinical Assessment of Gestational Age in the Newborn Infant, Journal of Pediatrics, vol. 77, p. 1–10, 1970, by permission.*)

Posture Observed with infant quiet and in supine position. Score 0: Arms and legs extended; 1: beginning of flexion of hips and knees, arms extended; 2: stronger flexion of legs, arms extended; 3: arms slightly flexed, legs flexed and abducted; 4: full flexion of arms and legs.

Square window The hand is flexed on the forearm between the thumb and index finger of the examiner. Enough pressure is applied to get as full a flexion as possible, and the angle between the hypothenar eminence and the ventral aspect of the forearm is measured and graded according to diagram. (Care is taken not to rotate the infant's wrist while doing this maneuver.)

Ankle dorsiflexion The foot is dorsiflexed onto the anterior aspect of the leg, with the examiner's thumb on the sole of the foot and other fingers behind the leg. Enough pressure is applied to get as full flexion as possible, and the angle between the dorsum of the foot and the anterior aspect of the leg is measured.

Arm recoil With the infant in the supine position the forearms are first flexed for 5 seconds, then fully extended by pulling on the hands, and then released. The sign is fully positive if the arms return briskly to full flexion (Score 2). If the arms return to incomplete flexion or the response is sluggish it is graded as Score 1. If they remain extended or are only followed by random movements the score is 0.

Leg recoil With the infant supine, the hips and knees are fully flexed for 5 seconds, then extended by traction on the feet, and released. A maximal response is one of full flexion of the hips and knees (Score 2). A partial flexion scores 1, and minimal or no movement scores 0.

Popliteal angle With the infant supine and his pelvis flat on the examining couch, the thigh is held in the knee-chest position by the examiner's left index finger and thumb supporting the knee. The leg is then extended by gentle pressure from the examiner's right index finger behind the ankle and the popliteal angle is measured.

Heel to ear maneuver With the baby supine, draw the baby's foot as near to the head as it will go without forcing it. Observe the distance between the foot and the head as well as the degree of extension at the knee. Grade according to diagram. Note that the knee is left free and may draw down alongside the abdomen.

Scarf sign With the baby supine, take the infant's hand and try to put it around the neck and as far posteriorly as possible around the opposite shoulder. Assist this maneuver by lifting the elbow across the body. See how far the elbow will go across and grade according to illustrations. Score 0: Elbow reaches opposite axillary line; 1: Elbow between midline and opposite axillary line; 2: Elbow reaches midline; 3: Elbow will not reach midline.

Head lag With the baby lying supine, grasp the hands (or the arms if a very small infant) and pull him slowly towards the sitting position. Observe the position of the head in relation to the trunk and grade accordingly. In a small infant the head may initially be supported by one hand. Score 0: Complete lag; 1: Partial head control; 2: Able to maintain head in line with body; 3: Brings head anterior to body.

Ventral suspension The infant is suspended in the prone position, with examiner's hand under the infant's chest (one hand in a small infant, two in a large infant). Observe the degree of extension of the back and the amount of flexion of the arms and legs. Note the relation of the head to the trunk. Grade according to diagrams.

Figure 8-3 Some notes on techniques of assessment of neurologic criteria. (*From L. M. S. Dubowitz, V. Dubowitz, and C. Goldberg, Clinical Assessment of Gestational Age in the Newborn Infant, Journal of Pediatrics, vol. 77, p. 1–10, 1970, by permission.*)

Determining Gestational Age from External Signs and Neurologic Exam A commonly used system for determining gestational age was described by Dubowitz et al.[11] The essentials of the observations to be made are shown in Figures 8-2 to 8-5. The conditions necessary for the observations have been defined by several authors. Amiel-Tison, who did much of the pioneering work on the neurologic tests used, states that if they are done immediately after birth, they should be repeated 2 or 3 days later, because of the changes in muscle tone which occur during the first 2 or 3 days.[12] She suggests that the infant should be wide-awake, but not agitated, as when extremely hungry. Lubchenco believes that observation of the resting position of the infant (posture) and recoil of the extremities are the best neurologic tests for use immediately after birth, with the complete neurologic battery being administered some hours later.[13] In the original work by Dubowitz et al., most of the examinations of infants were done in the first 24 hours after delivery, the remaining being completed within the first 5 days of extrauterine life.[14] They say that the state of the infant (awake, asleep) was of no consequence and that serial testing on the same infants showed no significant differences in comparing scores obtained in the first 24 hours with those done in the next 4 days. Scores obtained by different raters seem to be essentially the same. A skilled rater can complete the tests in 10 minutes or less. In using this system, the total score for both the neurologic examination and the observation of the external signs is obtained, and its position on the line of the graph in Figure 8-5 is determined. The gestational age is found by reading the age horizontally level with the point where the score falls on the line of the graph. The age and weight of the infant may then be plotted on the graph shown in Figure 8-1 so that a determination may be made as to the appropriateness of the weight of the infant for his or her gestational age.

THE PRETERM INFANT

There are several factors associated with spontaneous preterm delivery. More often than not, the infant is female, rather than male, and she is frequently a product of a pregnancy of an unmarried woman of lower socioeconomic station. The mother is most likely under 16 or over 35 years of age. Frequent pregnancies and a history of a previous preterm or stillborn infant are common, as are asymptomatic maternal bacteriuria and maternal cyanotic heart disease. Maternal diseases, especially metabolic disorders, are often associated with preterm delivery.

Physical Characteristics of the Preterm Infant

The preterm infant is easily recognized. The obviously diminutive size of the infant is striking. In addition, the proportionately larger head, the lack of musculature and subcutaneous fat deposits, the transparency of the skin, and the feebleness of response convey a sense of overall frailty. A typical infant of 32 weeks gestation would weigh approximately 1,600 g (3½ lb) and be approximately 42 cm (approximately 16¾ inches) in length, as compared with an infant of 40 weeks gestation, who would weigh nearly 3,200 g (approximately 7 lb) and be approximately 49 cm (approximately 19¼ inches) in length. The body of the 32-week infant would be well covered with lanugo and vernix. The skin would be a dark red color but rather transparent, with numerous veins visible on the abdomen. Edema of the extremities is usually present. Palpable breast tissue would be virtually absent, but the nipples would be well defined with a flat areola. The genitalia would be immature, with the testes undescended in the male and the labia majora small and widely separated in the female. The clitoris appears unusually large and prominent. The hair on the head is woolly in texture, and individual strands of hair are hard to identify. The ear is generally rather shapeless and the pinna is soft enough to stay folded when folded against the head. The sole of the foot is smooth, or perhaps has one anterior transverse crease. General muscle tone is poor, with only slight recoil in the legs and none in the arms. The abdomen may be distended, and the chest wall is poorly formed and very flexible. General neurologic responses to environment are poor and sluggish, with the exception of a good Moro reflex. (See Table 4-1 for a summary of characteristics of infants of 34 to 38, 38 to 42, and 42 weeks of gestation.)

Respiratory Function

Virtually all systems in the preterm infant are to some extent immature. Of critical importance, immediately, is the respiratory system. Surfactant, a substance which decreases the surface tension in the lungs (see discussion in Chapter 2, Establishment of Respiratory Function), is usually present in sufficient quantities so that normal respirations may be sustained by the thirty-fifth week.[15] (A younger infant *may* have sufficient quantities of surfactant to sustain respiratory function.) Difficulty in establishing and maintaining respirations may be experienced by a young infant due to poorly developed musclature of the thorax and great instability of the rib cage. The increased flexibility of the rib cage makes it difficult for the infant to maintain a satisfactory lung volume, since much of the respiratory effort results in a pulling inward of the soft structures of the thorax rather than inflation

External sign	Score*				
	0	1	2	3	4
Edema	Obvious edema of hands and feet; pitting over tibia	No obvious edema of hands and feet; pitting over tibia	No edema		
Skin texture	Very thin, gelatinous	Thin and smooth	Smooth; medium thickness. Rash or superficial peeling	Slight thickening. Superficial cracking and peeling especially of hands and feet	Thick and parchment-like; superficial or deep cracking
Skin color	Dark red	Uniformly pink	Pale pink; variable over body	Pale; only pink over ears, lips, palms, or soles	
Skin opacity (trunk)	Numerous veins and venules clearly seen, especially over abdomen	Veins and tributaries seen	A few large vessels clearly seen over abdomen	A few large vessels seen indistinctly over abdomen	No blood vessels seen
Lanugo (over back)	No lanugo	Abundant; long and thick over whole back	Hair thinning especially over lower back	Small amount of lanugo and bald areas	At least 1/2 of back devoid of lanugo
Plantar creases	No skin creases	Faint red marks over anterior half of sole	Definite red marks over > anterior 1/2; indentations over < anterior 1/3	Indentations over > anterior 1/3	Definite deep indentations over > anterior 1/3

Nipple formation	Nipple barely visible; no areola	Nipple well defined; areola smooth and flat, diameter < 0.75 cm	Areola stippled. edge not raised, diameter < 0.75 cm	Areola stippled, edge raised, diameter > 0.75 cm
Breast size	No breast tissue palpable	Breast tissue on one or both sides. < 0.5 cm diam-	Breast tissue both sides; one or both 0.5–1.0 cm	Breast tissue both sides; one or both > 1 cm
Ear form	Pinna flat and shapeless, little or no incurving of edge	Incurving of part of edge of pinna	Partial incurving whole of upper pinna	Well-defined incurving whole of upper pinna
Ear firmness	Pinna soft, easily folded, no recoil	Pinna soft, easily folded, slow recoil	Cartilage to edge of pinna, but soft in places, ready recoil	Pinna firm, cartilage to edge; instant recoil
Genitals	Neither testis in scrotum	At least one testis high in scrotum	At least one testis right down	
Female (with hips 1/2 abducted)	Labia majora widely separated, labia minora protruding	Labia majora almost cover labia minora	Labia majora completely cover labia minora	

*If score differs on two sides, take the mean.

Figure 8-4 Scoring system for external criteria. (*From L. M. S. Dubowitz, V. Dubowitz, and C. Goldberg, Clinical Assessment of Gestational Age in the Newborn Infant, Journal of Pediatrics, vol. 77, pp. 1–10, 1970, by permission.*)

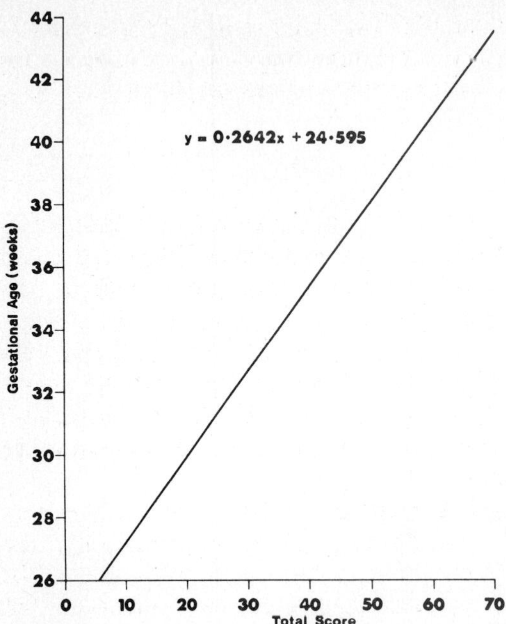

Figure 8-5 Graph for reading gestational age from total score. (*From L. M. S. Dubowitz, V. Dubowitz, and C. Goldberg, Clinical Assessment of Gestational Age in the Newborn Infant, Journal of Pediatrics, vol. 77, pp. 1–10, 1970, by permission.*)

of the lungs. In addition, many of the alveoli are thick-walled and because of this, very inefficient in gas exchange. Periodic respirations (alternate periods of breathing and pauses for a few seconds) further diminish gas exchange potentials. In general, then, the preterm infant must work much harder in order to accomplish the same degree of respiratory function as a term infant.

Thermoregulation

Like the term infant, the preterm infant needs to maintain body temperature within a relatively narrow range, though the preterm infant seems to function well at a slightly lower "set point" (see Chapter 2, Cold Stress and Metabolic Processes). Preterm infants are poorly equipped to cope with any degree of cold stress. They have much less adipose tissue (white fat) to function as insulation and less glucose to utilize in the metabolism of fats to prevent metabolic acidosis. At this time, the relative quantities of brown fat present in preterm infants are not available to this author, but it would seem likely that these too, would be less than are found in mature infants. In addition to these energy insufficiencies, cold stress and its accompanying metabolic increase also requires a great increase in use of oxygen if metabolic acidosis is to be avoided. To the preterm infant who may be having difficulty maintaining minimal oxygenation, the added cold stress is likely to be fatal.

Metabolic Function

The preterm infant differs metabolically from the term infant. Liver function is generally less mature, resulting in lowered glucose levels and glycogen stores. Hypoglycemia, thus, is frequently a serious problem in the preterm infant. Hypoproteinemia and hypoprothrombinemia are also thought to be a result of immature liver function. Due to deficiency in the production of glucuronyl transferase, the preterm infant cannot metabolize bilirubin effectively, resulting in hyperbilirubinemia. Jaundice in the preterm infant is most likely to peak at the end of the first week, rather than in the third day, as is true of the term infant.

Similarly, kidney function, which does not ordinarily reach mature levels until the second year after birth, may be greatly immature in the preterm infant. The kidney continues to add glomeruli until about the thirty-fifth week of gestation; hence, the preterm infant may not have a full complement of glomeruli. The immature kidney is less able to concentrate urine; thus dehydration is more likely. Its ability to clear metabolic products is likewise diminished, increasing the likelihood of metabolic acidosis and other toxic states. To further complicate the problem, the preterm infant is in a state of catabolism (tissue breakdown) for some time after birth, thus raising the blood levels of nonprotein nitrogen, potassium, and water.

Basically, the preterm infant seems to digest proteins and carbohydrates as well as a term infant, but fats are not digested well. This leads to losses of nutrition through diarrhea and failure to absorb most of the fat-soluble vitamins, notably vitamins A, D, E, and K. Vitamin C deficiencies are also common.

Immunity

Preterm infants are extremely susceptible to infection. As was discussed in Chapter 2, the preterm infant is especially handicapped by the inability to phagocytize organisms efficiently. Immunoglobulins which cross the placenta from the mother to the infant late in pregnancy are also notably lacking in the preterm infant. Antibody formation is similarly diminished, and it is thought that there may be additional factors in the tissues themselves which make the preterm infant more susceptible to invasion by hostile organisms.[16] The skin, which is a natural barrier to infection, is much thinner in the preterm infant, making that avenue of entry a much more likely one.

Hemostasis

Preterm infants are especially susceptible to intracranial and pulmonary hemorrhages. In addition to the difficulties in forming prothrombin experienced by the term infant, the preterm infant has diminished levels of some plasma-clotting factors, notably factors V, VII, and X, all of which react with thromboplastin to form thrombin. Decreased levels of platelets and diminished activity of the thromboplastin round out a picture of high susceptibility to hemorrhage.

NURSING CARE OF THE PRETERM INFANT

Specific disease conditions and their treatment will be discussed in Chapter 9. The care presented here will be focused on prevention of complications in otherwise healthy preterm infants.

Maintenance of Respirations

Because of the establishment and maintenance of respiratory function may be difficult for the preterm infant, nursing assistance may be required. In evaluating the respiratory efforts of the infant, the nurse should observe for bilateral expansion of the chest, cyanosis, retractions, flaring of the nares, and/or an expiratory "grunt." Usually tiny infants are monitored electronically for both heart and respiratory rates. If no difficulty is present, the infant's respiratory rate should remain below 60 respirations/minute.[17] If brief periods of apnea occur, respirations may be stimulated by gentle tactile stimulation or by gently lifting the abdominal musculature. If respirations are not established within 20 seconds, Brightman and Clattworthy recommend the institution of cardiopulmonary resusitation (CPR) and simultaneous notification of the physician.[18] To perform CPR, the infant should be placed on a hard surface (newer incubators have sufficiently firm mattresses) with the head slightly hyperextended and the airway cleared. Cardiac massage is administered with one or two fingers on the sternum at the rate of 40 to 60 beats/minute. A pause should be made in the cardiac compression at the end of each 10 beats for two quick inflations of the lungs, using a bag ventilator preferably, although mouth–to–mouth-and-nose resusitation is possible. If compression of the sternum occurs during inflation of the lungs, the lungs can be injured; hence, care should be taken to avoid that possibility when two persons are administering the CPR. The pressure used to inflate the lungs should be sufficient to cause a rise in the upper chest wall, but low enough to avoid rupture of the lungs. Short puffs of air from the nurse's mouth are sufficient to inflate the infant's lungs. If the abdomen rises with ventilation, the air is probably entering the stomach rather than the lungs, and the infant needs to be repositioned, or an airway device needs to be inserted. It is best in administering cardiopulmonary resuscitation for two people to work together and for someone to monitor the chest for the appearance of spontaneous respirations and/or spontaneous heart beat.

Suctioning

Suctioning may be necessary. While the procedure was described in detail in Chapter 4 (Maintaining and Supporting Normal Physiological Adaptations, Respiration), a few major points will be reiterated here. The mouth should be suctioned before the nose, since suctioning the nose may cause the infant to gasp and aspirate material from the mouth. When using a mechanical device, it is important to have the suction actually "pulling" only as the tube is withdrawn, in order to avoid tissue trauma. The catheter should be withdrawn gently but not too slowly, as the air in the respiratory passages is sucked out along with the mucus. Since passage of the catheter may stimulate the vagus nerve and cause bradycardia, as well as unavoidably traumatizing the tissues to some extent, it is important to avoid unnecessary suctioning. If the nurse is to be responsible for intratrachaeal suctioning, the procedure should be taught by a skilled clinician.

Positioning

If the infant is having difficulty maintaining respirations, positioning may be helpful. Raising the head of the mattress so that the infant's head is slightly higher than the rest of the body will take the weight of the abdominal contents off the diaphragm. In addition, a small blanket roll may be placed under the infant's shoulders to hyperextend the neck slightly to keep the respiratory passages open. Too much hyperextension may make it difficult for the infant to swallow his secretions, however; so, the nurse should observe very carefully for drooling or choking. Care should be taken to see that the infant's arms are positioned comfortably, but not on the infant's chest, as their weight would increase the work of respiration. If diapers are used, they should be fastened loosely so that they do not bind the abdomen, since the infant will probably need to use the abdominal muscles to aid respiratory efforts. Turning the infant from side to back to side every 1 to 2 hours will aid in drainage of fluids from the lungs. An infant having respiratory distress should never be placed in a prone position.

Administering Oxygen

Safe administration of oxygen to infants is at best a difficult procedure. The relative maturity of the lung, the type of equipment used, and the presence or absence of disease states, as well as the concentrations of oxygen administered all seem to affect the outcomes.[19,20] It should also be noted that humidification of the oxygen is essential to prevent mucosal drying.

Oxygen toxicity with resultant damage to the retina has long been known. Retrolental fibroplasia is a condition caused by too high concentrations of oxygen in the blood. The condition seems to occur only when the retina is not yet fully vascularized, as in preterm infants. When the Po_2 level is too high, constriction of the immature retinal vessels occurs. This vasoconstriction response is reversible if the oxygen concentration is lowered soon, but if the vasoconstriction continues for several hours, it seems not to be reversible. The vasoconstriction continues for the period of time the high levels of oxygen are present. After the oxygen level is lowered, new vessels grow into the retina. These new vessels are rather permeable, and edema and hemorrhages are likely to occur. The retina may then be detached from the back of the eye, and blindness results. There is apparently nothing that can be done to correct the condition once the retinal detachment occurs. The exact levels of oxygen which will cause retrolental fibroplasia are unknown for any specific infant. The condition may occur in ambient levels of oxygen lower than the 40 percent level generally accepted as "safe"; thus it is important to keep close watch on the Po_2 levels and to examine the eyes regularly.

There is also considerable evidence that prolonged high levels of oxygen may damage lung tissue. (Stern disagrees with this.[21] He believes that the severe damage often seen is more a result of the use of an intratracheal tube or of mechanical application of positive pressure to the respiratory system, or perhaps, both, rather than a direct effect of high concentrations of oxygen, per se.) The lung damage that is seen is esentially thickening of the tissue barrier between the gases in the alveoli and the blood in alveolar capillaries and an increase in respiratory vascular resistance to blood flow which can result in right ventricular hypertrophy and heart failure. If the infant survives the respiratory crisis which occurs, recovery from the lung changes tends to occur over a period of several months. In the meantime, the infant may have to be weaned from the oxygen very slowly and very carefully. Too abrupt discontinuation of oxygen may result in cyanosis and respiratory failure. Even after the arterial blood Po_2 level is satisfactory in room air, tachypnea may persist.[22]

In the administration of oxygen, several factors must be kept in mind. Klaus and Fanaroff recommend using a hood which fits inside the incubator and over the infant's head.[23] If a hood is used, the oxygen should be warmed to the temperature of the air inside the incubator and checked hourly to prevent cold stress, because the face is especially sensitive to cold. The flow of oxygen into the hood should be at least 5 liters/minute to prevent excessive CO_2 accumulation. Oxygen *must always be humidified* regardless of the route of administration to prevent excess drying of mucosal tissues. Klaus and Fanaroff recommend that hourly measurement of environmental oxygen concentrations be done if the infant is receiving supplemental oxygen and that the oxygen analyzer be calibrated to room air (20.94% O_2) and 100% O_2 to check its accuracy at least once every day.[24] They believe that frequent arterial Po_2 measurements should be taken if the infant is receiving high levels of supplementary oxygen (over 40 percent). The artery which should be used for these determinations is widely disputed, some feeling that the umbilical artery is best, and others favoring peripheral arteries. The arterial Po_2 level which is recommended by Llewellyn and Swyer is 60 to 90 mmHg.[25] Auld, on the other hand, recommends levels of 49 to 60 mmHg.[26] The goal is to ensure adequate oxygenation of the tissues while preventing toxic reactions. It should be kept in mind that it is the arterial concentrations of oxygen that influence the development of retrolental fibroplasia, rather than environmental levels. Environmental concentrations of less than 40 percent over a period as short as 3 days have been known to cause the disease, thus negating the old rule of thumb that any concentration of oxygen less than 40 percent is safe.[27] In some hospitals, ophthalmic examinations of the retina are done before, during, and after oxygen is administered to high-risk infants in an attempt to prevent eye damage. It is the environmental levels of oxygen which are suspect in lung toxicity, but the specific levels of oxygen concentration responsible, if indeed oxygen is the culprit, have not been established.

Auld proposes hourly adjustment of environmental oxygen concentrations to the level which will just eliminate cyanosis, with less frequent blood gas determinations than is recommended by others.[28] He feels that this method of control of oxygen is especially useful in hospitals where the highly sophisticated equipment and personnel found in neonatal intensive-care units are not available.

The nurse is the person who is primarily responsible for monitoring and regulating the flow of oxygen to the baby. Although the doctor orders the oxygen flow, the nurse must use judgment both in determining that the correct flow is being administered and in assessing the infant's condition to be sure that the ordered amount is still appropriate. In monitoring oxygen concentrations, attention should be paid not only to the numerical concentrations of oxygen present, but also to the response of the infant to the oxygen. The presence of generalized cyanosis, for instance, obviously means that the infant is not getting enough oxygen or is unable to utilize the oxygen. The absence of central cyanosis accompanied by increased activity and alertness may indicate that the oxygen should be decreased. Pertinent observations of these signs should be brought to the physician's attention without undue delay, as prevention of both hypoxia and oxygen toxicity is imperative. In monitoring the concentration of the oxygen, it is important to monitor the air-oxygen mixture that is actually taken into the lungs using such techniques as measuring the concentration at the level of the infant's nose, for instance. It is very important, also, to keep detailed records of the oxygen being administered, so that it is clear that the infant is actually receiving what is ordered. As with many other areas of infant care, meticulous attention to detail is imperative.

Maintaining Body Temperature

The importance of maintaining body temperature cannot be overstressed. The basic reasons for the provision of a thermoneutral environment have been discussed extensively in Chapters 2, 3, and 4. To reiterate the parameters of a thermoneutral environment, as defined by Heim, the air temperature inside an incubator should be maintained at 32 to 34°C (89.6 to 93.2°F), with the inner wall of the incubator registering the same temperature and a relative humidity of 50 percent.[29] If a servocontrolled incubator is used, the abdominal skin temperature of the infant should be maintained at 36 to 37°C (96.8 to 98.6°F). These criteria are useful as a guide. The nurse must maintain a flexible approach, however, with the goal of maintaining the optimal temperature of the individual baby. Concurrent checking of skin, rectal, and incubator air temperatures is probably advisable. A rectal temperature of 36 to 37°C is also generally considered to be satisfactory. A skin temperature higher than that indicates the possibility of too warm an environment. Air temperature more than 2 to 3°C lower than skin temperature indicates that the infant may be in too cold an environment.[30]

An infant kept in an incubator is usually neither dressed, nor diapered. The infant should not be removed from the incubator until it is established that body temperature can be maintained at room temperature. If access to the infant is required which cannot be provided in the incubator, the infant should be transferred to an open bed heated by an overhead radiant heater. To prevent heat loss during the transfer, the infant should be wrapped in warmed blankets before being removed from the incubator unless the institution of lifesaving measures precludes this precaution. It should also be remembered that too rapid warming of a cooled infant can result in periods of apnea.

Care of Incubators

The nurse may be the person responsible for seeing that the incubators are adequately maintained. In some institutions, the water reservoir under the bed of the incubator is kept filled with water to provide environmental humidity. If this is done, the nurse must be aware of the danger of the growth of Pseudomonas or other organisms that thrive in water. Pseudomonas infections are very difficult to treat and can easily cause the death of the infant. To prevent these infections, the water used in the reservoir should be distilled and sterilized and should be changed every 24 hours.

The reservoir should be cleaned before it is refilled, and silver nitrate added to the water (0.84 ml of 0.5 percent silver nitrate to 5 gallons of water).[31] All parts of the oxygenation system should also be changed every 24 hours, because of the moisture present in the system. Only sterile distilled water should be used in the oxygen humidifier, and that water should be changed every 8 hours to prevent the growth of organisms.[32] Cleaning the incubator varies somewhat from place to place. In many hospitals, the entire incubator is changed once a week to prevent the multiplication of pathogenic organisms. Cultures of various areas of the incubator may also be taken every 3 to 4 days to monitor its bacteriological safety. Special care should be paid to moist areas and to parts touched by personnel, such as the sleeves of the portholes. Such parts should be wiped daily with a disinfectant, with care taken to protect the infant from the disinfectant.

Preventing Hypoglycemia and Hypocalcemia

The fetus normally receives adequate supplies of glucose from the mother. At birth, this supply is cut off and the infant draws upon the glycogen stored in his or her liver, depleting the supply there in the first 2 or 3 hours after delivery. The infant then begins to metabolize fats (white fat) for glucose production until receiving glucose orally. A graph of glucose levels in normal term infants shows a rapid drop in blood levels during the first 2 hours after delivery, followed by a slight upward trend and a leveling off at 3 to 4 hours of age. A full-term infant usually shows levels of 50 to 60 mg/100 ml at 4 to 6 hours, with the levels 10 mg/100 ml lower if hypothermia is experienced. A level of 40 mg/100 ml is typical at 4 hours for low-birth-weight infants (compared with 50 to 60 mg/100 ml for the term infant). The glucose levels should stabilize at 40 mg or above after the third day of life.[33] A common definition of hypoglycemia is levels below 30 mg/100 ml in the first 3 days in term infants and below 20 mg/100 ml in preterm infants for the same time period. (After the first 3 days any level below 40 mg/100 ml is diagnostic.) Stern however, feels, that any infant with a glucose level below 40 mg/100 ml should receive treatment regardless of age, because in his experience, symptoms have occurred in infants with levels of 30 to 40 mg/100 ml.[34]

Preterm infants are more likely than term infants to experience hypoglycemia for several reasons. They have smaller stores of glycogen in the liver, their stores of white fat are much less than those of term infants, and they are likely to experience both hypothermia, which is associated with hypoglycemia, and respiratory distress (with an increased work of respiration), which increases the demand for energy. They are also less likely to tolerate early oral feedings, which could compensate to some degree for a lack of energy stores. In preventing hypoglycemia, all measures that decrease the energy demands on the infant are of value. Special attention should be paid to the organization of nursing care to conserve the baby's energy.

In many nurseries, Dextrostix determinations of blood glucose levels are done every hour for preterm infants in the first hours after birth. A heel stick is done and a drop of blood placed on the Dextrostix. To be most accurate, the heel from which the blood is obtained should be warmed briefly by holding it in the palm of the nurse's hand. This ensures adequate circulation so that freshly circulated blood is obtained rather than that which has been static in the capillaries for some time. The directions for performing the test must be followed *exactly,* especially with regard to the length of time the blood remains on the Dextrostix (exactly 60 seconds) before being rinsed off, and the resulting color must be read in adequate lighting. Even then, Wald feels that falsely high readings are likely to occur.[35] The doctor should be notified when a reading of 40 mg/100 ml or less is obtained.

Early oral feedings, sometimes begun immediately after delivery during the first period of reactivity, are useful in preventing hypoglycemia if the infant can tolerate them. If respiratory distress is present or if the infant is extremely weak and cannot suck, IV infusions of glucose may be started soon after delivery.

There are no specific symptoms of hypoglycemia, but generally, central nervous system symptoms such as tremors, convulsions, weakness, high-pitched cry, eye rolling, and poor muscle tone should alert the nurse to this possibility. Several other conditions, such as CNS damage, sepsis, congenital heart disease, and some metabolic disorders can cause the same symptoms, however. Of special importance is *hypocalcemia,* which is likely to accompany hypoglycemia.

Calcium is transferred from mother to fetus in the last weeks of pregnancy; hence, the preterm infant is likely to have inadequate stores. In addition, when glucagon is released by the pancreas to stimulate the conversion of glycogen to glucose, it also stimulates renal excretion of calcium. Stress experienced at the time of delivery or soon after also decreases serum levels of calcium, as does the administration of sodium bicarbonate to treat acidosis. In addition to this, formulas which are derived from cow's milk have a higher proportion of phosphorous than does breast milk, and since the level of calcium in the blood is affected by the ratio of phosphorous present, this, too, tends to decrease the serum calcium level. The addition of vitamin D to commercial formulas encourages bone deposits of calcium, but in doing so, again decreases the blood serum levels. A graph of calcium level changes would show a steep decline in calcium levels during the first 2 days, followed by a sharp rise in the third day (presumably due to the intake of milk), followed by a second decline on about the fifth day, especially in babies on commercial formulas. The incidence of clinical hypocalcemia is greatest in the first 2 days of life and between days 5 and 7.[36] The medical treatment for hypoglycemia and hypocalcemia will be discussed in Chapter 9.

Oral Feedings

Feeding the preterm infant is a vital nursing function. To be fed orally, the infant must not be experiencing respiratory distress and must have strong suck and swallow reflexes. The infant's ability to suck and swallow adequately are not necessarily related to age and size. Coordination of sucking and swallowing which closes the epiglottis at the appropriate time and is accompanied by an adequate gag reflex normally develops after the thirty-second week of gestation.[37] Infants born before this time are likely to aspirate oral feedings. In mature infants, there are prolonged periods of sucking with multiple swallows occurring simultaneously. In the immature infant a short period of sucking is either preceded or followed by swallowing. Because of the uncoordinated functioning of the various mechanisms, these infants may swallow sizable amounts of air with the formula. Regurgitation of milk into the lower esophagus is also common, due to poor sphincter tone at the lower end of the esophagus. Both the presence of air in the stomach and the presence of milk in the lower esophagus can add to respiratory distress.

The timing and composition of first feedings vary, depending on hospital policy and medical preferences. Generally, however, the trend is toward earlier milk feedings and/or early intravenous infusions to prevent hypoglycemia and hypocalcemia. Some institutions still give glucose for the first feeding, in spite of findings that when aspiration occurs, glucose irritates lung tissue as badly as does milk.[38] In other institutions, sterile water is preferred for early feedings to avoid such irritation.[39] In still others, early feedings are begun with formula with the understanding that care has been used in assessing the patency of the esophagus prior to feeding.[40]

For the infant who can suck well, breast-feeding may be a possibility. For those who have less strong suck reactions, bottle-feeding with a soft nipple may be preferable. If the mother wishes, breast milk may be obtained for these feedings. A plastic dropper or a syringe with a rubber tip may be substituted for the bottle and nipple for infants who tire too easily from sucking, but who can swallow well. The rubber tip on the syringe or dropper must be long enough (3 to 4 inches) to prevent the infant from *swallowing it* if it comes off. Sterile technique, of course, is used for all feedings.

In feeding the preterm infant, it is helpful to observe the baby's behavior. O'Grady has described five steps in the feeding process through which the baby progresses: "prefeeding behavior," "approach behavior," "attachment behavior," "consummatory behavior," and "satiety behavior."[41] The prefeeding behavior includes those behaviors which indicate the infant's hunger, such as body movements, stretching, crying, and sucking the fingers if the infant can get them to his mouth. Approach behavior includes rooting and turning the head toward the source of food. Some babies exhibit these behaviors when picked up for a gavage feeding. In such cases, it is felt that they will soon be ready for bottle-feeding. Attachment behavior includes the infant's attempts to take the nipple into his mouth and to grasp it securely. Some infants who are being tube-fed will try to mouth the feeding tube, again indicating partial readiness for bottle-feeding. Consummatory behavior is the coordinated sucking and swallowing which enables the infant to ingest the milk. Satiety behaviors are those which indicate that the infant is satisfied after feeding. Falling asleep is the most common of these.

When bottle-feeding an infant who is just learning to suck and to swallow, it is helpful to place most of the nipple in the baby's mouth as this seems to encourage sucking. Care should be taken to be sure the nipple is above the tongue, as these babies frequently hold their tongues touching the roofs of their mouths. Gently pressing the lower jaw against the nipple in a rhythmic motion will also encourage sucking. Young babies sometimes have difficulty in releasing the suction on the nipple and may not be able to get the milk because of a collapsed nipple. Gently rotating the nipple in the baby's mouth will help combat this problem. The student should not become discouraged if the first feedings of these tiny infants results in some of the formula being dribbled from the infant's mouth. Mothers often become upset by this phenomenon. Of course care should be taken to be sure that most of the formula is swallowed. If too much formula is lost or if the baby tires too easily during the bottle-feeding, gavage feeding may need to be reinstituted for a short time, or perhaps be used in addition to offering some formula by bottle. The baby should be observed for circumoral cyanosis, indicating the need to rest for a few minutes before continuing the feeding. The entire feeding period should not last longer than 20 minutes, however, to avoid tiring the baby. Patency of the nipple should be checked at the beginning of the feeding and during the feeding if the baby seems to be tiring. Tiring may be due to ineffective efforts to obtain milk through a clogged nipple.

An infant is able to maintain his or her body temperature, can be held in the nurse's arms for feedings. Otherwise, the infant should be cradled in the nurse's hands in the incubator, so that warmth of contact with the feeding person can be experienced. The parents should be encouraged to feed the infant just as soon as the condition permits. The infant should be observed for regurgitation and for periods of apnea after feeding. Babies who have just been fed should never be placed in a supine position.

The quantity of formula fed will vary according to the size and condition of the infant. Very young infants usually begin with quantities of 1 to 2 ml, with gradual increases being made as these are tolerated. If regurgitation occurs after feeding, the volume is probably too large, although simply not burping sufficiently can be a cause. Increases in formula volume should be made very slowly.

Gavage Feeding

For very young infants, gavage feedings are frequently necessary. Before inserting the tube, the infant should be placed on one side or in a supine position with the neck hyperflexed. The distance from the mouth to the ear lobe and down to the tip of the sternum is measured. The distance on the tube is marked with tape. The tube is lubricated with water and then passed through the mouth into the stomach. The tube may be left in place between feedings or removed. A small piece of tape to hold the tube in place will prevent the baby from accidentally removing it. Nonallergic paper tape should be used to prevent injury to the infant's tender skin.

The placement of the tube must be checked before *each feeding*. Ordinarily, if the tube goes into the trachea, the infant will react with coughing, increased activity, and cyanosis. It is therefore unlikely that the tube could be inadvertently misplaced, but the possibility should always be kept in mind. To check placement of the tube, 0.5 cm^3 of air may be injected into the tube while the nurse listens over the stomach with a stethoscope. The air can be heard as it rushes into the stomach. Air thus injected should be withdrawn prior to feeding to avoid regurgitation. The placement of the tube may also be tested by withdrawing stomach contents with a syringe. When this is done, the volume of fluid withdrawn should be measured as an indication of gastric motility. Sometimes the contents are returned to the stomach and the volume subtracted from the next feeding. The inability to withdraw stomach contents does not necessarily mean that the tube is in the trachea.

The feeding should be allowed to drip through the tube by gravity with the top of the liquid not more than *8* inches above the infant's head.[42] Tube feedings should not be rushed. The time required should be approximately the same as for a bottle feeding of the same volume. After the feeding, the tube may be rinsed with sterile water (1 to 2 ml) to prevent clogging of the tube. If the tube is to be removed, it should be rinsed with sterile water to prevent the possibility of milk dripping into the trachea as it is removed. At the time of removal, the open end of the tube should be pinched shut and the tube quickly pulled out. During the feeding the infant should be positioned so the head is slightly higher than the body. The baby should, in most cases, be turned to the right side after feeding and positioned to prevent aspiration if regurgitation occurs.

Intravenous Infusions

The regulation of infusion rates when tiny infants are being infused is a very important responsibility of the nurse. Most nurseries now use some type of infusion pump which can deliver minute amounts of solution continuously over a prolonged period of time. It should be noted, however, that such pumps do not cease functioning when the fluid goes into the tissue rather than into the veins and that some of them do not stop functioning when the fluid chamber is empty, thus pushing air into the system. Neither can the pump recognize signs of cardiac overload and heart failure.

The solutions used for infusions depend upon the needs of the infant. Sometimes dextrose and water or saline are the primary components; other times, a complete diet is infused, including amino acids (total parenteral alimentation or TPA). When these protein solutions are used, special precautions, such as frequent tubing changes, must be used to prevent the growth of organisms in the solutions. In some hospitals the tubes are changed every 24 hours regardless of the solution infused. Metabolic disturbances are also more likely when the amino acid mixtures are used, partly because their use indicates that other avenues of nutrition are not being employed. Any time infusions are being used, a strict intake-and-output chart should be kept for the infant. Weighing diapers or pads when they are placed under the infant and again after they are wet may be the best way to measure urinary output, especially for female infants. Twenty-four-hour urines may be collected for infants receiving TPA. If collections of urine can be made, they should be checked for the presence of glucose (indicating glucose overloads) and for specific gravity (to determine hydration status) as well as for volume. An infusion of TPA should never be "speeded up" if it is infusing at less than the ordered rate because of the danger of electrolyte imbalance and circulatory overloading.

Preventing Infection

All the precautions mentioned in the discussion of aseptic technique in the care of the term infant should be applied to the care of the preterm infant. (See Chapter 4.) Scrupulous attention to detail is vital to the infant's survival.

Of special importance is careful attention to hand washing and exclusion from the nursery of anyone with a skin or respiratory infection. Gowns usually are worn over scrub clothes if an infant is removed from the incubator. These gowns are usually discarded after use, or at least at the end of the shift, if they are reused. The precautions necessary for the protection of the infant, however, should not be reason to exclude parents from the nursery. Most parents are meticulous in following procedures once they understand them. Studies have shown repeatedly that the presence of parents in the nursery does not increase the infection rate.

The proper care of incubators has been discussed previously. Other nursery equipment in which water or water vapor are present should also receive special attention to prevent the growth of gram negative organisms, such as Pseudomonas. Such common devices as aerators on sink faucets may be sources of infection. The organisms may also grow in some of the disinfecting solutions such as benzalkonium (Zephiran).[43] Cultures should be obtained from various places in the nursery at regular intervals. The nurse is in the best position to supervise adequate surveillance of aseptic technique.

Preventing Hemorrhage

Just as the term infant needs vitamin K_1 to prevent postnatal hemorrhage, the preterm infant needs this vitamin, also. Besides an initial dose of vitamin K_1 soon after birth, preterm infants may need daily doses for a period of time. The dosage per kilogram of weight may be higher than that for the term infant. These daily doses are usually administered orally.[44] If injections are used, the injection site of choice in the preterm infant is the middle third of the anterior or lateral muscle of the thigh (see Figures 8-6 and 8-7). Gluteal muscles should never be used in these infants, since the muscle is very underdeveloped and danger of injury to the sciatic nerve is great.

General Nursing Observations

No part of nursing care of the preterm infant supersedes nursing observations in importance. It is largely through observation that the infant's condition is monitored. Vital signs are taken at intervals determined by the infant's condition. In addition, the infant is weighed daily by using a scale and sling apparatus that sits on top of the incubator. The sling fits under the

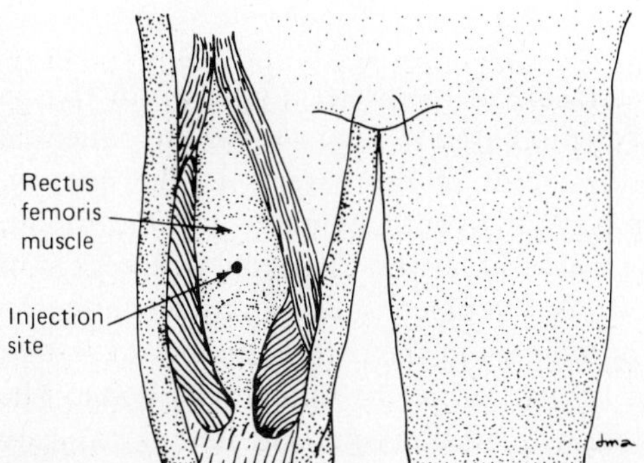

Figure 8-6 The middle one-third of the rectus femoris muscle is one injection site for an infant. *(From G. Scipien et al., Comprehensive Pediatric Nursing, McGraw-Hill, New York, 1975, p. 933, by permission.)*

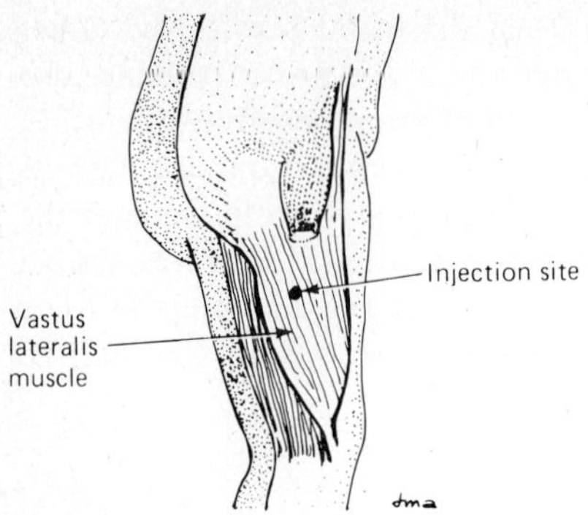

Figure 8-7 The middle one-third of the vastus lateralis muscle, anterior to the femur, is a good injection site for an infant. (*From G. Scipien et al., Comprehensive Pediatric Nursing, McGraw-Hill, New York, 1975, p. 933, by permission.*)

infant so that the infant does not have to be removed from the incubator. Other observations which are important are frequent observations of the infant's color, especially with regard to cyanosis and jaundice. The general activity level and "vigor" of the infant should be assessed at least every 8 hours, since a decrease in activity or the presence of limpness is an early sign of several disorders. The head circumference should be measured daily or every other day to detect the infrequent but possible development of hydrocephalus. With experience, the nurse can learn to differentiate the infant who is doing well from the one who simply "doesn't look right." Such a distinction is valid even when specific symptoms cannot be identified. A checklist, such as that shown in Figure 8-8 may be useful in ensuring systematic observations. Such a checklist would most often be a worksheet, not a part of the chart. The observations would be summarized in the nurse's notes.

Discharge Planning

An important component of nursing care of the preterm infant is discharge planning. Ideally, consideration for discharge is begun when the patient is admitted to the unit. From the first visit of the parents to the nursery, discharge planning should be a part of overall planning for the infant. Assessments of parental strengths and weaknesses, especially with regard to their teaching and emotional needs, is one place to begin this planning. As soon as possible parents should participate in the care of the infant so that affectional bonds are established firmly before the infant goes home. The parents should become comfortable with all the aspects of the infant's care for which they will be responsible *before* the infant is sent home. Frequently a predischarge home visit is made by a community-based nurse to be sure

FEEDING CHECK LIST
(front)

Addressograph

Feeding order: ______________________

Method of Feeding: Gavage ____ Dropper ____ Bottle ______

Time:	Amount Offered:	Amount Taken:	Amount Vomited:	Comments:
____	____	____	____	____
____	____	____	____	____
____	____	____	____	____
____	____	____	____	____

Check the following once each shift and more often as indicated.

Response: strong (s), weak (w), absent (a).	7-3	3-11	11-7	Comments
Reflexes: gag	____	____	____	____
suck	____	____	____	____
rooting	____	____	____	____
swallowing	____	____	____	____
Other: present (p), absent (a)				
hiccuping	____	____	____	____
drooling	____	____	____	____
regurgitation	____	____	____	____
projectile vomiting	____	____	____	____

Figure 8-8 Systematic observations may be facilitated by the use of checklists such as these.

FEEDING CHECK LIST
(back)

Feeding Behaviors: present (p), absent (a)	7-3	3-11	11-7
spontaneous prefeeding arousal	___	___	___
rooting, looking at feeder	___	___	___
grasps nipple, (mouths feeding tube)	___	___	___
coordinated suck and swallow (sucks tube)	___	___	___
relaxation and sleep after feeding	___	___	___

Parent Feeding Behaviors: present (p), absent (a)

Observes infant's feeding behaviors accurately ____

Comfortable in holding infant ____

Talks to baby ____

Attempts eye contact with baby ____

Deals appropriately with feeding problems ____

Other comments:

____

____

____

____

____

Suggestions for future planning: (Teaching needs of parents, techniques to use with baby, etc.)

Figure 8-8 *(Continued).*

FAMILY CARE

Addressograph

INFANT'S NAME	DATE OF BIRTH	SEX	ISOLETTE OR CRIB	OTHER CHILDREN

MOTHER'S NAME ____ AGE ____

DOES MOTHER HAVE SOMEONE AT HOME TO HELP HER CARE FOR INFANT?

DEMONSTRATIONS & DATE GIVEN

BATHING ____ CHANGING DIAPERS ____
FEEDING ____ CORD CARE ____
CIRCUMCISION CARE ____
READING THERMOMETER ____
GIVING VITAMINS ____

DOES MOTHER HAVE ADEQUATE SUPPLIES AT HOME TO CARE FOR INFANT?

OTHER COMMENTS REGARDING PARENT'S SITUATION OR REACTIONS - PLEASE DATE

Figure 8-9 Discharge planning is improved when it is arranged for systematically. (*Designed for use in the premature intensive care unit by Mary White, Head Nurse, and Joann Pritchard, Assistant Head Nurse, University of Cincinnati General Hospital, by permission.*)

that conditions in the home are adequate for safe care of the infant. Social workers and/or social service agencies may need to be consulted in order for some families to provide adequate care. In addition to predischarge planning, referrals for postdischarge follow-up are needed in many instances. These follow-ups are important for the necessary frequent health check-ups for the baby and for the parents to receive guidance as they care for the infant. Since the trend is toward earlier discharge of preterm infants (when they approach 2268 g [5 lb]), careful planning is a must. Figure 8-9 is an example of a form used for discharge planning by University of Cincinnati General Hospital.

REFERENCES

1 Lula O. Lubchenco, "Assessment of Gestational Age and Development at Birth," *Pediatric Clinics of North America,* February 1970, p. 126.

2 American Academy of Pediatrics, Committee on the Fetus and the Newborn, "Nomenclature for Duration of Gestation, Birth Weight, and Intra-Uterine Growth," *Pediatrics,* June 1967, p. 935.

3 Ibid., *Standards and Recommendations for Hospital Care of Newborn Infants,* American Academy of Pediatrics, Evanston, Ill., 1971, p. 19.

4 J. M. Tanner, "Standards for Birth Weight or Intra-Uterine Growth," *Pediatrics,* July 1970, pp. 1–6.

5 AAP Committee on the Fetus and the Newborn, "Nomenclature," p. 938.

6 Orvar Finnstrom, "Studies on Maturity in Newborn Infants, Part VI, Comparison between Different Methods for Maturity Estimation," *Acta Paediatrica Scandinavia,* January 1971, pp. 37–39.

7 Lubchenco, op. cit.

8 Ibid., p. 128.

9 Sheldon B. Korones, *High-Risk Newborn Infants: The Basis for Intensive Nursing Care,* Mosby, 1972, p. 12.

10 Ibid., p. 70.

11 Lilly M. S. Dubowitz, Victor Dubowitz, and Cissie Goldberg, "Clinical Assessment of Gestational Age in the Newborn Infant," *Journal of Pediatrics,* July 1970, pp. 1–10.

12 Claudine Amiel-Tison, "Neurological Evaluation of the Maturity of Newborn Infants," *Archives of Diseases of Children,* February 1968, p. 92.

13 Lubchenco, loc. cit.

14 Dubowitz, op. cit.

15 Korones, op. cit., p. 70.

16 Alexander J. Schaffer and Mary Ellen Avery, *Diseases of the Newborn,* Saunders, Philadelphia, 1971, p. 26.

17 Marshall Klaus and Avroy Fanaroff, "Respiratory Problems," in Marshall H. Klaus and Avroy A. Fanaroff (eds.), *Care of the High-Risk Neonate,* Saunders, Philadelphia, 1973, p. 128.

18 Jane M. Brightman and Stephanie Clatworthy, "Care of the High Risk Infant and His Family," in Joy Princeton Clausen, Margaret Hemp Flock, Bonnie

Ford, Marilyn A. Green, and Elsa S. Popiel (eds.), *Maternity Nursing Today,* McGraw-Hill, New York, 1973, p. 834.

19 Leo Stern, editorial comment in Klaus and Fanaroff, op. cit., p. 139.

20 Klaus and Fanaroff, op. cit., p. 139.

21 Stern, loc. cit.

22 Peter A. M. Auld, "Oxygen Therapy for Premature Infants," *Journal of Pediatrics,* April 1971, p. 706.

23 Klaus and Fanaroff, loc. cit.

24 Ibid.

25 Ann Llewellyn and Paul Swyer, "Assisted Ventilation," in Klaus and Fanaroff (eds.), op. cit., p. 161.

26 Auld, op. cit., p. 708.

27 Klaus and Fanaroff, op. cit., p. 140.

28 Auld, loc. cit.

29 Tibor Heim, "Thermogenesis in the Newborn Infant," *Clinical Obstetrics and Gynecology,* vol. 14, 1971, pp. 790–820.

30 Linda Lutz and Paul H. Perlstein, "Temperature Control in Newborn Babies," *Nursing Clinics of North America,* March 1971, pp. 15–23.

31 Brightman and Clatworthy, op. cit., p. 828.

32 Korones, op. cit., p. 213.

33 Michael K. Wald, "Problems in Chemical Adaptation," in Klaus and Fanaroff (eds.), op. cit., pp. 168–182.

34 Leo Stern, editorial comment in Wald, op. cit., p. 170.

35 Wald, op. cit., p. 170.

36 Ibid., pp. 175–176.

37 Avroy Fanaroff and Marshall Klaus, "Feeding and the Low-Birth-Weight Infant," in Klaus and Fanaroff (eds.), op. cit., p. 81.

38 Ibid., p. 83.

39 Gorham S. Babson, "Feeding the Low-Birth-Weight Infant," *Fetal and Neonatal Medicine,* October 1971, p. 689.

40 Leo Stern, editorial comment in Fanaroff and Klaus, op. cit., p. 83.

41 Roberta S. O'Grady, "Feeding Behavior in Infants," *American Journal of Nursing,* April 1971, p. 737.

42 Peggy L. Chinn, "Infant Gavage Feeding," *American Journal of Nursing,* October 1971, p. 1966.

43 Korones, op. cit., p. 196.

44 Samuel Gross and David K. Melhorn, "Hematologic Problems," in Klaus and Fanaroff (eds.), op. cit., p. 274.

BIBLIOGRAPHY

American Academy of Pediatrics, Committee on the Fetus and the Newborn: "Nomenclature for Duration of Gestation, Birth Weight, and Intra-Uterine Growth," *Pediatrics,* June 1967, pp. 35–39.

———: *Standards and Recommendations for Hospital Care of Newborn Infants,* American Academy of Pediatrics, Evanston, Ill., 1971.

Amiel-Tison, Claudine: "Neurological Evaluation of the Maturity of Newborn Infants," *Archives of Diseases of Children,* February 1968, pp. 89–93.

Auld, Peter A. M.: "Oxygen Therapy for Premature Infants," *Journal of Pediatrics,* April 1971, pp. 705–709.

———: "Use of Oxygen in Neonatal Units," *Journal of Pediatrics,* February 1972, pp. 317–318.

Babson, S. Gorham: "Feeding the Low-Birth-Weight Infant," *Fetal and Neonatal Medicine,* October 1971, pp. 694–701.

Brightman, Jane M., and Stephanie Clatworthy: "Care of the High-Risk Infant and His Family," in Joy Princeton Clausen, Margaret Hemp Flock, Marilyn A. Green, and Elsa S. Popiel (eds.), *Maternity Nursing Today,* McGraw-Hill, New York, 1973, pp. 820–867.

Chinn, Peggy L.: "Infant Gavage Feeding," *American Journal of Nursing,* October 1971, pp. 1964–1967.

Dubowitz, Lilly M. S., Victor Dubowitz, and Cissie Goldberg: "Clinical Assessment of Gestational Age in the Newborn Infant," *Journal of Pediatrics,* July 1970, pp. 1–10.

Fanaroff, Avroy, and Marshall Klaus: "Feeding the Low-Birth-Weight Infant," in Marshall H. Klaus and Avroy A. Fanaroff (eds.), *Care of the High-Risk Neonate,* Saunders, Philadelphia, 1973, pp. 77–89.

Farr, V., D. F. Kerridge, and R. G. Mitchell: "The Value of Some External Characteristics in the Assessment of Gestational Age at Birth," *Developmental Medicine and Child Neurology,* December 1966, pp. 657–660.

———, R. G. Mitchell, G. A. Neligan, and J. M. Parkin: "The Definition of Some External Characteristics Used in the Assessment of Gestational Age in the Newborn Infant," *Developmental Medicine and Child Neurology,* October 1966, pp. 507–511.

Finnstrom, Orvar: "Studies on Maturity in Newborn Infants, Part II, External Characteristics, and Part IV, Comparison between Different Methods for Maturity Estimation," *Acta Paediatrica Scandinavia,* January 1972, pp. 24–41.

Gross, Samuel, and David K. Melhorn: "Hematologic Problems," in Marshall H. Klaus and Avroy A. Fanaroff (eds.), *Care of the High-Risk Neonate,* Saunders, Philadelphia, 1973, pp. 270–286.

Heim, Tibor: "Thermogenesis in the Newborn Infant," *Clinical Obstetrics and Gynecology,* vol. 14, 1971, pp. 790–820.

Katz, Violet: "Auditory Stimulation and Developmental Behavior of the Premature Infant," *Nursing Research.* May–June 1971, pp. 196–201.

Klaus, Marshall, and Avroy Fanaroff: "Respiratory Problems," in Marshall Klaus and Avroy A. Fanaroff (eds.), *Care of the High-Risk Neonate,* Saunders, Philadelphia, 1973, pp. 119–151.

Korones, Sheldon B.: *High-Risk Newborn Infants: The Basis for Intensive Nursing Care,* Mosby, St. Louis, 1972.

Llewellyn, Ann, and Paul Swyer: "Assisted Ventilation," in Marshall H. Klaus and Avroy A. Fanaroff (eds.), *Care of the High-Risk Neonate,* Saunders, Philadelphia, 1973, pp. 152–167.

Lubchenco, Lula O.: "Assessment of Gestational Age and Development at Birth," *Pediatric Clinics of North America,* February 1970, pp. 125–145.

Lutz, Linda, and Paul H. Perlstein: "Temperature Control in Newborn Babies," *Nursing Clinics of North America,* March 1971, pp. 15–23.

O'Grady, Roberta S.: "Feeding Behavior in Infants," *American Journal of Nursing,* April 1971, pp. 736–739.

Roberts, Joyce E.: "Suctioning the Newborn," *American Journal of Nursing,* January 1973, pp. 63–65.

Schaffer, Alexander J., and Mary Ellen Avery: *Diseases of the Newborn,* Saunders, Philadelphia, 1971.

Segal, Sydney, "Oxygen: Too Much, Too Little," *Nursing Clinics of North America,* March 1971, pp. 39–53.

Tanner, J. M.: "Standards for Birth Weight or Intra-Uterine Growth" (commentary), *Pediatrics,* July 1970, pp. 1–6.

Wald, Michael K.: "Problems in Chemical Adaptation," in Marshall H. Klaus and Avroy A. Fanaroff (eds.), *Care of the High-Risk Neonate,* Saunders, Philadelphia, 1973, pp. 168–182.

Williams, Sandra L.: "Phototherapy in Hyperbilirubinemia," *American Journal of Nursing,* July 1971, pp. 1397–1399.

Chapter 9

The Infant in Need of Special Care

Of prime importance in the care of newborns is the identification of infants needing special care. The nurse is in a key position to effect such early identification of these infants.

THE DYSMATURE INFANT

The dysmature infant is one who is either small for gestational age (below the 10th percentile in body weight), large for gestational age (above the 90th percentile), or pre- or postterm. The preterm infant, discussed in detail in Chapter 8, will not be discussed here. The causes for dysmaturity are numerous and in many cases undetermined.

Small-for-Dates Infants

The small-for-dates baby suffers from intrauterine growth retardation, which may be caused either by some fetal incapacity for growth (exemplified by babies who have suffered intrauterine insults such as rubella infection) or by intrauterine malnutrition, which may be the result of poor maternal nutrition or some sort of placental dysfunction. It is important to identify these infants before birth, if possible, because they have, as a rule, sustained intrauterine deprivations of both glucose and oxygen which predispose them to intrapartal decompensation or death, especially if labor is prolonged or traumatic. Many of these fetuses have been in a state of distress for several days or even 2 or 3 weeks before delivery. It is not unusual to find greenish-yellow meconium staining of the nails, skin, and umbilical cord at birth. This staining indicates that meconium has been expelled from the gastrointestinal tract in utero—a reflex response to stress. Many infants who have this staining have already aspirated meconium particles into the lungs during reflex gasps taken in response to hypoxia. This phenomenon is called *massive aspiration syndrome.*

The prenatal identification of these infants can be hypothesized on the basis of maternal disease (toxemia, hypertension, advanced diabetes), reproductive history (previous fetal deaths, small-for-dates babies), or the course of the current pregnancy (lack of maternal weight gain in the last trimester or failure to increase uterine size, low maternal urinary levels of estriol). Special arrangements need to be made to provide complete fetal monitoring during labor and resuscitative assistance immediately after birth. Surgical intervention into the labor may also be needed in the event of severe fetal distress.

Postnatally, small-for-dates infants are predisposed to certain pathological conditions. Prominent among these is the tendency to develop hypoglycemia. The reasons for this tendency include a chronically poor nutritional state in utero, resulting in low glycogen stores, and the existence of a greater demand for glucose relative to weight because of the relatively normal (for age) development of such organs as the brain and kidneys, which utilize large quantities of glucose. To combat this tendency, many of these infants are started on glucose either intravenously or orally within 4 hours after birth. Close monitoring of blood glucose levels is vital. (See Chapter 8, Preventing Hypoglycemia and Hypocalcemia.)

Small-for-dates infants are also more likely to experience massive aspiration syndrome, described earlier. Pulmonary hemorrhage is a common problem, although the pathogenesis is not clear. General resuscitative and respiratory supportive measures are indicated.

Excessive postnatal heat loss is a problem for these infants because they usually have attained normal length for their gestational ages, giving them a relatively large surface area, but they do not have the insulating layers of muscle and subcutaneous fat found in normal infants. As has been emphasized throughout this book, excessive heat loss increases the need for oxygen, and it is associated with decreased levels of blood glucose.

These infants may also be polycythemic. It is hypothesized that the cause for the increased red blood cells is chronic intrauterine hypoxia, but the exact cause is not certain.[1] The infant may show no symptoms, or may develop distress related to increased blood viscosity, including respiratory symptoms (tachypnea, retractions, flaring of the nares, grunting), cardiac symptoms (tachycardia, congestive failure), cerebral symptoms (convulsions), or signs of vascular congestion (edema of the scrotum, erection of the penis). One would expect increased bilirubin levels in the days following delivery, also, as the red blood cell volume drops to a more normal level. This condition is usually treated if symptoms develop. Treatment may include decreasing the blood volume by removing some of the infant's blood, with or without fluid replacement, or a partial exchange transfusion.

Finally, any time small-for-dates infants are identified, they should be checked closely for evidence of intrauterine infection (which may still be communicable) and for the presence of hidden congenital anomalies, particularly those of cardiac or renal origin. Infants whose head circumference is small for gestational age are especially likely to have experienced intrauterine infections, such as rubella.

Large-for-Dates Infants

Large-for-dates infants are almost always the offspring of diabetic or prediabetic mothers. In addition to being heavier than expected for their gestational ages, these infants appear to be very fat and "puffy." (See Figure 9-1.) They may lack normal muscle tone, however, and often have a ruddy color. Many of them have fat pads over their upper backs not unlike those seen in Cushing's syndrome, although no increase in adrenal function has been demonstrated. Clinically, they are found to be comparatively dehydrated, having less water in proportion to body weight than their normal counterparts. Ironically, they may at the same time have pitting edema, as do preterm infants of comparable gestational ages. These infants are often delivered electively between 36 and 37 weeks of gestation in order to increase their survival rates. They react to extrauterine life with the same problems as would any infant of similar gestation.

Due to maternal hyperglycemia during pregnancy, these infants often show hyperplasia of the islets of Langerhans and subsequent hyperinsulinism. Although they frequently have elevated glucose levels at birth, the hyperinsulinism causes a precipitous fall in blood glucose, resulting in hypoglycemia which reaches its lowest levels at 2 to 4 hours of age. A depressed glucose level may persist for 24 hours. The infant may not show signs of hypoglycemia in spite of very low levels (below 20 mg/100 ml), however. Hypocalcemia may accompany the hypoglycemia.

Hyperbilirubinemia is also a greater problem for these infants than for their term counterparts. In this regard, they react much like other preterm infants, reaching peak jaundice levels between the fifth and seventh days.

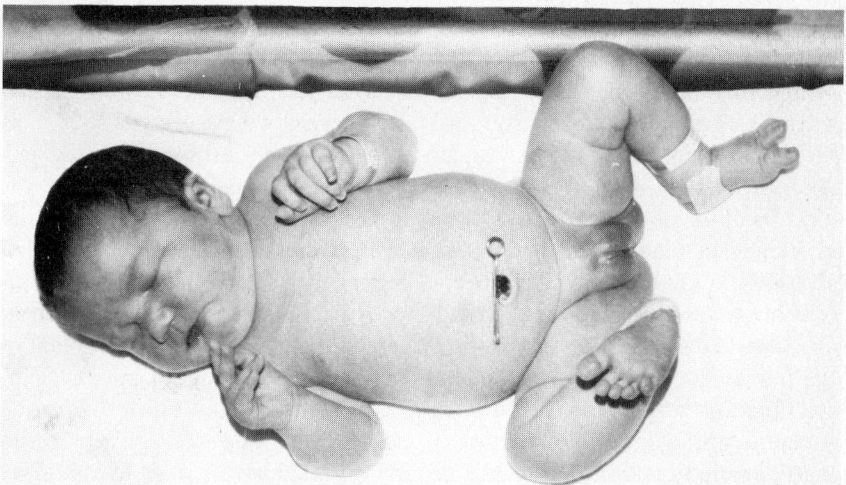

Figure 9-1 The infant of a diabetic mother has a characteristic "puffy" appearance. This infant at 40 weeks of gestation weighed 10 lb 13 oz. *(From G. Scipien et al., Comprehensive Pediatric Nursing, McGraw-Hill, New York, 1975, p. 297, by permission.)*

Another important problem of these infants is hyaline membrane disease. Since most of the infants are delivered by caesarean section, that may be a factor, but it is generally thought that the increased incidence of the disease is most closely associated with the low gestational age.

Congenital malformation is more likely in these infants, but the causative factors have not been defined. Placental pathology is common, being mostly of the degenerative nature (thrombosis and calcification of the vessels). Thrombosis of the infants' renal vessels is fairly common, also.

The prognosis for the infants is directly related to the severity of the maternal disease and the length of time it has been present. Approximately 50% of the infants have a normal postnatal course.[2] Once the infant survives the immediate postdelivery period, the prognosis is excellent, with the greatest problem being an increased incidence of diabetes later in life.

Treatment of the infants includes early and careful monitoring of blood glucose and calcium and the early institution of feedings and/or the use of intravenous fluids to supply needed glucose and fluids. Careful monitoring of respiratory function is a must. If hyaline membrane disease develops, it is treated as for any other infant. Bilirubin levels must be watched closely for several days. Renal function should be monitored, especially for the presence of protein and blood in the urine.

It is very important for the nurse to recognize that these infants are clearly high-risk infants and that in spite of their large size and "mature" appearance, they need careful attention.

The Postterm Infant

The infant born after 42 weeks gestation is designated postterm, or postmature, and has often suffered from placental dysfunction during the last weeks of gestation. As a result, an intrauterine weight loss is shown as evidenced by a loss of subcutaneous tissue. The infant's skin is dry and cracked, and vernix is absent. Often meconium staining is present, and it is thought that the infant has suffered some anoxia due to decrease in the efficiency of placental function. These infants are unusually wide-awake and alert, a characteristic which may reflect the chronic hypoxia.[3] The infant often has aspirated meconium before birth, and resuscitative measures are frequently required at delivery. Hypoglycemia is a common problem in the immediate newborn period. This, too, could be a result of poor placental function late in the gestational period. Most of the infants who die succumb during labor, a reflection of their chronic intrauterine hypoxic and malnourished condition. Labor is usually initiated by the obstetrician at 42 weeks, if it has not occurred spontaneously before that time. Treatment for the infants is focused upon resuscitative measures and respiratory support after birth and early feeding, if possible, to counteract hypoglycemia.

THE INFANT WITH RESPIRATORY DISTRESS

The first adaptation after birth is the establishment of adequate respirations. Similarly, the first responsibility of those who care for the infant is to assist in that adaptation.

Respiratory Depression at Birth

Failure to establish respirations at birth has numerous causes, the most common ones being occlusion of the airway and asphyxia during delivery. (Depression of the respiratory center due to maternal sedation is not considered to be a common occurrence.[4]) A definite pattern of behavior has been observed in newborn monkeys as they attempt to establish respiratory function.[5] First, there is a series of rapid gasps (these may occur in utero), which is accompanied by a thrashing of arms and legs. Following this period of activity (lasting about 1 minute) is a period of primary apnea, which also lasts approximately 1 minute. During primary apnea, spontaneous respirations can be stimulated by providing the monkey with sensory stimuli. Following the primary apnea is a period of spontaneous deep gasping which may last for 4 or 5 minutes, with the gasps becoming progressively weaker if oxygenation of the tissues does not occur. These gasps are followed by a period of secondary apnea which terminates in death unless artificial ventilation of the lungs occurs. It is thought that a similar sequence of events occurs in the human infant, though the periods may vary in timing somewhat from those of the monkey.[6]

Accompanying these behavior patterns are circulatory and biochemical changes. Blood pressure rises briefly, initially, and then falls until the asphyxia is corrected. Peripheral vasoconstriction occurs as a means of shunting blood to the brain, heart, and adrenal glands. The skin shows color changes which reflect this shunting of blood to the vital organs. It is at first dusky blue, then blotchy, and finally, pale. Biochemically, the infant changes from aerobic to anaerobic metabolism. Accumulation of lactic acid, a by-product of this anaerobic metabolism, results in metabolic acidosis. In addition, failure to aerate the lungs results in a rapid accumulation of carbon dioxide, which leads to respiratory acidosis as well. Hypoglycemia is not usually a concomitant of asphyxia, though it may be present due to some other cause, such as intrauterine malnutrition.

Asphyxia may be present at birth due to interference in normal placental function, or it may develop after birth due to failure to establish respiratory function. The severely asphyxiated infant is easily recognizable at birth. The infant is limp, cyanotic (or pale), unresponsive to stimuli, and is experiencing secondary apnea; vigorous resuscitative measures are mandatory. Nurses, other than those who have received special training in resuscitative techniques, do not usually do the actual resuscitation of these depressed babies, but they are responsible for providing appropriate supplies and equipment for assisting the physician or nurse specialist. (For those who desire a description of the procedure, see Klaus and Fanaroff pp. 11–12 or Korones pp. 52–58.) Generally, supplies needed include some means of visualizing the airway (lyringoscope), a means of clearing the airway (catheters, suction, plastic airways), a means of positive pressure ventilation, a source of oxygen which is humidified and warmed, drugs to counteract acidosis, cardiac stimulants (epinephrine) in case of cardiac arrest, and perhaps narcotic antagonists. A place must be provided for the resuscitation which will provide adequate lighting and work space for the examiner and at the same time protect the infant from cold stress. Some form of radiant heater is usually used. The surface on which the infant is lying should be firm enough to allow external cardiac massage if this is needed. The depressed infant will be positioned on his back with a blanket roll supporting the shoulders. The nurse should anticipate the need for the lyringoscope, first, with a suction apparatus being used as soon as the lyringoscope is positioned. (The batteries in a lyringoscope should be checked at the beginning of each shift to be sure that the light provided will be sufficiently bright to visualize the structures adequately.) If spontaneous respirations do not occur following suctioning of the airway, an endotracheal tube will be needed to provide for positive pressure ventilation of the lungs. (Experience will provide the nurse with the ability to anticipate the size of tubes that will be needed.) During assisted ventilation, the nurse should observe the infant's chest for bilateral expansion. (If the endotracheal tube is passed too deeply, the end will enter the right main stem bronchus and only the right lung will be expanded.) The nurse may also be asked to provide continuous auscultation of the chest for breath sounds and to assess the cardiac rate. If the rate falls below 100 beats/minute or if it does not increase after inflation of the lungs is begun, external cardiac massage is started. This procedure usually requires the coordinated efforts of two persons, one to inflate the lungs and the other to compress the sternum between lung inflations. (See Chapter 8, Nursing Care of the Preterm Infant, Maintenance of Respirations.) Prolonged resuscitative measures must include correction of acidosis as well as the other measures described above. Intravenous injections of sodium bicarbonate are usually used for this. The sodium bicarbonate is usually ordered on the basis of 3 meq/kg birth weight, diluted with water or dextrose and water and administered slowly through an umbilical vessel catheter. In some instances, a cardiac stimulant (epinephrine 1:10,000, for instance) may need to be administered either intravenously or directly into the heart.

For less depressed infants (those with Apgar scores of 3 to 6), the use of a lyringoscope and suctioning of the airway followed by oxygen administration for a short time will usually improve respiratory function. If apnea occurs in these babies, it is usually primary apnea and spontaneous gasping is expected. Recovery is rapid.

Later-Developing Respiratory Distress

Respiratory distress that develops after birth can be caused by many conditions. One study of 116 infants who developed respiratory distress within the first 4 hours after birth revealed that 80 of the infants, or 69 percent, had a transient respiratory problem which cleared with very little treatment; 12 of the infants, or approximately 1 percent, developed hyaline membrane disease, and 10 or 0.86 percent, had either massive aspiration syndrome or bronchopneumonia.[7]

The general principles for the care of all these infants includes the following points:

1 Minimize metabolic requirements.
2 Provide adequate ventilation and oxygenation to maintain a satisfactory arterial Po_2 level.
3 Correct metabolic acidosis with alkali. (It seems preferable to correct respiratory acidosis with assisted ventilation.)
4 Provide fluid and caloric needs by infusion during acute episodes.
5 Monitor vital signs and temperature continuously.

Minimize Metabolic Requirements The nursing care required to meet these objectives is quite detailed and demanding. To minimize metabolic requirements, one must maintain the infant in a truly thermoneutral environment (see Chapters 2, 3 and 4). This requires surveillance of air temperature inside and outside the incubator and of temperature of incubator walls and large surrounding objects, and an awareness of such factors as sunlight coming in the window and the presence of air conditioner vents. In addition, the temperature of the oxygen being administered to the infant (especially when a hood is used) must be monitored, and the infant's skin and core temperatures monitored and correlated with all the other factors. Every effort must be made to avoid stimulating the infant through excessive handling. Such stimulation, in addition to tiring the infant, is thought to increase apenic periods through changes in the excitatory state of the respiratory center.[8] Klaus and Fanaroff cite such simple maneuvers as taking rectal temperatures and cleaning the face as being associated with at least temporary clinical deterioration in seriously ill infants.[9]

Provide Adequate Ventilation In providing adequate ventilation, the nurse is in a key position to detect early apnea. Klaus and Fanaroff differentiate periodic breathing and apnea by two criteria.[10] Periodic breathing is a short cessation of breathing effort (less than 15 seconds) which is not accompanied by any functional changes such as cyanosis, hypotonia, or metabolic acidosis. Apnea is a cessation of breathing for more than 15 seconds or one of shorter duration which is accompanied by cyanosis, hypotonia, and/or metabolic acidosis. Small infants [less than 1,200 g (2 lb 10.5 oz)] may be harmed by cessation of breathing of from 5 to 10 seconds; hence the time period alone is not sufficient to judge the importance of the episode. Many electronic monitors are available to aid the nurse in recognizing apnea, but nothing can surpass the close attendance of a skilled nurse. In some hospitals, very sick infants are routinely "specialed" on a one-to-one basis for this reason. (Most intensive-care units use not more than a 1:2 or a 1:3 ratio for the very sick infants.) Gentle tactile stimulation will usually restore respiratory function when apnea occurs, but a bag resuscitator should be readily available for use with each infant. Stern recommends that the infant be resuscitated without increases in the percentage of oxygen already being administered, as raising the oxygen level increases the possibility of the infant's developing retrolental fibroplasia.[11] Similarly, others have recommended that the environmental oxygen concentration not be increased as a means of preventing simple apnea, because while this practice does seem to decrease the number of apneic episodes, it tends to increase the length of the periods.[12]

Positioning to increase ventilation has already been discussed in Chapter 8. Observations to evaluate the effectiveness of ventilation include watching for bilateral chest expansion and auscultation of the chest for breath sounds. (This is a clinical skill which can be learned by nurses who care for these infants regularly.) X-rays are frequently ordered to evaluate lung ventilation. When x-rays are done, the nurse should be sure adequate precautions are taken to protect the infant from exposure to infectious organisms and cold stress. Precautions are necessary, as well, to protect the infant and personnel from radiation hazards. Nursing care needed when assisted ventilation is used is discussed separately at the end of this section.

Precautions needed in the administration of oxygen have been discussed in detail in Chapter 8. To reiterate the most important points, the oxygen rate of flow and concentrations inside the hood or incubator should be checked hourly when concentrations over 40 percent are used, but use of concentrations of less than 40 percent are capable of causing retrolental fibroplasia in some infants. Measurements of arterial oxygen tension is essential in evaluating the infant's need for oxygen. The exact desirable level for arterial Po_2 is somewhat debatable, but the level should not exceed 90 mmHg in any event. In many hospitals, examination of the eyes for vasoconstriction of the retinal vessels is done at frequent intervals while oxygen is being administered. (Vasoconstriction is reversible if caught in time and if the oxygen concentration is lowered.) Oxygen must be warmed and humidified. The concentration of oxygen administered should be decreased slowly over a period of hours or days, never stopped abruptly. When lowering oxygen concentrations, the nurse should observe for tachypnea, tachycardia, pallor, a decrease in body temperature, or distension of the abdomen. All these signs indicate the need for blood gas determinations and a slight increase in ambient oxygen.

When blood gases are to be monitored over a period of time, catheterization of the umbilical artery is commonly done. While this is a medical procedure, the nurse is responsible for assisting and for supervising the care of the catheter once it is inserted. The procedure for insertion requires sterile technique and x-ray determination of placement of the catheter once it is in place. Complications of the procedure include the formation of thrombi, vascular spasm, occlusion of the artery, infection, and serious hemorrhage. If the leg of the infant blanches during insertion of the catheter, the doctor should be told at once, because the catheter needs to be removed immediately to restore circulation to that limb. Once inserted, the catheter is attached to a stopcock so that serial determinations of blood gases may be made. Although the stopcocks have locks to keep them closed, the possibility of serious hemorrhage must be kept in mind. When the catheter is removed, the stump of the umbilical artery must be sutured.

A new concern is developing regarding the use of plastics in circulatory catheters and containers of blood products (whole blood, plasma, etc.). A substance called a plasticizer, which maintains the flexibility of such equipment, is lipid-soluble and can be recovered from the tissues of infants receiving long-term cannalization, especially when they have received blood products stored in plastic bags. The consequences of these findings are not clear, but it has been noted that infants receiving exchange transfusions are more likely to develop necrotizing enterocolitis (to be discussed later) than infants not exchanged.[13] In a small series of infants studied by Hillman, three who died of enterocolitis had significant increases in the plasticizer content of their intestinal tracts.[14]

Correct Metabolic Acidosis In considering the administration of alkali, it is important to recognize that sodium bicarbonate, which is usually used, must be diluted and administered slowly. Too rapid injection of a hypertonic solution causes tissue fluid to enter the circulatory system, increasing the circulating volume and decreasing tissue hydration. There may be a rapid rise in pressure both in the circulation and in cerebrospinal fluid followed by a sharp fall in cerebrospinal fluid pressure.[15] Brain hemorrhage is one of the possible sequelae.

Provide for Fluid and Caloric Needs Fluid and caloric needs are usually met by infusion during acute respiratory distress. Oral or tube feedings risk the possibility of aspiration pneumonia and respiratory embarrassment from pressure of a full stomach on the diaphragm. Usually, during these periods, peristalsis is decreased, also, further necessitating the use of the parenteral route. Caloric requirements will probably increase during acute episodes because of the increased work of respiration, especially in hyaline membrane disease. Complete and accurate records of total intake and output should be maintained, and the rate and contents of infusions used should be noted frequently. The use of infusion pumps has simplified the regulation of these systems considerably, but careful personal observation is also needed.

Assisted Ventilation

There are times when the infant is unable to maintain adequate oxygenation of tissues even in 100 percent environmental oxygen. When this is true, some form of mechanical assistance is required. This assistance usually takes the form of apparatus that provides either positive pressures to the respiratory passages or negative pressures to the chest wall. Either of these approaches may be used either intermittently (the pressure changes with the respiratory cycle) or continuously (no change in pressure during the respiratory cycle). Positive pressure devices most often utilize either an endotracheal tube or a nasal device which intubates only the nares. If continuous positive pressure is used, the infant's blood pressure needs to be monitored because the pressure in the lungs may be translated to the pulmonary circulation and indirectly decrease cardiac output. Some authors advocate intubating the stomach and closing the mouth to prevent inflation of the gastrointestinal tract.[16] When negative-pressure devices are used, the infant's body is enclosed in a chamber which produces negative pressure on the body wall. If the chamber must be entered for any reason, it is necessary to remember that the effects of the chamber will be negated and that some other kind of ventilation assistance, such as a bag resuscitator, must be provided until the negative pressure can be reestablished. The introduction of air into the intestinal tract is common and may require intubation.

When a mechanical ventilator is in use, adequate monitoring of blood gases to determine changes in the infant's condition should be done. The endotracheal tube, if one is used, should be suctioned at least every 2 hours and more often if needed. Sterile technique should be used in suctioning. The infant's position should be changed every 4 hours. The ventilator and nebulizer tubings, if they are used, should be changed every 24 hours, and bacterial filters should be used if possible.[17] The concentration of oxygen actually going into the endotracheal tube should be checked frequently. The tubing should be checked for leaks, and mechanical and electrical failures should be guarded against. If the infant's condition suddenly deteriorates, the placement of the tube and its patency should be checked. The possibility of a pneumothorax exists when positive-pressure devices are in use. The possibility of an air leak, especially around the infant's neck, should be checked when a negative-pressure system is in use.

In weaning the infant from the respirator, it is important to change only one variable at a time. The mechanical device should not be removed simultaneously with the infant's placement in an environment which has a lower oxygen concentration than the infant was receiving with the ventilator, for instance. The infant should be tried on unassisted ventilation for a few hours before the endotracheal tube is removed, if one has been used. The tube is removed only after it has been established that the infant can maintain adequate oxygenation of tissues without mechanical assistance.

The mechanics involved in the use of ventilating devices are much too complex to be presented here. Let it suffice to say that any nurse responsible for the care of an infant who is receiving assisted ventilation should be completely familiar with the equipment used. Llewellyn and Swyer present an excellent discussion of assisted ventilation.[18]

Hyaline Membrane Disease

In considering specific causes of respiratory distress, the first condition that comes to mind is hyaline membrane disease (respiratory distress syndrome), since it is the most common of the life-threatening disorders. The etiology of the disease is not completely clear, but it seems to involve a decreased production or effectiveness of surfactant. (See Chapter 2, Surfactant.) This decrease may be associated with immaturity, since surfactant is not produced until the latter part of pregnancy. Sometimes associated with decreased surfactant in older infants (over 32 weeks of gestation) is the occurrence of intrauterine asphyxia, which results in hypoperfusion of the infant's pulmonary vessels with subsequent alveolar hypoperfusion. This, in turn, is thought to decrease the ability of alveolar cells to produce the surfactant. Concomitant to this alveolar damage is the effusion of fibrin into the airspaces, releasing a peptide that acts as a strong vasoconstrictor, thus further decreasing the blood supply to the alveolar vessels. The end result of surfactant deficiency is a greatly increased work of respiration, as described previously. In addition, the collapse of the alveoli in the expiratory phase of respiration results in atelectasis in parts of the lung and incomplete ventilation in others. The infant with hyaline membrane disease can be identified initially by an expiratory grunt when he or she is quiet. This may in fact be the only early sign that is present. An increasing respiratory rate, flaring of the nares, and cyanosis in room air are also common, however.

For differentiating infants with adequate and inadequate amounts of surfactant present, the "shake" test has been devised.[19] Amniotic fluid may be obtained by aspiration of the neonate's gastric contents (which include swallowed amnionic fluid) within 1 hour after birth or by amniocentesis before birth. The gastric aspirate or amnionic fluid is mixed with absolute alcohol in a specially provided test tube and the contents are shaken for 15 seconds. The presence of bubbles at the meniscus indicates the presence of substances in the amnionic fluid that reflect the presence of surfactant in the lungs. The absence of bubbles indicates inadequate surfactant. The presence of very tiny bubbles extending one-third of the circumference of the tube indicates borderline surfactant, and the presence of larger, more numerous bubbles establishes that sufficient surfactant is present to sustain normal respiratory function.

The infant with hyaline membrane disease may require assisted ventilation for several hours or days, and will surely require all the supportive measures discussed earlier in this chapter. The long-term outlook for these infants is generally good if they survive the first 2 or 3 days. A few of the small infants do show residual pulmonary problems after discharge, but most of these clear up by the time the child is 5 years old.[20]

Massive Aspiration Syndrome

Another condition which is fairly common is the massive aspiration syndrome, in which the infant aspirates amniotic fluid containing meconium. The meconium can be seen if the airway is visualized before suctioning, and it should be suspected any time meconium staining is present. Suctioning of the airway should always precede the administration of positive-pressure ventilation, as such use of pressure would push the solid particles further into the bronchial tree. The result of this syndrome is both mechanical blockage of the respiratory paths and chemical irritation and pneumonia. The lung can remove the meconium without assistance however, and recovery usually occurs after 48 hours. One complication that can occur is a sudden pneumothorax as a result of overexpansion of some parts of the lung. This should be suspected if an infant who is doing well suddenly deteriorates. The sudden occurrence of a distended abdomen is one sign which should alert the nurse to this possibility, also. A shift in the location of the apical pulse is another. To treat symptomatic pneumothorax, chest suction may be instituted. An emergency measure which may be life-saving is the administration of 100 percent oxygen for a brief period.[21] Because of changes which occur in concentrations of oxygen in tissue capillaries when 100 percent oxygen is administered, the total gas pressure in the tissues is decreased and the rate of absorption of the gas trapped in the pleural space is increased. The toxic effects of high concentrations of oxygen preclude the use of this treatment as any but an emergency measure, however.

Transient Tachypnea of the Newborn

Finally, a common respiratory problem of the neonate is the relatively innocuous transient tachypnea of the newborn. Most of the infants who develop this condition are term infants, the products of uneventful pregnancies and deliveries. Their primary symptom is an increased respiratory rate. Cyanosis is not usually present, and pH measurements are within normal limits. The disease runs its course in 4 to 5 days with spontaneous recovery. It is thought that the cause of this syndrome is slowness in absorption of the normal fluid found in the respiratory tract prior to birth.[22]

THE INFANT WITH HYPERBILIRUBINEMIA

A common problem in the neonatal period is moderate hyperbilirubinemia. The severe form of the condition is discussed separately in the section following this one.

Moderate Hyperbilirubinemia

When the red blood cell is hemolyzed, one of the by-products is bilirubin, which is carried in the blood in a fat-soluble form. Most of the serum bilirubin is carried in the blood bound to albumin molecules, and hence it is unable to leave the circulatory system. Only a tiny fraction of it is free of this albumin binding, and it normally diffuses into special cells in the liver where it is metabolized (conjugated) to a water-soluble form to be excreted as a component of bile into the intestinal tract. From there it is eliminated in the stools. Two substances, an enzyme, glucuronyl transferase, and a substrate, uridine-diphosphoglucuronic acid (UDPGA), are required for the conjugation of bilirubin in the liver.

Hyperbilirubinemia and bilirubin toxicity may result from increased hemolysis of red blood cells, from interference with albumin binding, from inadequate supplies of the enzyme or its substrate, or from interference with elimination of bile from the intestinal tract. In the newborn, particularly in the preterm infant, some or all of these conditions may be present, making hyperbilirubinemia a frequent occurrence.

Increased Rate of Hemolysis After birth, the rate of red blood cell hemolysis is initially increased due to the presence of polycythemia, especially when cord clamping is delayed until all pulsations have stopped and due to a shorter life span of the erythrocyte than is true for the adult. Hemolysis may also be caused by enzymes produced by bacteria in sepsis. Hemolysis of extravascular blood when large hematomas, extensive bruising, or numerous petechiae are present may also cause excess bilirubin to be formed.

Interference with Albumin Binding There are several substances which compete with bilirubin for the binding sites on the albumin molecule in the neonate. Of particular importance are free fatty acids, which tend to be increased after cold stress and hypoxia. Some drugs compete for the albumin sites, notably the sulfonamides, the salicylates, and high doses of vitamin K. Sodium benzoate, a common vehicle used in parenteral solutions, also competes for albumin binding sites. Bilirubin is also more readily released from albumin in the presence of acidosis.

Decreased Enzyme Function The enzyme glucuronyl transferase is generally thought to be somewhat deficient in neonates, particularly preterm infants. (Klaus disagrees with this conclusion, however.[23]) This deficiency is thought to decrease the ability of the liver to conjugate the bilirubin which is produced. UDPGA may also be reduced during hypoglycemia or hypoxia, as ample supplies of both are needed for its production.

Resorption from the Gastrointestinal Tract In the neonate there is a unique possibility of resorption of bile from the intestinal tract. In the fetal and neonatal intestine, the enzyme β-glucuronidase can convert conjugated (water-soluble) bilirubin excreted in the bile to a fat-soluble form which can then be reabsorbed into the circulatory system. The presence of normal intestinal bacteria flora inhibits this reconversion in the older infant, but the newborn's intestinal tract is sterile at birth and the inhibitory organisms are absent. Meconium contains a high concentration of bilirubin. Anything that slows elimination of meconium can therefore contribute significantly to increases in serum bilirubin levels. Hyperbilirubinemia is often associated with intestinal obstruction in the newborn, for instance. Congenital deformities that block the excretion of bile may also cause severe hyperbilirubinemia. Congenital atresia of the bile ducts is an example of one such condition.

Early Recognition Early recognition of hyperbilirubinemia is very important, as high levels can lead to *kernicterus*, a staining of brain tissues by bilirubin with serious neurologic sequelae. Jaundice is the first obvious sign of hyperbilirubinemia. The evaluation of skin jaundice has been discussed in Chapter 4. Later signs which occur are weakening of the Moro reflex, a decrease in sucking behavior or other feeding difficulties, a decrease in muscle tone, and a high-pitched cry. If these signs are not recognized and the hyperbilirubinemia is untreated, brain damage occurs and muscle rigidity, irritability, and opisthotonic posturing appear. Damage from kernicterus is not reversible; hence, the condition must be anticipated and prevented. It is especially important to remember that the appearance of jaundice in the first 24 hours of life usually portends the likelihood of significantly high bilirubin levels within hours. Later-appearing jaundice (after the first 24 hours) is less ominous, but worthy of close observation.

Treatment Treatment of hyperbilirubinemia is based upon measures to lower the blood level of bilirubin and correction of the cause, if possible. Phototherapy is often employed in moderate hyperbilirubinemia as a means of decreasing serum bilirubin levels (see Figure 9-2). This treatment has been discussed in Chapter 4 (Jaundice). Other forms of treatment may be attempted, also.

Albumin binding capacity may be increased by infusing the infant with extra supplies of albumin, especially just before an exchange transfu-

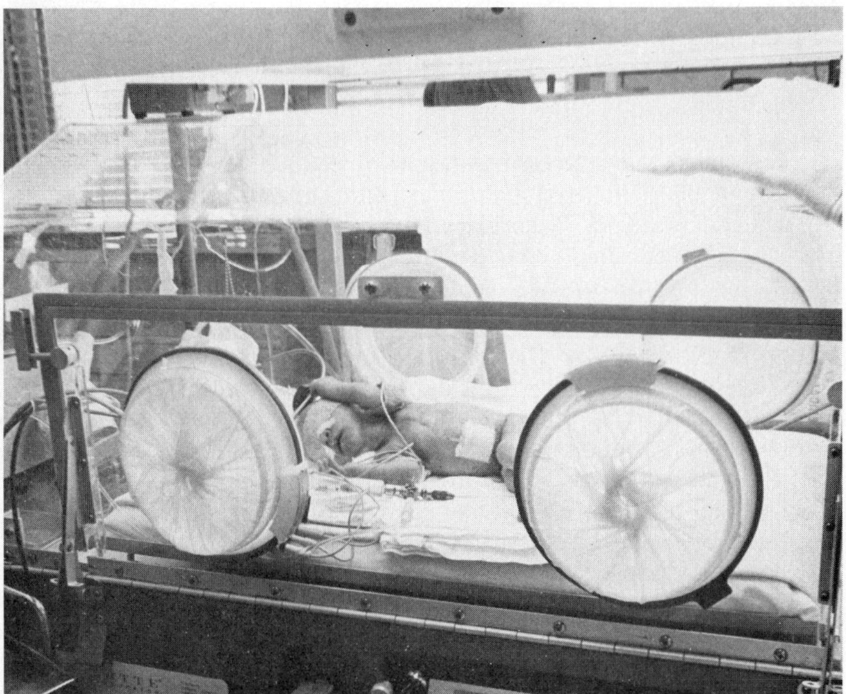

Figure 9-2 This seriously ill infant is receiving phototherapy. Note the blindfold. *(Photo: Penelope Ann Peirce.)*

sion, and by correcting conditions, such as acidosis, which decrease the binding capacity of albumin that is already present.

An attempt may be made to enhance enzyme function by providing for a thermoneutral environment and by ensuring adequate oxygenation and nutrition of tissues. In addition, it has been found that phenobarbitol administered either to the mother before delivery or to the infant after birth seems to enhance the activity of glucuronyl transferase and hence increases the functional capacity of the liver. The full effects of this treatment, however, have not been evaluated, and . t is used with caution.

Measures to evacuate meconium soon after birth, notably with early feedings of colostrum, which is thought to exert a laxative effect, are helpful. These early feedings also help in establishing the normal intestinal flora, which in turn prevents the conversion of the conjugated bilirubin to unconjugated bilirubin in the intestinal tract. The oral administration of agar to infants to hasten the elimination of meconium and to prevent reconversion of bilirubin have been tried with some success.[24]

Hemolytic Disease of the Newborn

Severe jaundice in the newborn is almost always a result of hemolytic disease of the newborn (formerly called erythroblastosis fetalis). This disease is essentially an antigen-antibody reaction caused by a difference in the blood types (ABO incompatibility) or, more commonly, in the Rh factor (Rh negative and Rh positive) between the fetus and the mother. The most severe reactions are seen in Rh incompatibility.

Rh-positive individuals have one of three or four Rh antigens attached to their erythrocytes, just as they may have antigens for blood types A or B. If blood cells with this Rh antigen enter the blood of a person with Rh-negative blood (who does not have the antigen), antibodies are produced. The antibodies eventually destroy the foreign erythrocytes.

When an Rh-negative woman is carrying an Rh-positive fetus, she may become sensitized to the Rh antigen. Although the placental barrier prevents wholesale mixing of fetal and maternal blood, occasional cells do cross the barrier, especially in late pregnancy when the tissue barrier thins. Almost always, at the time of delivery, when the placenta separates from the uterine wall, the mother receives into her blood stream some fetal blood from the placenta. If nothing is done at this time to prevent the formation of maternal antibodies, the mother becomes sensitized to that antigen. She will then manufacture large quantities of antibodies the next time the antigen enters her bloodstream. If the mother becomes pregnant with another child with the same antigen, there will usually be some antibodies present in her serum throughout the pregnancy and crossing of a few fetal cells into the maternal circulation will stimulate production of many more. The maternal antibodies cross the placenta readily and hemolyze the erythrocytes of the fetus.

The symptoms that occur in the fetus or infant depend upon when the antigen-antibody reaction begins and its strength. If it is initiated early in the pregnancy, the fetus may be born with severe disease or may be stillborn. If the process begins later, symptoms may not appear until after birth. In severe cases, fetal anemia in utero is severe due to destruction of red blood cells, and cardiac failure may occur as a result of the anemia. Severe edema (hydrops fetalis) and severe pallor are evident at the time of delivery. Usually the maternal and placental circulatory systems eliminate the fetal bilirubin that is produced by the destruction of the erythrocytes prior to delivery. When the fetus is severely affected before birth, that fact can be determined by following the antibody titer in the mother's blood. When indicated, intrauterine transfusions can be performed to counteract the anemia and prevent congestive failure. This procedure is seen infrequently now due to the use of Rh immune globulin to prevent sensitization of the mother. Early termination of the pregnancy is sometimes done to prevent intrauterine death.

If the reaction begins later in the pregnancy, the infant may appear normal at birth, only to show rapidly increasing levels of bilirubin in the first few hours afterward. For the infant who develops severe jaundice after birth, the procedure usually done is an exchange transfusion. Exchanges are usually done as the bilirubin level approaches 20 mg/100 ml. However, kernicterus has been known to occur at much lower levels (9 mg/100 ml) under certain conditions.[25] In an exchange transfusion, blood which will not be destroyed by the maternal antibodies is infused into the infant with alternate removal of small quantities of blood from the baby. In this way, the maternal antibodies are largely removed from the infant's bloodstream, and those that remain are greatly diluted. In addition, the infant is provided with blood cells that can carry on the normal functions of erythrocytes until fetal production of red blood cells can overcome the maternal antibodies remaining in his system.

Exchange Transfusion In preparing for an exchange transfusion, several points should be kept in mind. First, the blood to be used should be taken out of refrigeration about an hour before the exchange is to take place and allowed to warm slowly to room temperature. No artificial heat should be applied, however, because the cells closest to the outside of the container may become overheated and hemolyze. The exchange must be done in a thermoneutral environment. This is usually accomplished by using a radiant heater over an open bed or table. Resuscitative and respiratory support equipment should be available, also. The infant is usually kept NPO for about 3 hours prior to the exchange. If this is not possible, then intubation and gastric aspiration may be done to prevent vomiting and accidental aspiration into the lungs.

A glucose infusion will probably be started both for maintaining hydration and to combat hypoglycemia, which is a common problem. Hypoglycemia seems to accompany hemolytic disease of the newborn whether or not an exchange is done. It is hypothesized that glutathione, produced by the breakdown of red cells, stimulates insulin production before the infant is born, resulting in hyperplasia of the islets of Langerhans and hyperinsulinism at birth, which of course causes hypoglycemia to develop.[26] It is especially important to maintain normal glucose levels during an exchange because free fatty acids, which increase in hypoglycemia, compete with bilirubin for the albumin binding sites. (It should be recalled in this regard, also, that free fatty acids increase if hypothermia occurs.)

Hypoglycemia may be influenced by the blood used for the exchange. If heparinized fresh blood is used, there is no added glucose in the blood and free fatty acids are increased. Since the ratio of free fatty acids to glucose is inverse, adding a high level of free fatty acids to the blood may result in further lowering of its glucose level. When the blood used for the exchange has been preserved with an acid/citrate/dextrose mixture (ACD blood), as is true of blood stored in the blood bank, there is a high glucose level in the infused blood, and hypoglycemia during the exchange is not a problem. However, the high levels of glucose that result from the exchange will stimulate insulin production and may result in a drop in glucose levels approximately 2 hours after the exchange.

Acidosis contributes to a decrease in albumin binding of bilirubin. Infants who receive ACD blood are usually somewhat acidotic immediately after the exchange because of the acid used in preserving the blood. Ironically, they often become alkalotic a short time later because of excess sodium ions which are produced as the preservatives from the blood are metabolized. A buffer is usually added to the infused blood to prevent the acidosis, but several adjustments in blood pH may be necessary during and after the procedure.

When ACD blood is used, there may be also a problem of hypocalcemia due to depletion of calcium ions by the citrate used in the preservative. Frequent checks of blood calcium levels are necessary to prevent tetany and convulsions. Calcium gluconate should be readily available for infusion in case it is needed.

When blood is used that has been stored for more than 2 or 3 days, another hazard is introduced. Such blood is likely to have a high level of potassium ions due to hemolysis, which occurs during storage. The infant to be exchanged very likely already has elevated serum potassium due to hemolysis of his or her own cells. Since the dangers of adding potassium to the blood are especially great when calcium levels are low, these infants may be overwhelmed by hyperkalemia and death can result. The cardiac changes that result from hyperkalemia can best be diagnosed by the use of ECG tracings during the procedure.[77] Such tracings are also helpful in identifying hypocalcemia.

When heparinized blood is used, protamine sulfate is needed to neutralize the heparin during and/or following the exchange.

As the exchange is done, 10 to 20 ml of blood is withdrawn from the infant's circulation through an umbilical vein catheter and then an equal amount of donor blood is replaced until approximately 170 ml/kg body weight has been exchanged.[28] The first and last samples of blood withdrawn from the infant are sent to the laboratory for studies, particularly for bilirubin determinations. Vital signs are checked throughout the exchange, a careful record must be kept of volumes of blood withdrawn and infused, and venous pressure should be measured frequently to prevent cardiac overloading. Klaus recommends checking venous pressure after each 50 ml of exchange for a severely edematous infant because of the return of fluid into the circulatory system as the oncotic pressure rises during the exchange.[29] For nonedematous infants, venous pressure checks after every 100 ml of exchanged blood seem satisfactory. Frequent observations for signs of hypocalcemia (irritability, tachycardia, twitching) should be made when ACD blood is administered. If symptoms occur, intravenous calcium gluconate will be needed for slow infusion. The catheter will need to be rinsed with saline before and after the calcium infusion.

Complications that can occur from the exchange include cardiac overload and failure, cardiac arrest (thought to be due to overcooling the heart[30]), cardiac arrhythmias, electrolyte imbalances, bleeding from overheparinization, hypothermia and hypoglycemia, mechanical injury to the vessels or heart, the formation of air emboli or thrombi, and the possibility of infection.

Anemia is likely to occur in the second week after an exchange as the remaining maternal antibodies destroy more cells. It is thought that a contributing factor is that blood-producing tissues may be somewhat suppressed by the exchange.[31] This anemia is not usually treated unless the hemoglobin level falls below 7 to 8 mg/100 ml because it is not responsive to iron therapy, and it is thought that to transfuse again might further delay normal erythrocyte production.

In spite of the risk of several serious complications, exchange transfusion mortality rates are low. In one study, the mortality rate for the exchange and up to 6 hours afterward was less than 1 percent over a 6-year period.[32]

The best treatment for hemolytic disease, however, is prevention. In the early 1960s Rh immune globulin became available. This globulin prevents the sensitization of the mother at the time of delivery by inactivating the fetal antigens passively before they can stimulate antibody production in the mother. Clinical use of the immunoglobulin has all but eradicated the disease in mothers who receive the globulin within 72 hours of delivery.[33] The treatment must be repeated for each pregnancy and for any abortions that occur. It is possible for a mother to become sensitized during an abortion, just as she would be at the delivery of an infant.

THE INFECTED INFANT

No condition is so subtle, nor so difficult to identify, in the neonate as infection. The person most likely to note the earliest signs is the nurse because these signs are so insidious that only one who knows the infant well is likely to recognize them. Prominent among presenting symptoms is that the infant simply "doesn't look well" or is "doing poorly." Often, such a comment cannot be made more specific at first, so slight are the changes. A minute loss of muscle tone, a tiny decrease in alertness and activity, and refusal to feed or loss of eagerness for feeding are frequently the only observable signs of a fulminating infection. Temperature instability is common, but fever, the hallmark of infection in the older infant is not commonly seen in the neonatal period. Similarly, particular symptoms such as nuchal rigidity which accompanies meningitis and coughing which is normally seen in pneumonia in the older child are notably absent during the neonatal period.

Symptoms commonly seen in central nervous system infections during the neonatal period are either irritability or lethargy, seizures, bulging fontanels, and an increase or decrease in general muscle tone. It should be noted, however, that the infant may have meningitis without any of these symptoms.

Indications of respiratory infection may include all the signs of respiratory distress. Among signs of gastrointestinal infection are abdominal distention, poor feeding, and vomiting or diarrhea. Skin rashes may accompany septicemia, though not invariably. Jaundice and increased bleeding tendency are common indications of infection, as are changes in color and cardiac function (tachycardia, arrhythmias, hypotension). Almost any change in the condition of the infant may indicate the presence of an infection. Often, the diagnosis must be presumptive, based on slight physical findings and a knowledge of the history of the pregnancy and delivery and of the neonatal course.

Factors That Predispose to Infection

It is most helpful for the nurse to be aware of factors which are often associated with neonatal infections so that a high index of suspicion can be maintained during the infant's stay in the nursery. When two or more factors are combined, the infant is especially at risk for infection. Any maternal infections during pregnancy place the infant at risk. Of particular importance are rubella, herpes, and cytomegalovirus infections. Toxoplasmosis, syphilis, and bacterial infections of the urinary and intestinal tracts may also be important. All these infections may be passed to the fetus via the placenta before birth. Any sign of maternal infection at the time of delivery, such as fever, should also alert the nurse to the possibility of neonatal infection. Infection may also ascend the birth canal. This is most common when the amniotic membrane has ruptured more than 24 hours before delivery, though ascending infections have been known to occur when membranes are intact.[34] When the amniotic fluid becomes infected, the fetus becomes infected as the fluid is swallowed. If the fetus becomes hypoxic, it may gasp, as well, and aspirate the infected fluid. It is not uncommon for the organisms to enter the middle ear and the intestinal tract.

Trauma predisposes to infection, especially when the skin is broken or when large hematomas are formed. Resuscitative procedures and catheterizations of arteries and veins also increase the likelihood of infection. Preterm delivery is highly associated with neonatal infections for many reasons. The preterm infant is less able to defend against infection and more likely to require manipulation at birth or resuscitative measures. Males are more likely than females to develop infection. It is hypothesized that this tendency is a reflection of a genetic difference related to the X chromosome's influence on the synthesis of immunoglobulins.[35] The presence of congenital malformations and the necessity for surgery during the neonatal period also increase the likelihood of infection. Finally, it must be remembered that the nursery itself and the personnel who work there may constitute an infection hazard for the neonate. All aseptic techniques discussed previously should be observed scrupulously, especially hand washing and the barring of ill persons from the nursery.

Infectious Agents

The organisms which infect the newborn are typically different from those infecting older people. The bacteria most often culpable are those normally inhabiting the mother's intestinal and genital tracts, which are not usually pathogenic to older persons. Of special importance are the enteric organisms, *Escherichia coli* and *Klebsiella aerobacter,* and *Listeria monocytogenes,* often found in the genital tract of pregnant females. A second common important group of bacteria are those which thrive in water, of which Pseudomonas is the prime example. Group B hemolytic streptococcus and staphylococcus are the other most common bacterial agents. A variety of viruses may cause infections, the most important of which are found in congenital syndromes to be discussed later. Toxoplasmosis and congenital syphilis account for a few neonatal infections, though the incidence of congenital syphilis has dropped sharply since the middle 1940s.

Bacterial Diseases

Bacterial infections usually take the form of pneumonia, meningitis, septicemia, and gastroenteritis. A special syndrome, acute necrotizing enterocolitis, which has recently been identified, also includes an infectious process.

Pneumonia Pneumonia is the most common form of infection during the neonatal period. The presence of symptoms at birth or their development in the first 48 hours indicates an infection that was probably acquired in utero. The organisms most likely to be involved in such cases are the enteric organisms, such as *E. coli,* and streptococci or staphylococci. Infants with intrauterine-acquired infections usually require resuscitative measures at birth, and they may show indications of long-standing hypoxia. Retractions and apnea are common after respirations have been established.

Postnatally acquired pneumonia is more likely to be due to Pseudomonas infection. Its onset is usually more than 48 hours after delivery. Feeding difficulties and increasing respiratory distress are common symptoms.

Meningitis Meningitis is most often caused by enteric organisms. The most common symptom that would lead one to think of the central nervous system is bulging or fullness of the anterior fontanel. Other symptoms common to septicemia may also be present. Convulsions may or may not occur, as is true of loss of consciousness. Opisthotonic posturing is present in only about 25 percent of the infants with meningitis. Nuchal rigidity is notably absent. The diagnosis is made by spinal tap.

Septicemia Septicemia is a serious, though common form of infection in the neonate. The newborn's relative inability to localize infections (see Chapter 2, Defenses against Hostile Organisms) is thought to contribute to the frequency of this condition. The symptoms that occur may vary with the causative organisms. The first symptoms are so subtle that they are often overlooked by all but the most observant person. Indeed, it is the nurse best acquainted with the usual behavior of the infant who is most likely to identify the early signs. Feeding difficulties, vomiting, diarrhea, and abdominal distension may occur. Jaundice is often present, due to hemolysins produced by some bacteria.[36] Skin lesions are frequently helpful in diagnosing the causative organism. Abscesses of various types are most typical of streptococcal and staphylococcal infections. A purplish cellulitis is associated with pseudomonal infections. Respiratory distress, especially the sudden appearance of apenic periods, may indicate the presence of septicemia. Diagnosis is made upon physical findings and the culturing of offending organisms in the blood. The most common causative organisms in septicemia are the gram negative enteric organisms, especially *E. coli* and *K. aerobacter.*

Diarrhea Diarrhea was discussed in Chapter 4 in terms of the full-term infant. The same general recommendations should be followed for the high-risk infant. It is especially important in epidemic diarrhea that care be taken to contain the disease. Temporary closing of the nursery may be necessary to accomplish this task.

Acute Necrotizing Enterocolitis Acute necrotizing enterocolitis is a recently recognized disease. Barlow et al. hypothesize that this condition results from an insult (such as hypoxia, maternal hypotension, or vasospasm which might occur during umbilical artery catheterization) which causes blood to be shunted away from the gastrointestinal tract.[37] The infant's intestinal mucosal cells which are sensitive to loss of blood supply cease secreting mucus when this shunting occurs. Autodigestion of the mucosa occurs and bacterial invasion of the tissues follows. The bacteria which invade the tissues are carried via the lymphatics to the bloodstream, and sepsis results. An interesting observation, validated by animal studies, is that infants who are breast-fed immediately after birth or those who are begun on breast-feeding within the first 24 hours of life seem to be protected from this syndrome.[38] Animals died when they were exposed to certain organisms under specific stress conditions and were formula-fed for the first 48 to 72 hours of life and then switched to breast-feeding. Animals survived when exposed to the same experimental conditions but breast-fed for the first 24 hours of life and then switched to formula. The explanation for these remarkable observations lies in the concept of "local enteric immunity." Such immunity is absent at birth. It is thought that certain immunoglobulins (IgA and IgG) are needed to coat the lining of the intestine in order to protect the infant from bacterial invasion in the event of hypoxia. Breast milk contains both IgA and IgG and specific antibodies against *E. coli* which would prevent its invasion of the tissues. (It is a frequently found agent in the disease.) Active lymphocytes and macrophages can also be found in the milk. These help rid the intestinal tract of pathogenic organisms. Other components of breast milk enhance the growth of nonpathogenic normal intestinal flora, which of course would help prevent the growth of pathogenic species.

The implications of these findings upon management of early infant feeding could be very far-reaching. Would it be possible, for instance, to encourage all mothers to nurse their infants for 24 to 48 hours, even if they plan to bottle-feed after that time? If so, what measures would be needed to suppress lactation after that initial period? What about mothers who have negative feelings about breast feeding? Many such questions need to be considered. Nursing may have a unique contribution to make to the solution of this problem.

Treatment of Bacterial Infections The most important step in treating neonatal infections is to suspect their presence. Failure to notice the infection and subsequent failure to treat it may result in a mortality rate as high as 90 percent.[39] Neonatal infections also carry with them a high rate of permanent neurologic damage. When an infection is suspected, cultures should be taken of blood, spinal fluid, and urine *before* treatment is begun. It is important not to administer antibiotics before these cultures are done. Blood studies, including complete blood count, electrolytes, and glucose and serum bilirubin levels will probably be ordered, also. Chest x-rays are usually done, since symptoms are so nonspecific. After specimens for initial studies have been obtained, antibiotic therapy is started with antibiotics which are generally effective against the organisms thought to be most likely to be causing the infection. The specific antibiotics used vary from one hospital to another because of the development of resistant strains. As new antibiotics are developed, the less effective ones are used less frequently. It should be remembered in all antibiotic therapy that neonates generally metabolize drugs much less rapidly than do older infants and that adverse reactions to drugs, even those used with safety in older infants and children, are not uncommon. A summary of drug-related information is presented in Klaus and Fanaroff,[40] but students are encouraged to consult the most up-to-date pharmacology literature available to them.

Nursing Care in Infections It has been stated that once antibiotic therapy has begun, the infant's best ally is a knowledgeable nurse.[41] Nursing attention to *all* details of care, such as provision of a thermoneutral environment, are indeed crucial. Special attention should be paid to observations for progression of the disease or for symptoms that might pinpoint either the organism or the system involved. It is especially important to identify neurologic symptoms, because intrathecal administration of antibiotics is indicated in many forms of meningitis. The nurse may be called upon to make a judgment about the infant's ability to take nourishment by mouth. Special care, therefore, should be taken in feeding these infants and in observing their reactions to oral feedings. Respiratory supportive measures are indicated whenever respiratory distress is present. Alertness to increases in jaundice may be vital in preventing kernicterus. The nurse should be especially alert, also, to changes indicating disturbances in pH, hypoglycemia, and electrolyte imbalances, as prompt attention to these complications can change the course of the disease. Aseptic technique, of course, must be scrupulous.

Congenital Syndromes Caused by Viral Infections

Certain viral infections of the mother prenatally are known to cause identifiable syndromes in the neonate. Notable among these is rubella virus, herpes, and cytomegalovirus. The syndromes which result have been described extensively in the literature (see, especially, Korones, Klaus and Fanaroff, and Schaffer and Avery). Because treatment of these infants is primarily supportive after birth, no discussion of the syndromes will be presented here. It is vitally important for the female nurse of child-bearing age to realize, however, that many of these infants are infective for months after birth. Korones, in fact, recommends that any female nurse of child-bearing age who works in a nursery should be tested for her immune status against rubella, specifically, and receive rubella vaccine if she is not immune.[42] Unfortunately, there are presently no vaccines for the other viruses which may be contracted.

THE INFANT WITH HYPOGLYCEMIA AND HYPOCALCEMIA

Hypoglycemia and hypocalcemia are closely related phenomena, frequently occurring together (see Chapter 8). The treatment for hypoglycemia and hypocalcemia is the intravenous infusion of appropriate replacements. For hypoglycemia, 20 to 50 percent solutions of dextrose in water may be given initially, followed by maintenance infusions to meet caloric needs. If low levels of glucose persist, hydrocortisone may be added to the infusion. Hydrocortisone stimulates the production of glucose from protein metabolism, thereby raising the blood sugar level. It also blocks the action of insulin, thereby preventing it from further lowering the glucose level. Frequent determinations of blood glucose levels should be made while treatment is being carried out. It is important to taper the amount of glucose received by infusion to prevent a rebound reaction, which is likely to occur if the glucose is stopped abruptly.

In treating hypocalcemia, 10 percent calcium gluconate is infused at the rate of 1 ml/minute with a total volume of 10 ml for a full-term infant and 6 ml for a preterm infant.[43] Then, either intravenous or oral maintenance doses of calcium salts are given. If calcium chloride is used for oral administration, the strength of the solution given must not exceed 1 percent because stronger solutions can cause mucosal necrosis. When calcium chloride is given for more than 2 or 3 days, metabolic acidosis may occur. Calcium lactate and calcium glubionate are also available for oral administration. They do not cause the mucosal irritation nor the acidosis. The infant should be placed on a low-phosphorous formula. Breast milk is ideal, if it is available.

NEONATES REQUIRING EMERGENCY SURGERY

Occasionally, conditions are present at birth that require immediate surgery. The infants requiring surgery may be full-term infants or infants at high risk due to preterm or postterm delivery or intrauterine growth retardation. All the needs of the nonsurgical infant in each of these categories are present in these infants, with the additional problem of some major congenital anomaly. That so much can be done for these babies is the amazing fact. Critical to their survival, however, is the early recognition of the condition requiring surgical intervention. While it is beyond the scope of this book to deal with specific congenital anomalies, it is hoped that the following brief presentation will enable nursery personnel to assist in early identification of these tiny surgical patients. No attempt will be made to discuss specific care other than immediate measures that must be taken when a diagnosis is suspected, as the total care varies considerably with the extent of the anomaly present, and it is available elsewhere. (The reader is referred to any standard pediatric nursing or medical text for this information.) It is important to note, here, however, that the total needs of the infant and the parents should be considered. He or she is an *infant* with special problems, *not* a congenital anomaly!

Conditions That Interfere with Respiratory Function

Among the respiratory tract anomalies requiring immediate surgery are choanal atresia and diaphragmatic hernia. Choanal atresia is the obstruction of the posterior nares with either a membranous or a bony partition. Since the neonate is an obligatory nose breather, bilateral obstruction of the nares is life-threatening. The condition is suspected when the infant is cyanotic at rest, but whose color improves during crying. (Air enters the lungs as the infant gasps during crying.) Diagnosis is made by trying to pass a small catheter through the nares into the nasopharynx. If the bilateral obstruction is present, it is essential that an oral airway be put into place. This infant needs constant nursing attention to ensure that the airway remains patent until the infant "learns" to breathe through the mouth or until surgical intervention is done.

Diaphragmatic hernia is the result of incomplete embryonic development of the diaphragm. Abdominal viscera enter the chest cavity, decreasing the size of the thoracic cavity. The condition may be apparent due to extreme respiratory distress at birth, or it may become apparent only after the gastrointestinal tract becomes distended with swallowed air some hours after birth. The nurse may suspect the presence of this condition when the abdomen is unusually flat and the chest cavity bulging, and when bowel sounds can be heard in the chest cavity. The suspect infant should be placed in an upright position in an infant carrier and the physician notified immediately. Oral feedings should be withheld until a diagnosis can be established. Oxygen may help alleviate the respiratory distress.

Obstruction of the Gastrointestinal Tract

A tracheoesophageal (TE) fistula is one of several obstructive anomalies which may occur in the gastrointestinal tract. In the most common type, the upper end of the esophagus ends in a blind pouch. The cardiac end of the esophagus may be a blind pouch also, leading only a few centimeters from the stomach, or more commonly (87 percent of the cases[44]), it communicates directly with the trachea, making an open channel through which stomach contents may flow into the lungs when the infant is in a supine position. The infant with this most common type of TE fistula will be identified early by the presence of excessive "bubbly" mucus and drooling. If feeding is attempted, the infant may swallow once or twice and then begin choking. Before attempting to feed an infant with excessive mucus, however, the patency of the esophagus should be checked by trying to pass a feeding tube into the stomach. If an obstruction is felt, no force should be used, but the infant should be placed in an upright position and suctioned every few minutes until continuous suction of the blind pouch can be established. This defect should be suspected, also, when polyhydramnios is present. Since the fetus swallows amnionic fluid and digests it, an obstruction anywhere in the gastrointestinal tract may result in excess fluid accumulating in the amnionic sac. The type of surgery done and its extent will depend upon the specific defect present.

Another of the more common obstructive anomalies of the gastrointestinal tract is imperforate anus. In embryonic development, the hind gut and the external depression, the proctodaeum, which merges with it, must grow toward each other in order to form a continuous tube. Sometimes the tissue separating the two fails to disappear completely. In this case, a thin membrane or a section of tissue several centimeters wide then separates the hind gut from the external invagination that forms the anus. In either case, an obstruction of the lower bowel results. Sometimes, this obstruction is obvious at birth because of the absence of an anal opening. At other times, the external anus appears to be normal, hiding the obstruction from view. Some authorities advocate checking the patency of the anus immediately after birth; others prefer waiting 24 hours to see whether or not meconium is passed spontaneously. It is important to recognize the condition early so that surgery can be performed before the infant becomes debilitated. Surgery may be corrective, or a temporary colostomy may be done to relieve the obstruction until corrective surgery can be done at a later date. Not infrequently, a fistula is present between the rectum and either the vagina or the urinary tract. Embryonically, the anal and urogenital openings originate from a common aperture. Meconium may be passed through the fistula in these cases, but infection of the urinary tract is almost inevitable. A temporary colostomy is usually done to prevent such infections.

Cyanotic Heart Defects

Severe cyanosis that is present at birth or that develops soon afterward in spite of vigorous resuscitative measures should raise the suspicion of serious congenital heart disease. Temporary palliative surgery may be necessary to save the infant's life until corrective surgery can be done. These babies are usually recognized soon after birth when cyanosis persists after the usual resuscitative measures have been taken, or when marked cyanosis and exhaustion accompany attempts to feed the infant.

Obstruction of the Urinary Tract

Another surgical emergency is obstruction of the urinary tract. Failure of the infant to void within 12 to 24 hours or dribbling rather than voiding a strong stream of urine may indicate the presence of a partial or complete urinary tract obstruction.

Externalization of Internal Organs

The externalization of internal organs can occur in any of the systems. In general, the anomalies occur due to incomplete midline fusion of external tissues. Preoperative management of these infants includes protection of the exposed organs or sacs from trauma and infection. In many instances, it is necessary to cover the exposed organs with sterile saline-soaked pads to prevent excessive drying. Surgical intervention is often extensive.

REGIONALIZATION OF CARE

The newest trend in care of the high-risk infant is the establishment of regional centers for the treatment of the most seriously ill babies. With this trend goes the possibility of salvaging many of the infants who otherwise could not survive, and not just saving their lives, but preventing serious handicaps that might otherwise occur. With it also, however, goes greater nursing responsibilities. The nurses who work in such centers will of necessity become highly specialized and highly skilled. Nurses who work in general hospitals must also carry new responsibilities. They must become skilled in the early identification of suspect infants so that high-risk infants may be diagnosed early and transferred before their conditions deteriorate. Other nurses may be specially trained in the transport of these infants, so that they can receive the best possible care on their way to the treatment centers.

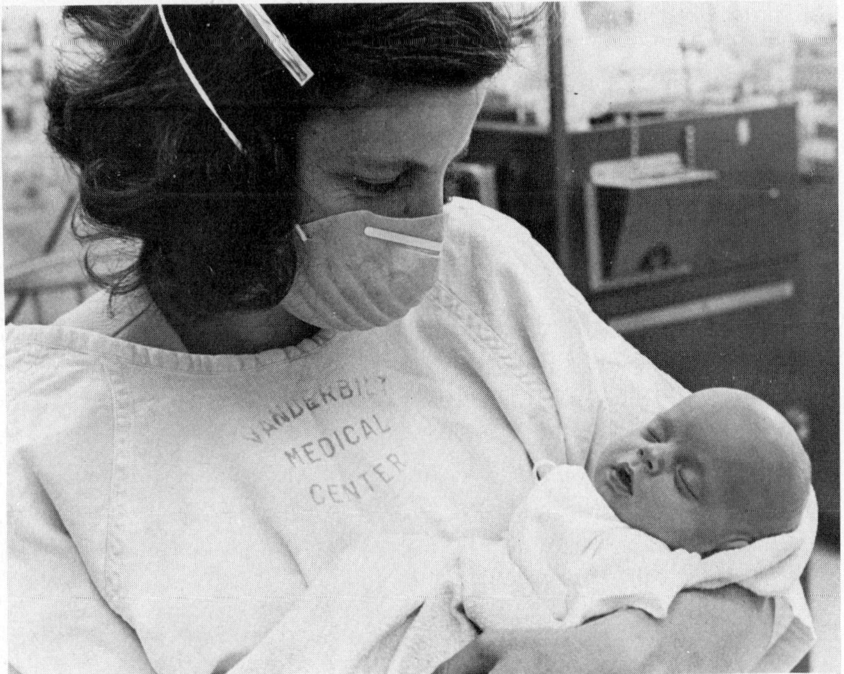

Figure 9-3 Mothers need to hold their preterm infants and learn to care for them before they are discharged from the nursery. (The use of masks has recently been discontinued at this nursery.) *(Photo: Penelope Ann Peirce.)*

All nurses who work with these babies must keep in mind that the removal of an infant from the hospital where his mother is a patient causes great stress for the parents. Special efforts must be made to maintain contact between the infant and the parents during the period of their separation. This may be especially difficult when geographic distances are great. Finally, special care must be taken to ensure that the infants are returned to hospitals close to the parents as soon as possible and that the parents are encouraged to assume a significant role in the infants' care as soon as their conditions permit.

REFERENCES

1 Avron Y. Sweet, "Classification of the Low-Birth-Weight Infant," in Marshall H. Klaus, and Avroy A. Fanaroff (eds.), *Care of the High-Risk Neonate,* Saunders, Philadelphia, 1973, p. 50.

2 Sheldon B. Korones, *High-Risk Newborn Infants: The Basis for Intensive Nursing Care,* Mosby, 1972, p. 184.

3 Ibid., p. 89.

4 David Fisher and Richard E. Behrman, "Resuscitation of the Newborn Infant," in Klaus and Fanaroff (eds.), op. cit., p. 14.
5 Ibid., p. 2.
6 Ibid., p. 3.
7 Marshall Klaus and Avroy Fanaroff, "Respiratory Problems," in Klaus and Fanaroff (eds.), op. cit., p. 129.
8 Ibid., p. 145.
9 Ibid., p. 133.
10 Ibid., p. 144.
11 Leo Stern, editorial comment in Klaus and Fanaroff, op. cit., pp. 145–146.
12 Klaus and Fanaroff, op. cit., p. 146.
13 Laura S. Hillman, Sally L. Goodwin, and William R. Sherman, "Identification and Measurement of Plasticizer in Neonatal Tissues after Umbilical Catheters and Blood Products," *The New England Journal of Medicine,* Feb. 20, 1975, p. 385.
14 Ibid.
15 Klaus and Fanaroff, op. cit., p. 140.
16 Gerard B. Odell, editorial comment in Ann Llewellyn and Paul Swyer, "Assisted Ventilation," in Klaus and Fanaroff (eds.), op. cit., p. 156.
17 Llewellyn and Swyer, op. cit., p. 163.
18 Ibid., pp. 152–167.
19 Jerry J. Evans, "Prediction of Respiratory-Distress Syndrome by Shake Test on Newborn Gastric Aspirate," *The New England Journal of Medicine,* May 22, 1975, pp. 1113–1115.
20 Judith Garvey, "Infant Respiratory Distress Syndrome," *American Journal of Nursing,* April 1975, p. 616.
21 Klaus and Fanaroff, op. cit., pp. 122–123, 143.
22 Ibid., p. 142.
23 Llewellyn and Swyer, op. cit., p. 185.
24 Leo Stern, "The Control of Hyperbilirubinemia in the Newborn," *Clinical Obstetrics and Gynecology,* September 1971, p. 864.
25 Gerald B. Odell, Ronald L. Poland, and Enrique M. Ostrea, Jr., "Neonatal Hyperbilirubinemia," in Klaus and Fanaroff (eds.), op. cit., p. 198.
26 Ibid.
27 Alexander J. Schaffer and Mary Ellen Avery, *Diseases of the Newborn,* Saunders, Philadelphia, 1971, p. 549.
28 Odell et al., op. cit., p. 194.
29 Ibid.
30 Schaffer and Avery, op. cit., p. 548.
31 Ibid., p. 549.
32 Odell et al., op. cit., p. 195.
33 Vincent J. Freda, John G. Gorman, William Pollack, and Edward Bowe, "Prevention of Rh Hemolytic Disease—Ten Years' Clinical Experience with Rh Immune Globulin," *The New England Journal of Medicine,* May 8, 1975, pp. 1014–1016.
34 Korones, op. cit., p. 194.

35 Schaffer and Avery, op. cit., p. 632.
36 Odell et al., op. cit. p. 189.
37 Barbara Barlow, Thomas V. Santulli, William C. Heird, Jane Pitt, William A. Blanc, and John N. Schullinger, "An Experimental Study of Acute Neonatal Enterocolitis—The Importance of Breast Milk," *Journal of Pediatric Surgery,* October 1974, pp. 587–595.
38 Ibid., p. 592.
39 "Infected from the Start," *Emergency Medicine,* September 1971, p. 23.
40 Klaus and Fanaroff, op. cit., pp. 216–217.
41 "Infected from the Start," p. 26.
42 Korones, op. cit., p. 206.
43 Michael K. Wald, "Problems in Chemical Adaptation," in Klaus and Fanaroff (eds.), op. cit., p. 176.
44 Mary Lou Moore, *The Newborn and the Nurse,* Saunders, Philadelphia, 1972, p. 169.

BIBLIOGRAPHY

Barlow, Barbara, Thomas V. Santulli, William C. Heird, Jane Pitt, William A. Blanc, and John N. Schullinger: "An Experimental Study of Acute Neonatal Enterocolitis—The Importance of Breast Milk," *Journal of Pediatric Surgery,* October 1974, pp. 587–595.

Clatworthy, H. William: "Special Problems in Surgery of Newborn Infants," *Surgical Clinics of North America,* August 1970, pp. 771–774.

"A Crying Need for Sugar," *Emergency Medicine,* March 1971, pp. 148–149.

Davis, Laura Albrecht: "Neonatal Respiratory Emergencies," *Nursing Clinics of North America,* September 1973, pp. 441–446.

Evans, Jerry J.: "Prediction of Respiratory-Distress Syndrome by Shake Test on Newborn Gastric Aspirate," *The New England Journal of Medicine,* May 22, 1975, pp. 1113–1115.

Fanaroff, Avroy, and Marshall Klaus: "Feeding the Low-Birth-Weight Infant," in Marshall H. Klaus and Avroy Fanaroff (eds.), *Care of the High-Risk Neonate,* Saunders, Philadelphia, 1973, pp. 77–89.

———: "Neonatal Infections," in Marshall H. Klaus and Avroy Fanaroff (eds.), *Care of the High-Risk Neonate,* Saunders, Philadelphia, 1973, pp. 205–227.

Fisher, David, and Richard E. Behrman: "Resuscitation of the Newborn Infant," in Marshall H. Klaus and Avroy Fanaroff (eds.), *Care of the High-Risk Neonate,* Saunders, Philadelphia, 1973, pp. 1–22.

Freda, Vincent J., John G. Gorman, William Pollack, and Edward Bowe: "Prevention of Rh Hemolytic Disease—Ten Years' Clinical Experience with Rh Immune Globulin" *The New England Journal of Medicine,* May 8, 1975, pp. 1014–1016.

Garvey, Judith: "Infant Respiratory Distress Syndrome," *American Journal of Nursing,* April 1975, pp. 614–617.

Hillman, Laura S., Sally L. Goodwin, and William R. Sherman: "Identification and Measurement of Plasticizer in Neonatal Tissues after Umbilical Catheters and Blood Products," *The New England Journal of Medicine,* Feb. 20, 1975, pp. 381–386.

"Infected from the Start," *Emergency Medicine,* September 1971, pp. 22–26.

Klaus, Marshall and Avroy Fanaroff, "Respiratory Problems," in Marshall H. Klaus and Avroy Fanaroff (eds.), *Care of the High-Risk Neonate,* Saunders, Philadelphia, 1973, pp. 119–151.

Korones, Sheldon B.: *High-Risk Newborn Infants: The Basis for Intensive Nursing Care,* Mosby, St. Louis, 1972.

Kumpe, Mary, and Leonard Kleinman: "Care of the Infant with Respiratory Distress Syndrome," *Nursing Clinics of North America,* March 1971, pp. 25–37.

Llewellyn, Ann, and Paul Swyer: "Assisted Ventilation," in Marshall H. Klaus and Avroy Fanaroff (eds.), *Care of the High-Risk Neonate,* Saunders, Philadelphia, 1973, pp. 152–167.

Miller, Richard C.: "Surgical Emergencies of the Newborn," *Journal of the Mississippi State Medical Association,* November 1970, pp. 585–593.

Moore, Mary Lou: *The Newborn and the Nurse,* Saunders, Philadelphia, 1972.

Odell, Gerald B., Ronald L. Poland, and Enrique M. Ostrea, Jr.: "Neonatal Hyperbilirubinemia," in Marshall H. Klaus and Avroy Fanaroff (eds.), *Care of the High-Risk Neonate,* Saunders, Philadelphia, 1973, pp. 183–204.

Rawson, John E.: "Respiratory Distress in the Newborn," *Journal of the Mississippi State Medical Association,* February 1971, pp. 57–64.

Robinson, Roger: "The Small-for-Dates Baby - II," *British Medical Journal,* November 1971, pp. 480–482.

"Safer Breath for Newborns," *Emergency Medicine,* April 1971, pp. 83, 87.

Santulli, Thomas V.: "Acute Necrotizing Enterocolitis: Recognition and Management," *Hospital Practice,* November 1974, pp. 129–135.

Schaffer, Alexander J., and Mary Ellen Avery: *Diseases of the Newborn,* Saunders, Philadelphia, 1971.

Stern, Leo: "The Control of Hyperbilirubinemia in the Newborn," *Clinical Obstetrics and Gynecology,* September 1971, pp. 855–868.

Sweet, Avron Y.: "Classification of the Low-Birth-Weight Infant," in Marshall H. Klaus and Avroy Fanaroff (eds.), *Care of the High-Risk Neonate,* Saunders, Philadelphia, 1973, pp. 36–57.

Wald, Michael K.: "Problems in Chemical Adaptation," in Marshall H. Klaus and Avroy Fanaroff (eds.), *Care of the High-Risk Neonate,* Saunders, Philadelphia, 1973, pp. 168–182.

Index

Index

C